# Clinical Management of Diabetic Neuropathy

# CONTEMPORARY ENDOCRINOLOGY

P. Michael Conn, SERIES EDITOR

8. ***Clinical Management of Diabetic Neuropathy,*** edited by *ARISTIDIS VEVES,* 1998
7. ***Gastrointestinal Endocrinology,*** edited by *GEORGE H. GREELEY JR.,* 1998
6. ***G Proteins, Receptors, and Disease,*** edited by *ALLEN M. SPIEGEL,* 1998
5. ***Natriuretic Peptides in Health and Disease,*** edited by *WILLIS K. SAMSON AND ELLIS R. LEVIN,* 1997
4. ***Endocrinology of Critical Diseases,*** edited by *K. PATRICK OBER,* 1997
3. ***Diseases of the Pituitary:*** *Diagnosis and Treatment,* edited by *MARGARET E. WIERMAN,* 1997
2. ***Diseases of the Thyroid,*** edited by *LEWIS E. BRAVERMAN,* 1997
1. ***Endocrinology of the Vasculature,*** edited by *JAMES R. SOWERS,* 1996

# Clinical Management of Diabetic Neuropathy

*Edited by*

ARISTIDIS VEVES, MD
*Beth Israel Deaconess Medical Center*
*and Harvard Medical School, Boston, MA*

HUMANA PRESS
TOTOWA, NEW JERSEY

999 Riverview Drive, Suite 208
Totowa, New Jersey 07512

For additional copies, pricing for bulk purchases, and/or information about other Humana titles, contact Humana at the above address or at any of the following numbers: Tel: 973-256-1699; Fax: 973-256-8341; E-mail: humana@humanapr.com or visit our website at http://humanapress.com



This publication is printed on acid-free paper. ∞
ANSI Z39.48-1984 (American National Standards Institute)
Permanence of Paper for Printed Library Materials.



Printed in the United States of America. 10 9 8 7 6 5 4 3 2 1

Clinical management of diabetic neuropathy/edited by Aristidis Veves.
p. cm.—(Contemporary endocrinology; 8)
Includes bibliographical references and index.
ISBN 0-89603-528-4 (alk. paper)
1. Diabetic neuropathies. II. Veves, Aristidis. II. Series: Contemporary endocrinology (Totowa, NJ); 8
[DNLM: 1. Diabetic Neuropathies—therapy. 2. Diabetes Mellitus—complications. WK 835 C641 1998]
RC422.D52C55 1998
616.4'62—dc21
DNLM/DLC
for Library of Congress 97-49683
CIP

# PREFACE

Diabetic neuropathy is one of the most common long-term complications of diabetes and can affect almost every organ or system of the human body. Peripheral somatic neuropathy is directly related to foot problems and, along with peripheral vascular disease, is the main cause for foot ulceration and lower extremity amputation, the commonest reason for hospital admission among diabetic patients. On the other hand, autonomic neuropathy is involved in the development of silent cardiac ischemia and cardiac arrhythmia and can be a major contributory factor in the increased cardiovascular morbidity and mortality observed in diabetic patients.

Although the majority of practicing physicians are aware of the above effects of diabetic neuropathy, other features of the disease may remain unrecognized despite their significant impact on the patient's daily life activities. Impotence can affect up to half of the diabetic male population and can have a severe impact not only on patients' lives, but also on the lives of their partners. However, since both patients and physicians may feel uncomfortable in discussing this problem, it is not surprising that it is often left untreated despite the ready availability of inexpensive, uncomplicated, and easily accessible therapeutic options. Finally, a variety of gastrointestinal conditions that are related to autonomic neuropathy can also cause significant problems that may ultimately require hospitalization and intensive treatment.

*Clinical Management of Diabetic Neuropathy* has been written for the greater audience of physicians who are treating diabetic patients, and who encounter neuropathy-related problems in their daily practice. The family practitioner, internist, endocrinologist, podiatrist, cardiologist, neurologist, urologist, and gastroenterologist are all members of the team that cares for diabetics and may greatly benefit from *Clinical Management of Diabetic Neuropathy*. It was therefore felt that this volume could only be successful if it concentrated more on the clinical aspects of diabetic neuropathy and its current management, and concisely detailed the causes that are, or are presumed to be, responsible for the various clinical syndromes. Special emphasis is also given to the detailed description of treatments that are currently available, or are expected to become available in the near future. The detailed bibliography at the end of each chapter will, it is hoped, prove helpful to the reader who would like a more detailed picture of any specific topic discussed.

I would like to express my gratitude to the authors, all internationally distinguished in their field, who accepted my invitation to contribute to this project. I am also indebted to Ms. Paula Smakowski, MS, PT, for her valuable editorial assistance. Finally, my sincere thanks also go to Humana Press and the series editor, Dr. P. Michael Conn, for their trust in my ability to realize such a project.

***Aristidis Veves, MD***

# CONTENTS

# CONTRIBUTORS

CAMERON M. AKBARI, MD, *Division of Vascular Surgery, Beth Israel Deaconess Medical Center, Harvard Medical School, Boston, MA*

ANDREW J. M. BOULTON, MD, FRCP, *The University Department of Medicine, Manchester Royal Infirmary, Manchester, UK*

EDWARD J. BOYKO, MD, MPH, *Department of Medicine, University of Washington School of Medicine, VA Puget Sound Health Care System, Seattle, WA*

JAMES S. CHRZAN, DPM, *Division of Podiatry, Beth Israel Deaconess Medical Center, Harvard Medical School, Boston, MA*

EFTHYMIOS N. DELIARGYRIS, MD, *Department of Cardiology, University of North Carolina Hospitals, Chapel Hill, NC*

EVA L. FELDMAN, MD, PHD, *Department of Neurology, University of Michigan Medical Center, Ann Arbor, MI*

ROGER A FIELDING, PHD, *Department of Health Sciences, Sargent College of Health and Rehabilitation Sciences, Boston University, MA*

ROY FREEMAN, MD, *Autonomic and Peripheral Nerve Laboratory, Department of Neurology, Beth Israel Deaconess Medical Center, Harvard Medical School, Boston, MA*

ROBERT G. FRYKBERG, DPM, MPH, *Deaconess Joslin Foot Center, Beth Israel Deaconess Medical Center, Harvard Medical School, Boston, MA*

DAVID A. GELBER, MD, *Department of Neurology, Southern Illinois University School of Medicine, Springfield, IL*

JOHN M. GIURINI, DPM, *Division of Podiatry, Beth Israel Deaconess Medical Center, Harvard Medical School, Boston, MA*

DOUGLAS A. GREENE, MD, *Division of Endocrinology and Metabolism, University of Michigan Medical Center, Ann Arbor, MI*

GEOFFREY M. HABERSHAW, DPM, *Division of Podiatry, Beth Israel Deaconess Medical Center, Harvard Medical School, Boston, MA*

NATHAN K. LEBRASSEUR, MSPT, *Department of Health Sciences, Sargent College of Health and Rehabilitation Sciences, Boston University, MA*

FRANK W. LOGERFO, MD, *Division of Vascular Surgery, Beth Israel Deaconess Medical Center, Harvard Medical School, Boston, MA*

THOMAS E. LYONS, DPM, *Division of Podiatry, Beth Israel Deaconess Medical Center, Harvard Medical School, Boston, MA*

JUAN-R. MALAGELADA, MD, *Digestive System Research Unit, Hospital General Vall d' Hebron, Autonomous University of Barcelona, Spain*

RICHARD W. NESTO, MD, *Department of Cardiology, Beth Israel Deaconess Medical Center, Harvard Medical School, Boston, MA*

MICHAEL PFEIFER, MD, *Department of Internal Medicine, Southern Illinois University School of Medicine, Springfield, IL*

BARRY I. ROSENBLUM, DPM, *Division of Podiatry, Beth Israel Deaconess Medical Center, Harvard Medical School, Boston, MA*

GERARD SAID, MD, *Service de Neurologie, Hôpital de Bicêtre, Université Paris XI, France*

JONATHAN E. SHAW, MRCP, *The University Department of Medicine, Manchester Royal Infirmary, Manchester, UK*
ANDERS A. F. SIMA, MD, PHD, *Departments of Pathology and Neurology, Wayne State University, School of Medicine and Detroit Medical Center, Detroit, MI*
MARTIN J. STEVENS, MD, *Division of Endocrinology and Metabolism, University of Michigan Medical Center, Ann Arbor, MI*
SOLOMON TESFAYE, MD, MRCP, *Department of Medicine, Royal Hallamshire Hospital, Sheffield, UK*
THOMMEY THOMAS, MD, *Division of Endocrinology and Metabolism, University of Michigan Medical Center, Ann Arbor, MI*
ARISTIDIS VEVES, MD, *Department of Medicine, Beth Israel Deaconess Medical Center, Harvard Medical School, Boston, MA*
JOHN D. WARD, MD, FRCP, *Department of Medicine, Royal Hallamshire Hospital, Sheffield, UK*
LYNNE WEBSTER, MB, CHB, MSC, FRCPSYCH, *Department of Psychiatry, Manchester Royal Infirmary, Manchester, UK*
DAN ZIEGLER, MD, *Diabetes Research Institute, Heinrich Heine University, Düsseldorf, Germany*

# 1 The Epidemiology of Diabetic Neuropathy

*Edward J. Boyko, MD, MPH*

*CONTENTS*



## INTRODUCTION

Peripheral neuropathy is a devastating complication of diabetes mellitus because of the debilitating symptoms it causes, or associated higher risk of other complications, in particular those involving the lower extremities. The epidemiology of diabetic neuropathy is not as well-understood as other complications of this metabolic disorder, including retinal, renal, and coronary artery disease. Different peripheral nerves may be damaged through a variety of pathologic processes as described in other chapters of this book. This chapter will review the prevalence, incidence, and risk factors for different types of diabetic neuropathy. The natural history of diabetic neuropathy will be briefly described with regard to foot complications.

There are six major types of diabetic neuropathy: distal symmetric polyneuropathy, autonomic neuropathy, nerve entrapment syndromes, proximal asymmetric mononeuropathy (also known as diabetic amyotrophy), truncal radiculopathy, and cranial mononeuropathy. This chapter will focus mainly on the first two types of neuropathy. Little is known regarding the epidemiology of the remaining types, probably because, with the exception of nerve entrapment syndromes, these occur infrequently.

From: *Contemporary Endocrinology: Clinical Management of Diabetic Neuropathy*
Edited by: A. Veves © Humana Press Inc., Totowa, NJ

## EPIDEMIOLOGIC PRINCIPLES RELEVANT TO THE STUDY OF DIABETIC NEUROPATHY

In order to understand published research on the epidemiology of diabetic neuropathy, certain principles of epidemiologic study design must be taken into consideration. These principles guided this author in the selection of relevant citations and data presentation. Only cross-sectional or case-control studies conducted in a population-based sample (such as a defined community or health plan enrollment) were considered for this chapter based on review of MedLine citations using the keywords "epidemiology," "diabetes," and "neuropathy" from 1966 to March, 1997, review of bibliographies of the articles obtained from the MedLine search for relevant citations, and review of the author's files. Nine published studies met this criterion. Clinic-based cross-sectional or case-control studies have not been considered except in two instances, because of the potential problem of selection bias associated with these study designs *(1)*. All 11 prospective studies were considered. Prospective research is less likely to be biased because of differences in probability of subject selection based on disease (neuropathy) and risk factor presence. Prospective research is a stronger study design with regard to inferring the possibility of causation, since the presence of risk factors may be determined prior to neuropathy onset.

The problem of measurement error in the assessment of the presence or absence of diabetic neuropathy is well-recognized. Nerve conduction velocity, arguably the most objective and accurate test available for the diagnosis of this complication, is known to sometimes result in erroneous classification. For example, nerve conduction velocity may be normal in diabetic subjects with symptoms of distal symmetric polyneuropathy *(2)*. This misclassification problem becomes even more problematic when a test result is used to formulate a clinical plan for an individual patient, as compared to epidemiologic analysis where population statistics are the result of interest. When misclassification of neuropathy or risk factor status occurs nondifferentially (randomly), the net result is bias of any observed difference towards the null value *(1)*. Therefore, observed differences found in an epidemiologic analysis of risk factors for diabetic neuropathy validly reflect potential causative factors for this complication, but probably underestimate the magnitude of the risk increase. Epidemiologic studies may draw valid conclusions regarding risk factors for diabetic neuropathy even if the techniques used to measure either neuropathy or the potential risk factor are known to be inaccurate.

## DISTAL SYMMETRIC POLYNEUROPATHY— PREVALENCE AND RISK FACTORS (CROSS-SECTIONAL RESEARCH)

Dyck et al. examined the prevalence of neuropathy among all clinically diagnosed diabetic subjects who resided in Rochester, Minnesota *(3)*. Only 380 of 870 eligible subjects (44%) agreed to participate, possibly caused by concern about the lengthy neurodiagnostic study protocol. Neuropathy was defined if two criteria were satisfied: abnormal nerve conduction in more than one nerve or abnormal test of autonomic function (low heart-rate variation in response to breathing or the Valsalva maneuver); and neuropathic symptom or sign or abnormal quantitative sensory testing. Median duration of diabetes was 14.5 yr for insulin-dependent diabetes mellitus (IDDM) and 8.1 yr for noninsulin-dependent diabetes mellitus (NIDDM) subjects. Although the prevalence of neuropathy was high (Table 1), most subjects with neuropathy were asymptomatic (~71%).

**Table 1**
**Distal Symmetric Polyneuropathy: Prevalence, Incidence, and Risk Factors From Cross-Sectional Research Studies**

| *Reference* | *Subjects* | *Prevalence* | *Significant Risk Factors* | *Odds Ratio (95% CI)* |
|---|---|---|---|---|
| *(3)* | 100 IDDM | 54% | Not reported | |
| | 259 NIDDM | 45% | | |
| *(4)* | 277 NIDDM | 27% | Age, 5-yr increase | 1.2 (1.0–1.4) |
| | 89 IGT | 11% | Male gender | 2.2 (1.2–4.1) |
| | 496 NGT | 4% | Diabetes duration, 5-yr increase | 1.3 (1.0–1.6) |
| | | | Glycosylated hemoglobin, 2.5% increase | 1.3 (1.0–1.8) |
| | | | Insulin use | 2.7 (1.4–5.2) |
| *(6)* | 363 IDDM | 34% | Diabetes duration, 10-yr increase | 1.2 (1.1–1.2) |
| | | | Glycosylated hemoglobin, 1% increase | 1.4 (1.2–1.7) |
| | | | HDL cholesterol, 0.13 m*M* decrease | 1.2 (1.1–1.3) |
| | | | Current smoking | 2.2 (1.3–3.8) |
| | | | Any macrovascular disease | 2.3 (1.0–5.4) |
| *(10)* | 2405 DM | 30% IDDM | Diabetes duration | not reported |
| | 20,037 non-DM | 38% NIDDM | Hypertension | not reported |
| | | | Poor glucose control | not reported |
| *(11)* | 1084 DM | 14% | Age at diagnosis | not reported |
| | | | Diabetes duration | not reported |
| | | | Plasma creatinine | not reported |
| | | | Insulin dose | not reported |
| | | | Orthostatic blood pressure fall | not reported |
| *(12)* | 1077 (20% IDDM, 80% NIDDM) | 17% | IDDM | |
| | | | Height (1-cm increase) | 1.06 (1.00–1.13) |
| | | | Retinopathy | 9.0 (7.7–10.3) |
| | | | NIDDM | |
| | | | Height (1-cm increase) | 1.06 (1.03–1.08) |
| | | | Age (1-yr increase) | 1.02 (1.00–1.05) |
| | | | Alcohol "units"/wk (1-unit increase) | 1.03 (1.00–1.05) |
| | | | HbA1c (1% increase) | 1.2 (1.1–1.4) |
| | | | Retinopathy | 2.1 (1.7–2.6) |
| *(13)* | 375 DM (78% IDDM) | [a] | IDDM | |
| | | | Age | not reported |
| | | | Diabetes duration | not reported |
| | | | NIDDM | not reported |
| | | | Height | |
| *(14)* | 137 NIDDM, 139 non-diabetic controls | 53–63%, depending on the test | Not reported | |

[a] Not reported, since all persons with diabetes were not included in this survey.

A community-based study in San Luis Valley, Colorado, measured prevalence of neuropathy in a bi-ethnic (Hispanic and Anglo) population *(4,5)*. Neuropathy was defined if two of three criteria were satisfied: neuropathic discomfort in feet and legs; abnormal Achilles tendon reflexes; and inability to feel an iced tuning fork on the dorsum of the foot (test of thermal sensation). Subjects with NIDDM had the highest prevalence of neuropathy, whereas subjects with impaired glucose tolerance (IGT) defined according to World Health Organization criteria had a prevalence about midway between normal glucose tolerance (NGT) and NIDDM (Table 1). No IDDM subjects were included in this study. Significantly higher prevalence of neuropathy was found in relation to greater age, diabetes duration, and glycosylated hemoglobin; male gender; and insulin use. Factors not associated with neuropathy prevalence included blood pressure, height, smoking, prior alcohol use, ankle-arm index, and serum cholesterol, lipid, and lipoprotein levels.

The Pittsburgh epidemiology of diabetes complications study included 363 subjects with IDDM over 18 yr of age in a defined community (Allegheny County, Pennsylvania) *(6–8)*. Two of three of the following criteria had to be satisfied to fulfill the definition of neuropathy: abnormal sensory or motor signs on clinical examination; neuropathic symptoms; and abnormal tendon reflexes. Overall neuropathy prevalence was 34% (18% in 19–29 yr olds, and 58% in those 30 yr of age or older) (Table 1). Higher prevalence of neuropathy was associated with longer diabetes duration, higher glycosylated hemoglobin, lower HDL-cholesterol, smoking, and presence of peripheral vascular, coronary artery, or cerebrovascular disease (Table 1). Another analysis of the Pittsburgh population explored the association between physical activity and distal symmetric polyneuropathy among 628 IDDM subjects between 8–48 yr of age *(9)*. Male subjects who reported higher historical levels of leisure-time physical activity (adjusted for diabetes duration, age, and current activity levels) had a significantly lower prevalence of neuropathy. No association between historical levels of physical activity and neuropathy prevalence was seen in females.

Data from the United States National Health Interview Survey were used to generate neuropathy prevalence statistics on a nationwide sample of diabetic subjects *(10)*. A total of 2405 self-reported diabetic and 20,037 self-reported nondiabetic subjects were surveyed for the presence of symptoms of neuropathy in the extremities (numbness, pain, decreased hot or cold sensation). Prevalence of symptoms was more than three times greater in diabetic vs nondiabetic subjects (Table 1). Among subjects with NIDDM, higher prevalence of symptoms was associated with longer diabetes duration, hypertension, and self-reported frequent high blood glucose, whereas age, gender, height, insulin treatment, and smoking were unrelated to this outcome.

A population-based survey in Western Australia included 1084 diabetic subjects, estimated to be 70% of the total who resided in this geographic area *(11)*. Sensory neuropathy was defined as a bilateral reduction in pinprick sensation in the feet during a sensory exam performed by endocrinologists. Neuropathy was found in 14% of subjects, and was related to greater age at diabetes diagnosis, diabetes duration, plasma creatinine, insulin dose, and orthostatic blood pressure difference (Table 1).

In a survey of 10 general practices in an English community, 1077 diabetic subjects were identified and screened for neuropathy *(12)*. Two of the following five criteria fulfilled the definition of neuropathy: neuropathic foot symptoms; loss of light touch sensation; impaired pinprick sensation; absent ankle jerk reflexes; and vibration perception threshold greater than 97.5% of an age-standardized value. A total of 16.8% of diabetic subjects fulfilled these criteria, as compared to 750 nondiabetic controls drawn from the same general practices. Risk factors associated with higher neuropathy prevalence are shown in Table 1.

A survey of diabetic subjects in a defined community in Sweden yielded 375 subjects between the ages of 15–50 with diabetes (78% IDDM) *(13)*. A vibrameter was used to assess vibration threshold and pain sensation was evaluated with application of an electric current to the foot. Among IDDM subjects, neuropathy presence was associated with greater, age, diabetes duration, and height, although the association with height disappeared in multivariate analysis after adjustment for gender. Among subjects with NIDDM, neuropathy was associated with greater height only.

A survey of NIDDM subjects in a Dutch community revealed a high prevalence of neuropathy, but also found that a substantial proportion of nondiabetic controls also tested positive for neuropathy, probably because of the high median age of the population (70 yr) *(14)*. Proportion of diabetic and control subjects with abnormal results by test is as follows: temperature 63 vs 49%, vibration (128-Hz tuning fork) 53 vs 33%, and absent tendon reflexes 62 vs 21%. Analysis of risk factors for neuropathy was not performed.

Another community-based study that was conducted in two municipalities in Sicily will be mentioned but not discussed in detail, since only subjects who responded affirmatively to questions regarding the presence of symptoms of neuropathy were evaluated further by a neurologist *(15)*. This method likely led to considerable underascertainment of neuropathy prevalence.

Although not community-based, two other cross-sectional studies are worthy of mention because of their large sample sizes and, in one case, multinational composition. The EURODIAB IDDM complications study (A cross-sectional clinic-based study of complications from 16 European countries) examined prevalence of neuropathy, defined if two or more of the following were present: symptoms, absence of two or more ankle or knee reflexes, abnormal vibration perception threshold, and abnormal autonomic function (postural systolic blood pressure fall of 30 mmHg or more or loss of heart-rate variability as demonstrated by an RR ratio $< 1$) *(16)*. The factors positively correlated with neuropathy prevalence were age, diabetes duration, HbA1c, weight, current smoking, severe ketoacidosis, macroalbuminuria, and retinopathy. The UK Prospective Diabetes Study examined the association between neuropathy and potential risk factors among 2337 newly diagnosed subjects with NIDDM *(17)*. Neuropathy was defined as absence of two or more reflexes in the knees and ankles (5% of subjects), or vibration sensation greater than two standard deviations from the age-corrected mean when measured with a biothesiometer (7% of subjects). Neuropathy was significantly related to ischemic skin changes of the foot (smooth or hairless skin), but unrelated to HbAlc, fasting plasma glucose, smoking, serum lipid and lipoprotein levels, and the albumin/creatinine ratio.

Of the five community-based cross-sectional studies reviewed of NIDDM subjects that presented data on risk factors for neuropathy, three reported a higher prevalence of this outcome with longer diabetes duration and higher glycosylated hemoglobin, and two found neuropathy prevalence correlated with age and height. The remaining risk factors reported were not reproduced by other investigators. Only three community-based cross-sectional studies addressed neuropathy prevalence in IDDM subjects in association with risk factors. Two of these investigations reported a correlation between diabetes duration and neuropathy prevalence. No other significant risk factor was reported by more than one IDDM community-based study. Cross-sectional research affirms the importance of intensity and duration of hyperglycemia as potential risk factors for neuropathy, but also suggests other possible etiologies, as shown in Table 1.

## DISTAL SYMMETRIC POLYNEUROPATHY—INCIDENCE AND RISK FACTORS (PROSPECTIVE RESEARCH)

The most important epidemiologic study of diabetic neuropathy performed to date is the Diabetes Control and Complications Trial (DCCT). Although designed to answer a therapeutic question, this trial provides much valuable information regarding the incidence of diabetic neuropathy and its relation to glycemic control. This clinical trial included 1161 patients with IDDM who were followed for 5 yr for the development and progression of neuropathy *(18)*. Subjects were randomized to intensive or control treatment groups, after being initially divided into a primary (diabetes for 5 yr or less, no microalbuminuria, no retinopathy) or secondary prevention (diabetes for 15 yr or less, moderate or less nonproliferative retinopathy, urinary albumin excretion less than 200 mg/24 h) subgroups, depending on the presence of end-point complications at baseline. Clinical neuropathy was defined as two of the three following conditions: neuropathic symptoms; sensory deficit to light touch, position, temperature, or pinprick; and abnormal deep tendon reflexes. Confirmed clinical neuropathy was defined as an abnormal clinical exam plus either abnormal nerve conduction in two or more nerves or abnormal response to autonomic testing. After 5 yr follow up, the cumulative incidence of clinical neuropathy, confirmed clinical neuropathy, and abnormal nerve conduction was lower in the intensively treated vs control groups, irrespective of presence of complications at baseline (Fig. 1). Among controls, the cumulative incidence of clinical neuropathy was 15–21%, depending on presence of baseline complications. Cumulative incidence of abnormal nerve conduction was very high among controls (40–52%). These data demonstrate the crucial role of hyperglycemia in the development of distal symmetric polyneuropathy, but also suggest that neuropathy will continue to develop even in intensively treated subjects exposed to milder degrees of hyperglycemia.

Several other prospective studies were designed to specifically define the incidence of and risk factors for diabetic neuropathy. Of 288 veterans with diabetes but no neuropathy, 20% developed neuropathy after 2 yr follow up *(19)*. Neuropathy was defined as insensitivity to the 5.07 monofilament at one or more of nine sites on either foot. Risk factors for incident neuropathy in multivariate logistic regression analysis included (OR, 95% CI): height, 2.5 cm increase 1.2 (1.1–1.4); previous foot ulcer 2.1 (1.0–4.1); age, 1 yr increase 1.04 (1.00–1.08); glycohemoglobin, 1% increase 1.2 (1.0–1.3); CAGE alcohol score *(20)*, four questions answered positively vs none 7.0 (1.7–29.0); current smoking 0.2 (0.1–0.7); and serum albumin level adjusted for serum creatinine, 1 mg/dL increase 0.3 (0.1–0.8).

Another investigation followed 231 NIDDM subjects free from distal symmetric neuropathy at baseline for a mean follow-up period of 4.7 yr to assess risk factors and incidence of this outcome *(21)*. Distal symmetric neuropathy was defined as described above for the San Luis Valley cross-sectional study *(4,5)*. Incidence of this outcome was 6.1/100 person-years (95% CI 4.7–7.8). In a logistic-regression model that included age, NIDDM duration, insulin treatment, glycohemoglobin, smoking, Hispanic ethnicity, gender, history of myocardial infarction, and angina, the following factors were

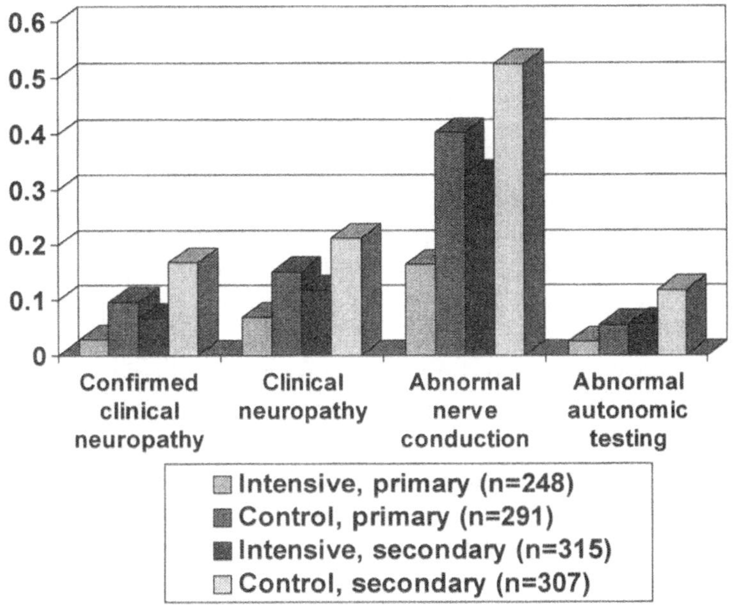


**Fig. 1.** Cumulative incidence of neuropathy after 5-yr follow up in intensively treated and control subjects enrolled in the Diabetes Control and Complications Trial (DCCT). Definitions of neuropathy and primary and secondary cohorts are provided in the text. Intensive treatment consisted of three or more insulin injections/d or an insulin pump, compared to two injections of insulin daily in the control group.

independently related to neuropathy incidence: NIDDM duration (5 yr increase) (OR 1.3, 95% CI 1.0–1.6); current smoking (OR 2.2, 95% CI 1.0–4.7), and history of myocardial infarction (OR 3.5, 95% CI 1.2–9.7). Insulin treatment (OR 2.0, 95% CI 0.9–4.4) and female gender (OR 1.7, 95% CI 0.9–3.3) were associated with neuropathy incidence at borderline statistical significance.

Data from a cohort of IDDM subjects seen within 1 yr of diagnosis at Children's Hospital of Pittsburgh were analyzed after 4 yr of follow up to assess the incidence of neuropathy in relation to baseline glycemic control, defined as poor (glycosylated hemoglobin 11% or greater, $n = 220$) or fair (<11%, $n = 438$) *(22)*. Distal symmetric polyneuropathy was defined as presence of two of three criteria: neuropathic symptoms, decreased or absent tendon reflexes, or signs of sensory loss. Four-year cumulative incidence of this outcome in this cohort of subjects with a mean age of 28 yr, all of whom were diagnosed prior to age 17, was 13%, with an approximately threefold higher risk in poor vs fair control groups (RR 3.2 $p < 0.001$).

Newly diagnosed Finnish NIDDM subjects ($n = 133$) were followed for 10 yr for the development of peripheral neuropathy defined on the basis of nerve conduction velocity and clinical symptoms *(23)*. At baseline, 4.5% of subjects had polyneuropathy, whereas after 10 yr of follow up this proportion increased to 20.9%. Higher cumulative incidence of neuropathy was related to higher baseline fasting plasma glucose, lower fasting serum insulin, and lower serum insulin 1 and 2 hours following a 75-g oral glucose load. Baseline age, smoking, alcohol use, serum lipid values, urinary albumin excretion, and use of antihypertensive medication were unrelated to incidence of polyneuropathy after 10 yr.

A sample of 444 younger onset (diagnosed with diabetes before 30 yr of age and taking insulin) and 406 older onset diabetic subjects without neuropathy from an 11 county area in Wisconsin were followed for up to 10 yr for the development of self-reported loss of tactile sensation or temperature sensitivity *(24)*. Higher glycosylated hemoglobin was related to higher incidence of symptomatic neuropathy, even after adjustment for age, duration of diabetes, and gender in a multivariate model.

The only other prospective study of risk factors for diabetic neuropathy that enrolled more than 100 subjects compared baseline measures of HbA1c, age, diabetes duration, and height in relation to change in thermal, vibration, and monofilament perception of the feet over 2 yr of follow up in 201 medical clinic patients with NIDDM (30% African American, 67% Hispanic) *(25)*. Subjects were divided into an upper fiftieth percentile change for all sensory tests vs those with change below the fiftieth percentile for all tests. The comparisons of baseline measures by this classification did not show significant differences for any potential risk factor.

Four other small prospective studies have been performed on risk factors for diabetic neuropathy. An IDDM cohort ($n = 96$) enrolled in a randomized control trial of intensive glucose control was followed for development of neuropathy defined as two or more abnormal lower extremity nerve conduction velocities or abnormal vibration or thermal sensation *(26)*. No association was found between baseline HbA1c and incidence of neuropathy over 5 yr of follow up, although higher HbA1c during follow up was significantly related to this outcome, except for change in vibration sensation, which was related to diabetes duration only. In another IDDM cohort, 77 subjects ages 25–34 years without clinical neuropathy at baseline were followed for 2 yr for the development of clinically overt neuropathy (as previously defined for the Pittsburgh epidemiology of diabetes complications study) *(27)*. Nephropathy (defined as an albumin excretion rate greater than 200 μg/min on at least 2 of 3 occasions) and higher vibration perception threshold at baseline independently predicted the development of neuropathy, which occurred in 9% of subjects. Change in vibration sensation was measured over 5 yr in a cohort of 71 newly diagnosed subjects with NIDDM *(28)*. Mean fasting blood glucose over the 5-yr period, male gender, age, and body mass index positively correlated with change in vibration sensation threshold. A study of 32 newly diagnosed subjects with IDDM followed for 5 yr found poorer glucose control (HbA1c of 8.3% or greater) related to diminished nerve conduction and decreased thermal (but not vibration) sensation *(29)*.

One large cohort study is worthy of mention for historical purposes. Pirart followed 4400 patients with diabetes in a Belgian clinic for the development of complications from 1947 to 1973 *(30)*. The cumulative incidence of neuropathy was 50% after 25 yr of follow up, and was found to occur more frequently in subjects with poorer glucose control by urine and blood testing. Although the sample size of this study is impressive, its methodology is compromised by a vague definition of neuropathy and outdated methods for measurement of glycemic control.

Prospective research on the risk of distal symmetric polyneuropathy confirms its relationship to poorer glycemic control as reflected by fasting plasma glucose or HbA1c at baseline, as reported by five of the seven largest (more than 100 subjects) and two smaller (less than 100 subjects) cohort studies. Two prospective studies reported age as a risk factor for neuropathy, whereas the following potential risk factors were reported in one prospective study: male gender, height, increase in body mass index, nephropathy, high CAGE alcohol use score, low serum albumin level, insulin treatment, history of myocardial infarction, diabetes duration, nonsmoking, fasting and stimulated serum insulin levels. However, another prospective study produced contradictory results by finding female gender and current smoking associated with neuropathy *(21)*. Whether these discrepant results arise from differences in neuropathy definition, dissimilar patient populations, or both, cannot be determined at the current time.

## PREVALENCE, INCIDENCE, AND RISK OF AUTONOMIC NEUROPATHY

Diabetic autonomic neuropathy has been the subject of fewer research investigations as compared to distal symmetric polyneuropathy. In a community-based cross-sectional study of 168 subjects with IDDM, abnormal autonomic function, as measured by the E:I ratio and the mean circular resultant, was associated with female gender, high LDL cholesterol, and hypertension *(31)*. In addition, abnormal E:I ratio was related to low HDL cholesterol, whereas abnormal mean circular resultant was associated with higher serum triglyceride. Definitions for abnormal E:I ratio or mean circular resultant were not provided in this publication.

Several prospective studies of autonomic neuropathy risk have been reported. The DCCT found mixed results regarding the association between intensive glucose control and 5-yr cumulative incidence of autonomic neuropathy defined as R-R variation with breathing less than 15/min, Valsalva ratio less than 15 with R-R variation with breathing less than 20/min, or orthostatic blood pressure drop of 10 mmHg or more with a blunted catecholamine response (Fig. 1) *(18)*. Greater R-R variation with breathing was seen with intensive treatment in the primary prevention cohort only at the end of follow up, whereas Valsalva ratio did not differ by intensive treatment in either cohort. A Finnish cohort of 133 newly diagnosed NIDDM subjects was followed for 10 yr for the development of parasympathetic neuropathy defined as an E:I ratio of 1:10 or lower, and sympathetic neuropathy, defined as an orthostatic systolic blood pressure decline of 30 mmHg or more *(32)*. At baseline, 4.9% of NIDDM subjects had parasympathetic neuropathy, whereas apparently none had sympathetic neuropathy. After 10 yr of follow up, rates of these neuropathies were 65.0% and 24.4%, respectively. In a stepwise logistic regression model that considered as independent variables age, gender, body mass index, systolic blood pressure, fasting plasma insulin and glucose, and ischemic ECG changes, only fasting plasma insulin (OR 3.1, 95% CI 1.3–7.6) and female gender (OR 3.4, 95% CI 1.2–9.8) were independently and significantly related to cumulative incidence of parasympathetic neuropathy. In a similar logistic model for sympathetic neuropathy cumulative incidence that considered all these factors plus use of diuretic medication, only diuretic use entered the model at $p < 0.05$ (OR 2.9, 95% CI 1.0–8.2). The previously mentioned Stockholm clinical trial followed 96 IDDM subjects for changes in autonomic function as measured by respiratory sinus arrhythmia, Valsalva maneuver, and orthostatic blood pressure fall *(26)*. Baseline HbA1c was unrelated to change in autonomic function, but HbA1c during 5 yr of follow up was significantly related to this outcome. The remaining prospective study was small in size ($n = 32$ subjects with IDDM), and found poorer glucose control (HbA1c > 8.3%) related to diminished heart-rate variability at rest and during deep breathing over 5 yr of follow up *(29)*.

The literature on risk factors for diabetic autonomic neuropathy can be characterized as smaller in size and less consistent compared to that available for distal symmetric polyneuropathy. The only risk factor reported in more than one study was female gender, found to be associated with higher risk by two authors. The absence of a consistent relationship between glucose control and autonomic neuropathy risk raises the possibility that the course of this complication is set soon after diabetes develops and is not amenable to change thereafter, or that available research, including the DCCT, may have been statistically underpowered for the detection of this association.

## OTHER DIABETIC NEUROPATHIES

Little information exists on the prevalence of entrapment or focal neuropathies associated with diabetes. In a cross-sectional survey based in Rochester, Minnesota, asymptomatic carpal tunnel syndrome was found in 22% of those with IDDM and 29% of those with NIDDM, whereas the corresponding prevalence for symptomatic cases was 11% and 6%, respectively *(33)*. Ulnar and femoral cutaneous entrapment was found in 2% of IDDM and 1% of NIDDM subjects. Cranial mononeuropathy and truncal radiculopathy were not observed in the Rochester population, whereas proximal asymmetric polyneuropathy was identified in 1% of IDDM and NIDDM subjects *(33)*. No incidence data are available for any of these types of neuropathy.

No information exists on associations between potential risk factors and diabetic nerve entrapment, mononeuropathies, or proximal asymmetric polyneuropathy from community-based cross-sectional or prospective studies.

## NEUROPATHY AS A RISK FACTOR FOR DIABETIC FOOT ULCER

A key factor in the pathogenesis of diabetic foot complications is presence of neuropathy. Prospective studies demonstrate a higher risk of foot ulcer in association with sensory lower-limb neuropathy as measured with the 5.07 monofilament or by vibration perception threshold. Diabetic American Indians ($n$ = 356) unable to feel the 5.07 monofilament had a 9.9-fold increase in risk of incident foot ulcer over a mean of 2.7 yr of follow up *(34)*. Higher vibration perception threshold ($>$ 25 V) as measured with a biothesiometer was associated with a nearly sevenfold increase in foot-ulcer risk among 469 diabetic patients followed for at least 3 yr *(35)*. A prospective study of 728 United States veterans followed for a total of 1800 person-years found higher foot-ulcer risk independently associated with both insensitivity to the 5.07 monofilament (RR 3.0, 95% CI 1.6–5.4) and orthostatic blood pressure drop of 30 mmHg, a measure of sympathetic neuropathy (RR 2.0, 95% CI 1.2–3.2) *(36)*. Impaired sensation and autonomic dysfunction may independently contribute to diabetic foot-ulcer pathogenesis.

## IS IMPAIRED GLUCOSE TOLERANCE A RISK FACTOR FOR DIABETIC NEUROPATHY?

The San Luis Valley study demonstrated a higher prevalence of distal sensory neuropathy among subjects with IGT as compared to NGT (11.2 vs 3.5%) *(4)*. This finding was not supported in a study of 51 Swedish subjects with persistent IGT for 12–15 yr who were compared to 62 age-matched nondiabetic controls *(37)*. Nerve conduction velocities did not significantly differ between the IGT and the NGT groups. Abnormal heart-rate variation with breathing was more common in IGT vs NGT subjects (29% vs 8%, $p < 0.01$), suggesting that IGT may increase the risk of developing autonomic neuropathy. Whether IGT increases risk of diabetic sensory or autonomic neuropathy cannot be determined from available data.

## IMPLICATIONS FOR FUTURE EPIDEMIOLOGIC RESEARCH

Research on the epidemiology of diabetic neuropathy is at an early stage compared to other diabetic complications. Considerable advances would occur in this field if standardized definitions were developed and used in multiple investigations, although care should be taken to avoid protocols that would be burdensome to study participants, because these would increase the likelihood of bias caused by unacceptably low participation rates. Also, measurement methods should be used that easily translate into clinical practice. Important potential confounding variables must be considered in future studies, including alcohol consumption in particular, height, and possibly nutritional factors as well. Further investigation of the association between hyperlipidemia and risk of neuropathy is warranted to examine the possibility that this complication may have, in part, a macrovascular etiology. Prospective studies of large cohorts of diabetic subjects would likely yield the best quality information concerning potential causative risk factors for diabetic neuropathy. Because of the low frequency of occurrence of diabetic focal neuropathies, the case-control approach would be best suited to identify risk factors for these outcomes. Hopefully these efforts will lead to better methods to prevent this difficult-to-manage complication of diabetes mellitus.

## REFERENCES

1. Rothman KJ. Modern Epidemiology. Little, Brown, Boston, 1986.
2. Oh SJ. Clinical Electromyography. University Park, Baltimore, MD, 1984.
3. Dyck PJ, Kratz KM, Lehman JL, Karnes JL, Melton LJ, O'Brien PC, Litchy WJ, Windebank AJ, Smith BE, Low PA, Service FJ, Rizza RA, Zimmerman BR. The Rochester Diabetic Neuropathy Study: design, criteria for types of neuropathy, selections bias, and reproducibility of neuropathic tests. Neurology 1991;41:799–807.
4. Franklin GM, Kahn LB, Baxter J, Marshall JA, Hamman RF. Sensory neuropathy in non-insulin-dependent diabetes mellitus. Am J Epidemiol 1990;131:633–643.
5. Franklin GF, Shetterly SM, Cohen JA, Baxter J, Hamman RF. Risk factors for distal symmetric neuropathy in NIDDM. Diabetes Care 1994;17:1172–1177.
6. Maser RE, Steenkiste AR, Dorman JS, Nielsen VK, Bass EB, Manjoo Q, Drash AL, Becker DJ, Kuller LH, Greene DA, et al. Epidemiological correlates of diabetic neuropathy. Report from Pittsburgh Epidemiology of Diabetes Complications Study. Diabetes 1989;38:1456–1461.
7. Maser RE, Nielsen VK, Bass EB, Manjoo Q, Dorman JS, Kelsey SF, Becker DJ, Orchard TJ. Measuring diabetic neuropathy. Assessment and comparison of clinical examination and quantitative sensory testing. Diabetes Care 1989;12:270–275.
8. Orchard TJ, Dorman JS, Maser RE, Becker DJ, Ellis D, LaPorte RE, Kuller LH, Wolfson SK Jr, Drash AL. Factors associated with avoidance of severe complications after 25 yr of IDDM. Pittsburgh Epidemiology of Diabetes Complications Study I. Diabetes Care 1990;13:741–747.
9. Kriska AM, LaPorte RE, Patrick SL, Kuller LH, Orchard TJ. The association of physical activity and diabetic complications in individuals with insulin-dependent diabetes mellitus: the Epidemiology of Diabetes Complications Study—VII. J Clin Epidemiol 1991;44:1207–1214.
10. Harris M, Eastman R, Cowie C. Symptoms of sensory neuropathy in adults with NIDDM in the US population. Diabetes Care 1993;16:1446–1552.
11. Knuiman MW, Welborn TA, McCann VJ, Stanton KG, Constable IJ. Prevalence of diabetic complications in relation to risk factors. Diabetes 1986;35:1332–1339.
12. Walters DP, Gatling W, Mullee MA, Hill RD. The prevalence of diabetic distal sensory neuropathy in an English community. Diabetic Med 1992;9:349–353.
13. Bergenheim T, Borrssen B, Lithner F. Sensory thresholds for vibration, perception, and pain in diabetic patients aged 15–50 years. Diabetes Res Clin Prac 1992;16:47–52.
14. Verhoeven S, van Ballegooie E, Casparie AF. Impact of late complications in Type 2 diabetes in a Dutch population. Diabetic Med 1991;8:435–438.
15. Savettieri G, Rocca WA, Salemi G, Meneghini F, Grigoletto F, Morgante L, Reggio A, Costa V, Coraci MA, Di Perri R. Prevalence of diabetic neuropathy with somatic symptoms: a door-to-door sur-

vey in two Sicilian municipalities. Sicilian Neuro-Epidemiologic Study (SNES) Group. Neurology 1993;43:1115–1120.

16. Tesfaye S, Stevens LK, Stephenson JM, Fuller JH, Plater M, Ionescu Tirgoviste, C., Nuber A, Pozza G, Ward JD. Prevalence of diabetic peripheral neuropathy and its relation to glycaemic control and potential risk factors: the EURODIAB IDDM Complications Study. Diabetologia 1996;39:1377–1384.
17. UK Prospective Diabetes Study 6. Complications in newly diagnosed type 2 diabetic patients and their association with different clinical and biochemical risk factors. Diabetes Res 1990;13:1–11.
18. The Diabetes Control and Complications Trial Research Group. The effect of intensive diabetes therapy on the development and progression of neuropathy. Ann Intern Med 1995;122:561–568.
19. Adler AI, Boyko EJ, Ahroni JH, Stensel V, Forsberg RC, Smith DG. Risk factors for diabetic peripheral sensory neuropathy: results of the Seattle prospective diabetic foot study. Diabetes Care, 1997;20:1162–1167.
20. Ewing JA. Detecting alcoholism: the CAGE questionnaire. JAMA 1984;252:1905–1907.
21. Sands ML, Franklin GM, Shetterly SM, Hamman RF. Incidence of distal symmetric (sensory) neuropathy in NIDDM. Diabetes Care 1997;20:322–329.
22. Lloyd CE, Becker D, Ellis D, Orchard TJ. Incidence of complications in insulin dependent diabetes mellitus: a survival analysis. Am J Epidemiol 1996;143:431–441.
23. Partanen J, Niskanen LK, Lehtinen J, Mersvaala E, Siitonen O, Uusitupa MIJ. Natural history of peripheral neuropathy in patients with non-insulin-dependent diabetes mellitus. N Engl J Med 1995;333:89–94.
24. Klein R, Klein BEK, Moss SE. Relation of glycemic control to diabetic microvascular complications in diabetes mellitus. Ann Intern Med 1996;124(1 pt 2):90–96.
25. Sosenko JM, Kato M, Soto R, Bild DE. A prospective study of sensory neuropathy in patients with Type 2 diabetes. Diabetic Med 1993;10:110–114.
26. Reichard P. Risk factors for progression of microvascular complications in the Stockholm Diabetes Intervention Study (SDIS). Diabetes Res Clin Pract 1992;16:151–156.
27. Maser RE, Becker DJ, Drash AL, Ellis D, Kuller LH, Greene DA, Orchard TJ. Pittsburgh Epidemiology of Diabetes Complications Study. Measuring diabetic neuropathy follow-up study results. Diabetes Care 1992;15:525–527.
28. Hillson RM, Hockaday TDR, Newton DJ. Hyperglycemia is one correlate of deterioration in vibration sense during the 5 years after diagnosis of Type 2 (non-insulin-dependent) diabetes. Diabetologia 1984;26:122–126.
29. Ziegler D, Mayer P, Muhlen H, Gries FA. The natural history of somatosensory and autonomic nerve dysfunction in relation to glycemic control during the first five years after the diagnosis of type 1 (insulin-dependent) diabetes mellitus. Diabetologia 1991;34:822–829.
30. Pirart J. Diabetes mellitus and its degenerative complications: a prospective study of 4,400 patients observed between 1947 and 1973. Diabetes Care 1978;1:168–188.
31. Maser RE, Pfeifer MA, Dorman JS, Kuller LH, Becker DJ, Orchard TJ. Diabetic autonomic neuropathy and cardiovascular risk. Pittsburgh Epidemiology of Diabetes Complications Study III. Arch Intern Med 1990;150:1218–1222.
32. Toyry JP, Niskanen LK, Mantysaari MJ, Lansimies EA, Uusitupa MIJ. Occurrence, predictors, and clinical significance of autonomic neuropathy in NIDDM. Ten-year follow-up from diagnosis. Diabetes Care 1996;45:308–315.
33. Dyck PJ, Kratz KM, Karnes JL, Litchy WJ, Klein R, Pach JM, Wilson DM, O'Brien PC, Melton III LJ, Service FJ. The prevalence by staged severity of various types of diabetic neuropathy, retinopathy, and nephropathy in a population-based cohort: the Rochester Diabetic Neuropathy Study. Neurology 1993;43:817–824.
34. Rith-Najarian SJ, Stolusky T, Gohdes DM. Identifying diabetic patients at high risk for lower-extremity amputation in a primary health care setting. Diabetes Care 1992;15:1386–1389.
35. Young MJ, Breddy JL, Veves A, Boulton AJM. The prediction of diabetic neuropathic foot ulceration using vibration perception thresholds, a prospective study. Diabetes Care 1994;17:557–560.
36. Boyko EJ, Ahroni JH, Stensel V, Forsberg R, Smith DG. A prospective study of risk factors for diabetic foot ulcer. Diabetes 1996;45(suppl 2):194A.
37. Eriksson KF, Nilsson H, Lindgarde F, Osterlin S, Dahlin LB, Lilja B, Rosen I, Sundkvist G. Diabetes mellitus but not impaired glucose tolerance is associated with dysfunction in peripheral nerves. Diabetic Med. 1994;11:279–285.

# 2 Pathogenesis of Diabetic Neuropathy

*Martin J. Stevens, MD, Eva L. Feldman, MD, Thommey Thomas, MD, and Douglas A. Greene, MD*

***Contents***



## INTRODUCTION

Diabetic peripheral neuropathy (DPN), which is characterized by nerve fiber atrophy and loss *(1)*, is a multifactorial disorder resulting from complex interrelated metabolic and vascular defects. It is common, frequently underdiagnosed, and has been reported to be present in 39% of healthy insulin-dependent diabetic patients (in the Diabetes Control and Complications Trial [DCCT]) *(2)* and may afflict over 50% of diabetic subjects after 25 yr of diabetes *(3)* or 44% of diabetic subjects between 70–79 yr of age *(4)*. Although the DCCT has definitively implicated hyperglycemia in its pathogenesis and progression *(2,5)*, the resulting defects in glucose metabolism underlying diabetic neuropathy remain to be identified, and their interaction with other elements in the diabetic milieu (e.g., deficiencies of insulin and other growth-factors, oxidative stress, and so on) remain uncertain. Moreover, the precise cellular localization of the deficits remains highly speculative *(6–8)*.

Glucose-related or "gluco-toxic" metabolic pathogenetic mechanisms include activation of the aldose reductase (AR) pathway *(6,7,9)*, which alters cellular redox potential, promotes intracellular sorbitol and fructose accumulation, and exacerbates oxidative stress *(6,10)*. In diabetic nerves, sorbitol accumulation has been proposed to lead to compensatory osmotic depletion (and metabolic insufficiency) of other nonionic organic osmolytes such as myo-inositol (MI) *(1,6,11)* and the β-amino acid taurine *(12)*, with resultant effects on signal-transduction pathways, $Na^+$-$K^+$-ATPase activity, and antioxidative capacity. In turn, increased oxidative stress may have heretofore unantici-

From: *Contemporary Endocrinology: Clinical Management of Diabetic Neuropathy*
Edited by: A. Veves © Humana Press Inc., Totowa, NJ

pated effects on nerve osmolyte levels and nerve growth factor metabolism. These metabolic defects may directly damage specific critical cellular components of complication-prone tissue, e.g., peripheral nerve axons or Schwann cells, or they may contribute to end-organ dysfunction and damage indirectly through functional and/or structural defects involving supporting mesenchymal elements such as the extracellular matrix or microvasculature *(13,14)*. Alternatively, a reduction in nerve blood flow has been invoked to be of primary etiological importance *(8)* and has been attributed to systemic or localized rheological abnormalities *(15,16)* and alterations in vasoactive agents including endothelium-derived nitric oxide (NO) *(17,18)*, eicosanoids *(19)* and endothelin-1 *(20,21)*.

Increasingly, the complex interdependent nature of the metabolic and vascular defects is emerging. Aldose reductase inhibitors (ARIs) that, for example, prevent organic osmolyte depletion and decrease oxidative stress also correct nerve blood flow deficits potentially through effects on both NO and eicosanoid metabolism *(22)*. Vasoactive agents including NO and the prostaglandins in-turn regulate $Na^+$-$K^+$-ATPase activity differentially within the vasculature and the nerve *(23,24)*. Recently, increased optimism has emerged that an effective and safe treatment for DPN is not just a distant dream as studies have demonstrated that a new generation of potent ARIs, preserve nerve conduction velocity (NCV), prevent nerve-fiber loss, and promote nerve-fiber regeneration in human DPN *(25,26)*. This review will explore the current seemingly divergent hypotheses that have been invoked in the pathogenesis of diabetic neuropathy and attempt to demonstrate their interdependence.

## ALDOSE REDUCTASE

Glucose metabolism through AR is concentration-dependent but phosphorylation-independent and AR, the rate-limiting enzyme that reduces glucose to sorbitol, and sorbitol dehydrogenase (SDH), the second enzyme in the AR pathway that oxidizes sorbitol to fructose (Fig. 1), are both abundantly expressed in tissue prone to the chronic complications of diabetes *(6,7,9,22)*. Hyperglycemia activates the AR pathway primarily by mass action, since carrier-mediated glucose uptake into these tissues is relatively insulin-independent. Moreover, since AR employs NADPH as its reductant, and SDH employs $NAD^+$ as its oxidant, AR pathway flux alters the cytoplasmic redox state of these adenine nucleotide couples as it increases steady-state sorbitol levels and converts glucose to fructose *(6,22)* (Fig. 1).

### *Evidence Implicating the Aldose-Reductase Pathway in the Pathogenesis of DPN*

Studies with specific ARIs increasingly implicate this metabolic pathway in the pathogenesis of DPN (and perhaps other diabetic complications) *(7,25,26)*. In experimental diabetic neuropathy in the rat, ARIs prevent, reverse, or moderate various defects in NCV *(7,12,22)* and ameliorate morphologically evident nerve-fiber damage and loss *(27)*. More importantly, potent ARIs improve NCV in diabetic patients with DPN *(25,26)*. In multicenter placebo-controlled clinical trials in patients with DPN, doses of potent ARIs that lower sural nerve sorbitol content by 80–85% also reverse the histological loss of myelinated sensory-nerve fibers (expressed as the density [D] of myelinated nerve fibers [MNF] = MNF/$mm^2$ cross-sectional area in serial sural nerve biopsies) *(26)*. The yearly improvement in NCV and MNFD with effective ARI treat-

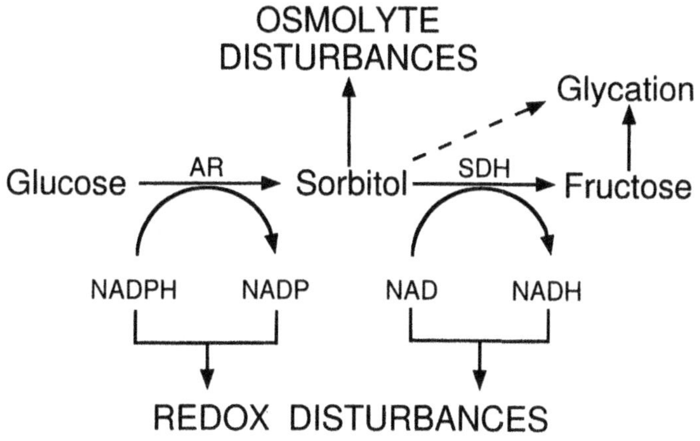


**Fig. 1.** Pathological effects of polyol-pathway activation.

ment exceed the magnitude of the yearly loss of MNFD and NCV in untreated diabetic subjects, and approximate the magnitude of change deemed clinically evident and significant *(26)*.

The success of recent clinical trials has therefore resulted in the importance of high polyol pathway flux in the pathogenesis of DPN becoming generally recognized. In contrast however, the precise mechanisms whereby these beneficial effects are achieved remain controversial. This controversy results from the ability of ARIs to correct many of the known functional deficits in experimental diabetic neuropathy (EDN), including impaired axonal transport *(28,29)*, nerve osmolyte depletion *(12,22)*, redox disturbances *(22,30)*, increased oxidative stress *(10,22)*, depressed nerve $Na^+$-$K^+$-ATPase activity *(22,31)*, depletion of vasoactive agents *(32)*, and nerve blood-flow deficits *(32,33)*. "Osmolyte disturbances" for example, as shown in Fig. 1, comprise only one limb of AR pathway effects and indeed MI depletion comprises only one segment of the "osmolyte disturbance" limb. Other metabolically important osmolytes such as taurine may be equally depleted by sorbitol accumulation *(12)*. Redox disturbances resulting from shifts in adenine nucleotide cofactor couples, and nonenzymatic glycation/glycoxidation resulting from fructose production (Fig. 1) comprise the two other principal pathogenetic pathways that may contribute to the deleterious effects of AR pathway activation.

### *Aldose-Reductase-Related Osmolyte Disturbances*

Activation of AR has been viewed as a critical link between hyperglycemia, cellular osmotic dysregulation, and tissue damage in diabetes *(6,7,34)*. In the renal medulla, AR is now known to play a physiologic role in intracellular osmoregulation during antidiuresis *(35)*. Indeed, the observation that the expression of the AR gene is strongly and specifically induced by extracellular hyperosmolality *(36)* has led to a "compatible osmolyte hypothesis" that argues that a class of nonionic and therefore, "nonperturbing" *(34)* osmotically active compounds such as sorbitol, MI, and taurine, function as alternative organic intracellular osmolytes responding coordinately to changes in external osmolality, thereby buffering otherwise injurious shifts in the intracellular electrolyte and water composition *(34–38)*. On exposure to hypertonic stress, AR promotes the intracellular accumulation of sorbitol *(34–36)*; induction of other stress-response proteins such as the $Na^+$-taurine cotransporter *(38)* and $Na^+$-myo-inositol cotransporter (SMIT) *(37)*, promote accumulation of taurine and MI, respectively. Osmotic induction of these genes is widespread and may occur in response to much smaller osmotic shifts than previously suspected. Hyperglycemia-induced isotonic sorbitol accumulation is unaccompanied by osmotic induction of other osmoresponsive genes *(39,40)*. Indeed the subtle osmotic effects of intracellular sorbitol accumulation (producing a "relative" extracellular hypotonic state) are thought to downregulate the other $Na^+$-osmolyte cotransporters at the transcriptional and/or posttranscriptional level *(41,42)*. Moreover, since the compatible osmolytes exit through a single shared "volume-sensitive organic anion channel" (VSOAC) *(43)*, the osmotic consequences of sorbitol accumulation may also activate MI and taurine efflux. Therefore in diabetes, inappropriate sorbitol accumulation may cause compensatory depletion of other intracellular osmolytes rendering them rate-limiting for normal intracellular metabolism *(6,11,12)*.

Although initially regarded as metabolically inert, these alternative organic osmolytes are now thought to have important metabolic as well as osmoregulatory roles *(6,11,12,22,44,45)*. Thus, MI may become limiting for phosphoinositide (PI) signaling *(11)*, and taurine depletion may exacerbate oxidative stress and lead to disruption of intracellular calcium homeostasis *(44,45)*. Given the osmoregulatory and metabolic importance of taurine and MI under isomolar as well as hypertonic conditions, abnormal expression of osmoresponsive genes (e.g., AR, taurine transporter, or SMIT) may exaggerate the deleterious effects of trivial osmolar or metabolic stress in diabetes predisposing to complications. Indeed, evidence links increased AR enzyme activity and/or protein abundance and the presence of diabetic complications *(46,47)*. However ascribing nerve osmolyte depletion entirely to the osmotic stress resulting from exaggerated accumulation of intracellular sorbitol appears to be an oversimplification as levels of nerve MI and taurine can be changed in diabetic and nondiabetic nerves independently of nerve sorbitol levels.

### *Sorbitol and the Myo-inositol Depletion Hypothesis*

Nerve MI depletion has been invoked as an important mediator of the effect of sorbitol pathway activation on NCV slowing in acute experimental diabetes *(1,6,48–50)*, although this view has now been challenged *(8,32,51,52)*. Oral 1% MI supplementation, whether given in chow *(53)* or synthetic diet *(12,48,49,53,54)*, corrects sciatic-nerve MI depletion and reproduces the beneficial effects of ARI treatment on slowed NCV *(6,12,29,49)*, reduced nerve blood flow *(55)* and the development of paranodal axonal swelling *(56)* in the steptozotocin-induced diabetic (STZ-D) and spontaneously diabetic Bio-breeding (BB) rat models of experimental diabetic neuropathy (EDN). The oral dose of MI appears critical, since 3% MI supplementation is not efficacious, and produces some slowing of MNCV in nondiabetic rats *(32)*. This may reflect depletion of other compatible osmolytes such as taurine *(12)*. Thus the action of ARIs on the acute and rapidly reversible slowing of nerve conduction in experimental diabetes is thought to be mediated in part by correction of sorbitol-pathway-induced MI depletion *(6)*. Depletion of intracellular MI has been thought to render it rate-limiting for membrane PI synthesis and turnover *(6,11)* necessary for phospholipase-C-mediated G protein-associated signal transduction. This has been speculated to lead to diminished PI-derived diacylglycerol (DAG) and impaired activation of protein kinase C (PKC), which may link altered MI metabolism to defective $Na^+$-$K^+$-ATPase regulation *(6,48)* in diabetic nerves. This assertion is based on the observations that $Na^+$-$K^+$-ATPase activity *(23,24,31,48)*, arachidonyl-DAG *(57)* and PKC activation *(54)* are diminished in diabetic nerves and that dietary MI supplementation in vivo *(6,22)*, or exogenous PKC agonists in vitro *(58)* correct impaired nerve $Na^+$-$K^+$-ATPase activity. In addition, MI depletion through its effects on signal-transduction pathways and fatty acid metabolism, may impair NO synthase activity *(23,59)* and/or lipoxygenase/cyclooxygenase pathways *(60)*, resulting in widespread metabolic and vascular deficits through the disruption of NO and prostaglandin metabolism at the level of the sympathetic ganglia, peripheral neuron, or endoneurial vasculature. The ability of a competitive inhibitor of SMIT to reproduce the functional deficits of EDN in nondiabetic rats, and the ability of dietary MI supplementation to overcome these deficits *(61)*, underlines the functional significance of MI depletion and its consequences in EDN.

### *Taurine Depletion as a Mediator of Gluco-toxicity in Diabetes*

Glucose-induced activation of the AR pathway results in depletion of the β-amino acid taurine (2-aminoethanesulfonic acid) *(12,42,45,62,63)* in complication-prone diabetic tissues, including the peripheral nerve *(12)*. The effect of glucose-induced MI depletion on PI signaling is well-known *(11)*, but the role of taurine depletion has only recently been appreciated. Taurine is a potent antioxidant *(64,65)*, calcium modulator *(44,66–68)*, and neurotransmitter *(69,70)*, so that its intracellular depletion could promote chronic cytotoxicity in diabetes by interaction with a complex matrix of biochemical mechanisms.

Like vitamin E, taurine inhibits oxidant-generating biochemical cascades rather than scavenging free radicals. Hypotaurine, its immediate precursor and taurine transporter substrate *(71)* is, however, a potent hydroxyl-radical scavenger *(72)*. High taurine concentrations are found in tissues subject to oxidative stress *(12,45)*. For example, in diabetic rat lens, increased malonyldialdehyde (MDA) levels can be reversed by ARI *(73)*, which normalizes taurine levels *(45)*, or by media supplementation with physiological concentrations of taurine, which prevents cataractogenesis *(62)*. In the kidney in vitro, taurine can reproduce the effects of vitamin E by reversing the inhibitory effects of high glucose and advanced glycosylation end products (AGEs) on mesangial-cell growth *(74)* and can reduce glucose-stimulated mesangial-cell collagen production *(63)*. Taurine's effects on cell growth are analogous to those of superoxide dismutase, catalase, and glutathione, which correct the prolonged replication time of cultured human endothelial cells in high glucose *(75)*. In the sciatic nerve, taurine levels are depressed in diabetic rats *(12)* and nerve taurine replacement partially prevents deficits in nerve blood flow and NCV in EDN (Pop-Busui and Stevens, unpublished observations), suggesting an important modulatory role for taurine on nerve function (Fig. 2). In additional to its antioxidant effects, taurine modulates intracellular $Ca^{2+}$ *(44,66–68)* and PKC activation *(67)*. Taurine lowers cytosolic $Ca^{2+}$ by stimulating mitochondrial uptake *(66,67)*, inhibiting PI turnover *(67)*, and by decreasing internal $Ca^{2+}$ flux *(66)*, thereby inhibiting $Ca^{2+}$-dependent PKC activation *(67)*. Thus, intracellular taurine depletion in diabetes may contribute to the glucose-induced activation of PKC that has been invoked in the pathogenesis of diabetic complications *(76,77)* including DPN. In

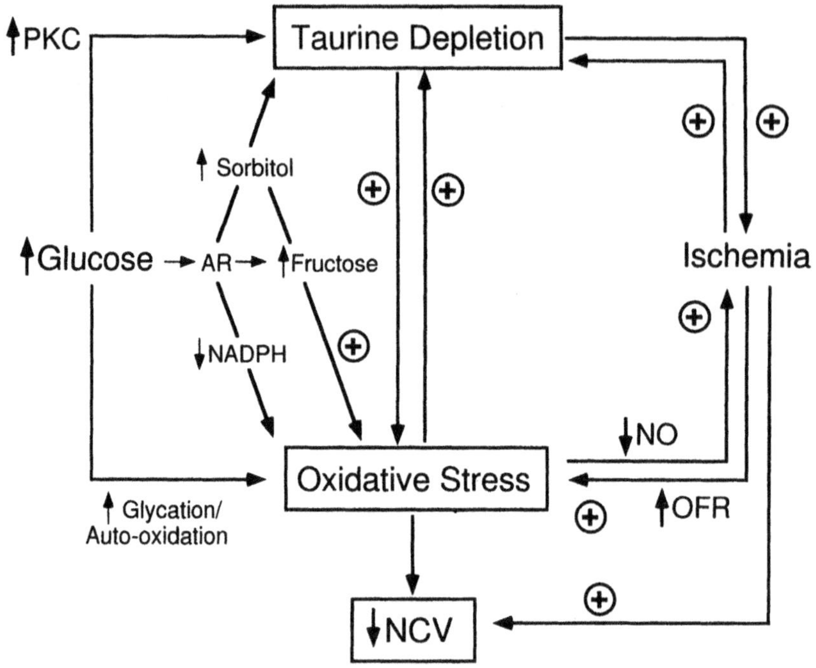


**Fig. 2.** Potential mechanisms linking taurine depletion to oxidative stress and NCV slowing in experimental diabetic neuropathy. Hyperglycemia may exacerbate oxidative stress by both AR-related and AR-unrelated mechanisms. Firstly, glucose-induced activation of the AR pathway results in intracellular sorbitol accumulation leading to compensatory depletion of taurine, alteration of cellular redox potential, and the generation of the potent glycosylator fructose. By AR-unrelated mechanisms, high glucose may activate PKC, which inhibits taurine-transporter activity and leads to taurine depletion and/or stimulates nonenzymatic protein glycation and auto-oxidation of glucose. Taurine depletion may increase oxidative stress directly and indirectly by aggravating nerve ischemia, which in, turn generates oxygen free radicals (OFRs). Reciprocally, oxidative stress may consume taurine, and quench nitric oxide (NO), thereby further exacerbating nerve ischemia. Both nerve ischemia and oxidative stress may result in NCV slowing.

addition, neuronal and glial taurine *(78)* is thought to function as an osmoregulator, neuromodulator, or inhibitory neurotransmitter *(35,38,69,70,79)* as well as neurotrophic agent *(80,81)*. Taurine may also modulate neuronal hyperexcitability by producing hyperpolarization *(82)* or by inhibiting $Ca^{2+}$/calmodulin-dependent protein kinases and its depletion may therefore play a role in the pathogenesis of painful neuropathy *(12)*.

### *Aldose Reductase and Oxidative Stress*

Increasingly, oxidative stress, has been implicated in the development of chronic diabetic complications *(83–86)* including DPN *(8,87)*. Malonyldialdehyde, a degradation product of lipid hydroperoxide, is increased in experimental *(88)* and human diabetes *(89)*. Reduced levels of circulating antioxidants including ascorbic acid, platelet vitamin E, and taurine in human *(90–92)* and experimental diabetes *(88,93,94)* have been ascribed to increased antioxidant consumption from increased oxidative stress, or to transition metal-catalyzed glucose "auto-oxidation" *(84,85)*. Increased oxygen-free-

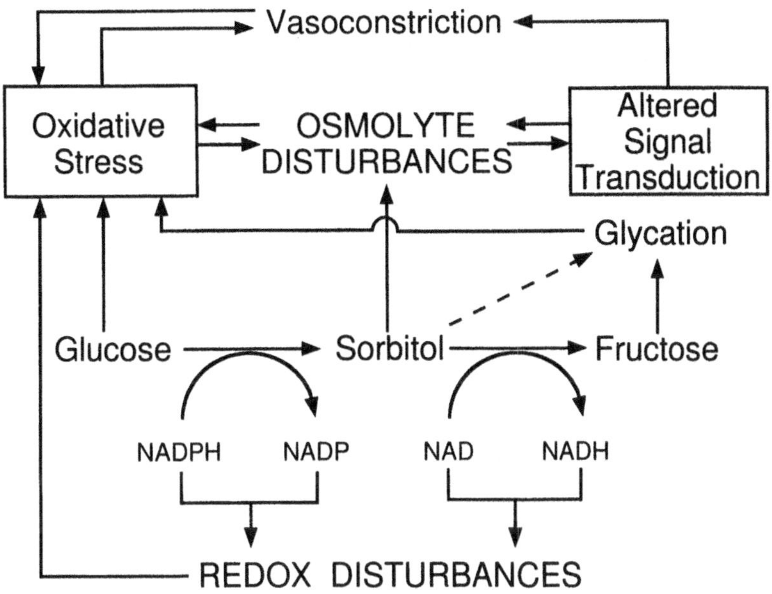


**Fig. 3.** Potential interrelationships between polyol-pathway activation, oxidative stress, and alterations in signal-transduction mechanisms.

radical activity in diabetes is reversed by insulin *(95,96)* or ARIs *(30,97)*, and has been ascribed to glucose–protein interactions *(84,98)*, to auto-oxidation of glucose *(84–86)*, and to glucose-induced activation of the AR pathway *(10,30,97,99)* (Fig. 3).

In EDN, nerve blood flow is decreased, hypoxia may be present and reducing equivalents are increased *(8,100)*. In STZ-D rats, levels of conjugated dienes are increased and superoxide dismutase (SOD) levels decreased after 1 mo of diabetes compared to aged matched nondiabetic control animals *(100)*, and levels of nerve glutathione *(101)* are decreased. Hypoxia may exacerbate oxidative stress by the generation of oxygen free radicals by the xanthine–xanthine oxidase reaction *(102)*. The impairment of the blood–nerve barrier *(103,104)*, reduced nerve norepinephrine *(105)* content, and decreased SOD *(106)* supports the existence of increased nerve oxygen free radicals. Conversely, in diabetes, increased oxidative stress may, in part, be responsible for the reduction in nerve blood flow (Fig. 2). Increased oxidative stress in diabetic vasculature *(85,89,98)* has been implicated in elevations in DAG and PKC *(76)*, which may contribute to vascular dysfunction and proliferation *(76,77,107)*. Oxidative stress can perturb prostanoid synthesis *(88,108)* and NO synthesis *(109,110)* in diabetes and impaired endothelium-dependent relaxation in hyperglycemic rabbits can be corrected by the antioxidant probucol *(111)*.

Support for a role of oxidative stress in EDN is provided by the ability of antioxidants and pro-oxidants to prevent or provoke, respectively, functional nerve deficits. Lipid-soluble antioxidants *(87,101,112)* such as probucol, the free-radical scavenger and glutathione precursor *N*-acetylcysteine *(113)*, glutathione itself *(101)*, the chain-breaking antioxidant lipoic acid *(114)*, and natural antioxidant vitamins C, E, and β carotene *(115)* prevent vascular defects and NCV slowing in diabetic animals. The advanced glycosylation end-product (AGE) inhibitor aminoguanidine prevents motor and sensory NCV deficits *(116,117)* in diabetic rats and prevents the reduction in nerve blood flow *(117)*. Conversely, aggravation of oxidative stress with primaquine in nondiabetic rats partially reproduces diabetic nerve dysfunction *(87)*.

Amelioration of oxidative stress may emerge as the principal mechanism of action of the ARIs *(10,97)*. Advanced glycation is exacerbated by high polyol pathway flux as fructose is a more potent glycating agent than glucose, as are the intermediates and products of the hexose-monophosphate shunt that generates NADPH for AR *(118)*. High flux through the polyol pathway may consume NADPH, which is required for the reduction of glutathione, which is involved in glutathione-peroxidase-catalyzed removal of peroxide formed by the scavenging action of SOD on oxygen free radicals *(87)*. A number of observations suggest that the beneficial effects of ARIs in diabetes may involve decreasing oxidative stress by a mechanism that may involve direct antioxidant effects as oxygen free-radical scavengers or via effects on cellular redox, glutathione, or taurine concentrations *(98)*. The ARIs sorbinil and rutin *(119)* inhibited collagen-linked fluorescence *(10)* and increased vascular permeability in diabetic animals. In diabetic patients, the ARI tolrestat decreases plasma oxygen free-radical levels *(99)*. ARIs may also work partly by binding free copper ions, thus blocking copper-catalyzed ascorbate oxidation *(98)* and by preventing depletion of the endogenous antioxidant taurine *(12)*. Therefore, accumulating evidence implicates a central role for increased oxidative stress in the pathogenesis of EDN. The availability of a plethora of naturally occurring and synthetic antioxidants should also accelerate the instigation of clinical trials to evaluate their efficacy in humans.

### *Nonenzymatic Glycation*

Nonenzymatic formation of Schiff-base residues between glucose and the amine groups of proteins with subsequent Amadori rearrangement, yields glycosylated proteins including hemoglobin *(84–86,118)*. More complex heterocyclic carbohydrate-protein adducts (AGEs) in diabetes lead to protein–protein cross-links and liberation of highly reactive free radicals that structurally alter extracellular matrix and promote cytotoxicity, NO quenching and macrophage activation via the "AGE" receptor *(120)*, a cascade central to current theories regarding the pathogenesis of diabetic complications. Involvement in the pathogenesis of DPN is suggested by evidence that glucose–protein adducts on laminin reduce its support of neurite outgrowth in vitro *(121)*, and that aminoguanidine (which impedes the formation of complex sugar–protein adducts among other actions) ameliorates some of the characteristic defects of EDN *(116,117)*. Recent studies, however, suggest that glucose has a particularly low glycosylation potential among sugars, especially compared to fructose and its metabolites *(118)*. In particular, a novel metabolic pathway that enzymatically phosphorylates fructose (and possibly sorbitol) leading to fructose-3-phosphate (and possibly sorbitol-3-phosphate), which subsequently degrades to 3-deoxyglucosone (3dG), a particularly potent glycosylating agent *(122)*. Thus, AR pathway flux, that converts glucose with its low glycosylating potential, into fructose and sorbitol, phosphorylation by a 3-phosphokinase *(122)*, and subsequent degradation to 3dG, would radically accelerate the formation of complex heterocyclic carbohydrate–protein adducts known as AGE.

### *The Sorbitol-Redox Hypothesis*

In diabetes, the sorbitol-redox hypothesis proposes that the flux of glucose through AR and sorbitol dehydrogenase stochiometrically oxidizes NADPH/$NADP^+$ and reduces NADH/ $NAD^+$ ratios, respectively. Polyol pathway activation in diabetes could, therefore, produce redox disturbances if the capacity of the cell to buffer redox shifts is otherwise compromised or overwhelmed (Fig. 3). Increased oxidative tissue damage in diabetes has been proposed to result from oxidation of NADPH/$NADP^+$ and resulting depletion of reduced glutathione *(100,101)*. Depletion of NADPH may also limit NADPH-dependent synthase reactions, including those responsible for the synthesis of NO, a potent vasodilator and neuromodulator. Thus could lead to NO depletion with secondary effects on nerve blood flow and energy reserve, which could further impair redox-buffering capacity and other energy-requiring processes, e.g., $Na^+K^+$ATPase *(23)*. The metabolic oxidation of glucose-derived sorbitol to fructose by sorbitol dehydrogenase and the consequent reduction of the NADH/$NAD^+$ couple has been suggested to reproduce the redox effects of hypoxia *(123)*, a metabolic pseudohypoxia *(124)* and has been critically implicated in the pathogenesis of diabetic neuropathy *(124)*. The resultant shifts in cytoplasmic NADH/$NAD^+$ would divert glycolytic intermediates to the synthesis of phospholipid precursors such as α-glycerophosphate, phosphatidic acid, DAG, and cytidine-diphospho-diglyceride (CDP-DG), while at the same time interfering with β-oxidation of long-chain fatty acids *(124)* that accumulate in diabetic nerve. The tissues most at risk from this stress may be those with limited oxidative capacity such as the erythrocyte or renal medulla, or in tissues in which oxygen delivery is compromised in diabetes. These relationships are currently being assessed in both cell culture and animal models. Support for the metabolic pseudohypoxia hypothesis has been provided by the ability of millimolar concentrations of pyruvate, which should oxidize the NADH/$NAD^+$ redox couple, to block glucose toxicity *(124)*. However in cell culture, pyruvate has been shown to enhance $Na^+$-dependent MI transport rather than correct a putative alteration in cytoplasmic redox, providing an alternative explanation for the beneficial effects of pyruvate *(125)*. This is another demonstration of the importance of nonosmotic factors in the regulation of nerve osmolyte levels, and suggests the possibility that ischemic hypoxia, by reducing pyruvate levels, could exacerbate MI depletion under some circumstances.

## SIGNAL TRANSDUCTION PATHWAYS AND $NA^+$-$K^+$-ATPASE ACTIVITY

### *Antiparallel Effects of Glucose on PKC Activity*

Glucose-induced alterations of signal transduction pathways are thought to play a critical role in the development of diabetic complications including DPN. However, there appears to exist a heterogeneous and cell-specific relationship between ambient glucose and intracellular signaling. Physiological hyperglycemia has been speculated to alter PI signal transduction by two separate mass-action mechanisms with antiparallel effects *(126)*. In peripheral nerve, glucose-induced, AR-catalyzed sorbitol accumulation and reciprocal MI depletion diminish PI synthesis and turnover, and the subsequent release of PI-derived arachidonyl-DAGs *(6)*, with the net result that PKC activity is decreased (Fig. 4). However, this is in direct contrast, with for example, the vascular tissues in which the predominant effect of elevated concentrations of glucose appears to be PKC activation *(76,77)*. In order to explore the etiology of these tissue-specific phenomena, elements of this pattern of metabolic glucotoxicity have recently been studied in tissue culture *(11,127)*. In cells with high AR gene expression and activity *(11,128)*,

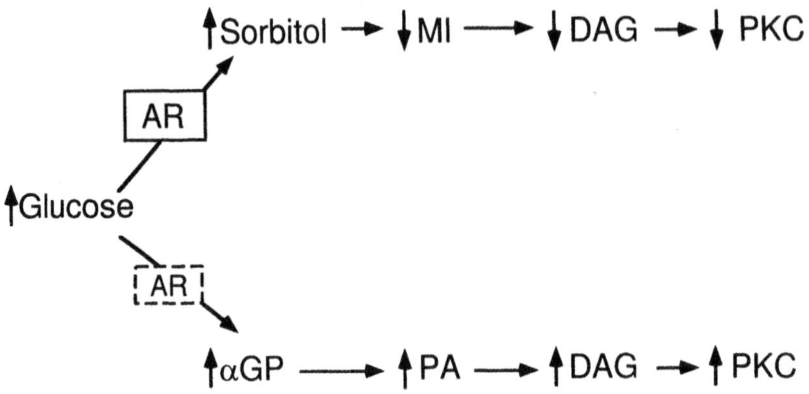


**Fig. 4.** Bidirectional effects of glucose on PKC activity. GP (glycero-phosphate), PA (phosphatidic acid).

including retinal pigment epithelial cells *(11,39,40)* and retinal microvascular pericytes *(127)*, basal and/or agonist-stimulated PI turnover and release of inositol phosphates and/or DAG is diminished after exposure to 20–25 m*M* glucose. In low AR-expressing retinal pigment epithelial cells *(11)*, and other incubated cells and tissues with relatively low AR expression *(128)* such as retinal microvascular endothelial cells *(129)* and isolated renal glomeruli *(130)*, elevated glucose increased DAG precursors such as α-glycerophosphate and phosphatidic acid, which are thought to increase *de novo* synthesis of DAG, in an AR-independent fashion. Thus, there appears to be two distinct metabolic responses that reflect the level of AR gene expression and activity, and the presence or absence of MI depletion (Fig. 4).

The existence of cell-specific AR-mediated heterogeneity of the effects of glucose on DAG is intriguing given the varied cellular composition of most tissues prone to diabetic complications including the retina *(131)*, the renal glomerulus *(132)*, the arterial wall *(128)*, and peripheral nerve *(133)*. For example, discordant effects of glucose on DAG levels and molecular species in retinal pericytes *(127)* and endothelial cells *(129)* could produce simultaneous but diametrically opposite or at least divergent *(134)* effects on growth factor responsiveness and the cell cycle, promoting the simultaneous pericyte loss and endothelial cell replication characteristic of early diabetic retinopathy. Also, the reported beneficial effects of dietary essential-fatty-acid supplementation *(135,136)* or prostaglandin analogs *(33)* on nerve function in STZ-D rats could be explained by amelioration of AR-mediated reductions in arachidonyl-DAG and related molecular species in diabetic nerve. By these constructs, ARIs would offer the potential to convert the biochemical response to hyperglycemia from one pattern to the other in a tissue-specific manner, which would be dependent upon the intrinsic level of AR activity, the degree and site of AR inhibition, and the propensity to increase *de novo* synthesis of PI-related compounds from glucose. The importance of glucose-induced activation of PKC in some tissues prone to diabetic complications has received some support by the recent demonstration that a specific PKC β 1 inhibitor could correct diabetes-induced retinal and renal dysfunction in the STZ-D rat *(137)*. As the effects of activation or inhibition of PKC can be expected to have divergent tissue-specific regulatory effects, e.g., on $Na^+$-$K^+$-ATPase activity and NO synthase activity, tissue-nons-

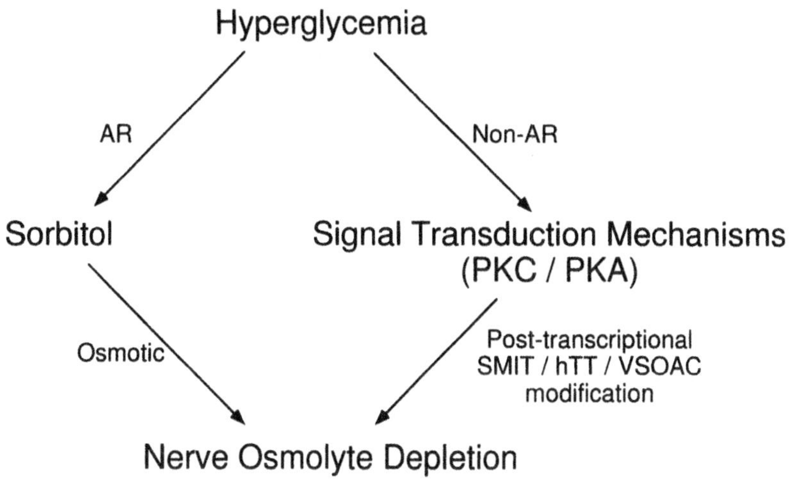


**Fig. 5.** Osmotic and nonosmotic regulation of nerve-osmolyte levels.

elective pharmacological blockade (or activation) of PKC isoforms could be expected to ameliorate the effects of hyperglycemia in some tissues, but may aggravate glucotoxicity in others. Indeed, the effects of PKC β 1 inhibition on tissues that differ from the retina and kidney in the signal-transduction response to hyperglycemia such as the peripheral nerve were not reported *(137)*.

### *Reciprocal Effects of Signal Transduction Pathways on Nerve Osmolyte Levels*

Depletion of nerve osmolytes in diabetes has previously been proposed to result from osmotic compensation for glucose-induced sorbitol accumulation *(6)*. The recent demonstration that nerve acetyl-L-carnitine replacement in STZ-D rats can correct nerve MI levels independently of polyol pathway activity *(138)* and the reported ability of cyclo-oxygenase (COX) blockage to decrease nerve MI levels in nondiabetic rats *(139)*, suggests that nonosmotic metabolic factors may also regulate nerve organic osmolyte levels in EDN. Intracellular levels of MI and taurine are regulated by transmembrane transport mediated by their $Na^+$-dependent cotransporters (regulating cellular uptake) *(37,38)* and VSOAC (regulating cellular efflux) *(43)*. These transport mechanisms are critically regulated by signal-transduction pathways (Fig. 5). In cell culture systems, PKC activation appears to have parallel effects on transmembrane transport of MI and taurine, as it inhibits active uptake *(140)* and stimulates efflux *(43)*. However, in contrast activation of PKA appears to selectively stimulate MI uptake alone *(141*, Stevens unpublished observations). Thus in diabetes, glucose-mediated activation of PKC or inhibition of PKA or altered nerve-energy balance may mediate a major component of the rapid depletion of MI and, possibly, taurine observed in diabetic rodents *(6,12,49)* (Fig. 5). Moreover, therapeutic interventions that have a major impact on signal-transduction pathways (e.g., prostaglandin analogs, PKC antagonists/agonists) may have unanticipated effects on nerve osmolyte levels that may not always be beneficial. Therefore, the heretofore unforeseen and divergent effects of polyol pathway-independent

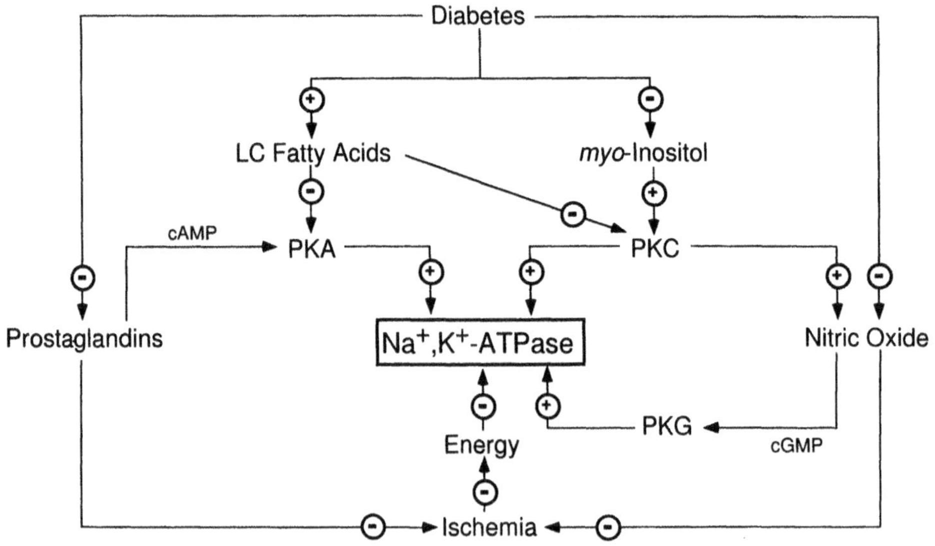


**Fig. 6.** Regulation of nerve $Na^+$-$K^+$-ATPase activity

metabolic interventions on nerve osmolyte levels indicates that careful consideration will need to be given these effects in the selection of future therapeutic agents.

## *Regulation of the NA$^+$-K$^+$-ATPase*

The Na-$K^+$-ATPase has emerged as a possible mechanism for nerve conduction slowing in acutely and chronically diabetic rats as many interventions that prevent nerve dysfunction correct $Na^+$, $K^+$-ATPase activity *(6)*. Decreased $Na^+$, $K^+$-ATPase activity may reflect altered energy metabolism *(142)* and voltage-clamp studies have documented decreased resting axolemmal membrane potential and a four- to five fold increase in intra-axonal [$Na^+$] *(143)*. This ATP-dependent $Na^+$-$K^+$-antiporter also maintains the $Na^+$ gradient that is necessary for the transmembrane transport of MI and taurine. Support for the importance of $Na^+$, $K^+$-ATPase activity in the maintenance of nerve function is provided by recent studies in which pharmacological manipulation of nondiabetic rats with agents that decreased nerve $Na^+$-$K^+$-ATPase activity reproduced diabetic NCV slowing *(23)*. Cyclo-oxygenase products appear to play an important role in the tonic maintenance of nerve $Na^+$, $K^+$-ATPase activity as COX-inhibition potentially decreases ouabain-sensitive activity *(139)* (Fig. 6). Moreover, in EDN, PGE1 analogs *(33)* and cilostazol (a phosphodiesterase inhibitor) *(144)* correct the reduced cAMP levels and prevent the decrease in $Na^+$, $K^+$-ATPase activity in STZ-D rats. The potency of COX-inhibition to disrupt nerve $Na^+$, $K^+$-ATPase activity contrasts with its lack of effect on $Na^+$, $K^+$-ATPase activity in vascular tissue *(24)* (and lack of effect on systemic blood pressure). Moreover, in cultured rat vascular smooth-muscle cells, elevated glucose has been proposed to inhibit $Na^+$, $K^+$-ATPase activity by sequential activation of PKC and PLA2, thereby increasing the production of arachidonic acid and PGE2 *(145)*. These effects diametrically contrast to those of NO, which potently regulates vascular $Na^+$, $K^+$-ATPase activity *(24)* and blood pressure *(23)*, but appears less critical in the direct maintenance of the nerve $Na^+$, $K^+$-ATPase activity *(23)* (specific NO synthase inhibitor takes 3 mo to decrease nerve $Na^+$, $K^+$-ATPase activity) *(23)*. In diabetes, disruption of prostanoid and NO metabolism may have synergistic effects on decreasing nerve $Na^+$, $K^+$-ATPase activity, via both direct metabolic and indirect vascular (ischemic) mechanisms (Fig. 6).

The importance of impaired $Na^+$, $K^+$-ATPase activity in mediating the early decrease in motor NCV in EDN is debated, as ouabain-sensitive $Na^+$, $K^+$-ATPase activity is not detectably decreased before 4 wk of diabetes and some therapies correct its activity without ameliorating MNCV slowing *(138)*. This discordance may reflect differences in fiber type and/or differences in α isoform of the $Na^+$, $K^+$-ATPase (or phosphorylation of its regulatory domain), which principally contribute to these measurements. For example, MNCV is determined by rapidly conducting large myelinated fibers, in which significant concentrations of $Na^+$, $K^+$-ATPase enzyme may be limited to the paranodal Schwann cell processes and the nodal axolemma *(143,146)*. In these fibers (and their Schwann cells) *(146)*, the predominant isoform may be the α 1 *(147)*, which in rodents, is highly ouabain resistant *(147–149)*. In contrast, much of the measured composite ouabain-inhibitible $Na^+$-$K^+$-ATPase activity in whole sciatic nerve may reside in the ouabain-sensitive α2 and α3 isoforms *(147,148)* of the unmyelinated nerve fibers *(149)* that contribute little to the measured MNCV. Alternatively, composite $Na^+$, $K^+$-ATPase correction may be necessary but not sufficient alone to correct MNCV slowing.

The $Na^+$-$K^+$-ATPase is a heterodimer comprised of an α ($M_r$ 112-kDa) subunit, which contains the catalytic subunit and the ATP and ouabain-binding site *(150,151)*, and is the substrate for protein kinases *(152)*, and a α subunit ($M_r$ 35 kDa) that may be important for membrane binding *(153)*. Three different isoforms of the α subunit have been identified (α1, α2, α3) *(148,154)*, with α1 predominating in peripheral nerve and the Schwann cell *(148)*. In STZ-D, a marked and rapid insulin-sensitive reduction in the α1 subunit has been demonstrated by Western analysis after 3 wk of diabetes (a time point at which $Na^+$, $K^+$-ATPase activity is not typically changed) the reductions of the other subunits being delayed *(147)*. PKC activation may itself have bidirectional, tissue- and species-specific effects on $Na^+$, $K^+$-ATPase activity. A reduction in arachidonyl-containing DAGs and PKC activity has been demonstrated in diabetic rat sciatic nerve *(57,58)* and exogenous PKC agonists correct impaired nerve ouabain-sensitive energy metabolism and $Na^+$, $K^+$-ATPase activity in vitro *(155)*. Moreover, PKC activation is without effect on the phosphorylation state of the α subunit in nerves from non-diabetic rats *(148)*, whereas in the STZ-D rat, increased α subunit$^{32}$p labeling was observed with PKC activation. This suggests that in this model, tonic endogenous PKC-mediated $Na^+$-$K^+$-ATPase phosphorylation exists, which is diminished by diabetes. However PKC activation has been associated with diminished $Na^+$-$K^+$-ATPase activity in peripheral nerve in the chronically diabetic mouse, which has low AR levels *(156)*. This may suggest that chronic stimulation of PKC could potentially lead to compensatory up- or downregulation of its action in this animal model.

## DISRUPTION OF VASOACTIVE AGENTS AND NERVE ISCHEMIA IN DIABETES

Increasing evidence suggests that a reduction of nerve blood flow plays a central role in the pathogenesis of diabetic neuropathy and that nerve ischemia may result from metabolic disruption. Hemodynamic and oximetric measurements in anesthetized rats suggest reduced endoneurial blood flow and oxygen tension in chronically diabetic rats

*(8,51)*, which may occur as early as 1 wk after the induction of diabetes *(51)* (although this contention has been disputed) *(157)*. In normal rat sciatic nerve, the nutritive component has been reported to comprise 55% of resting flow, a proportion that is unaffected by diabetes *(32)*. In EDN, endoneurial nutritive flow has been reported to be reduced by 45%, and nonnutritive flow by 48% *(32)*. A wide variety of vasoactive agents partially or completely correct NCV slowing in diabetic rats including those with direct vasodilatory actions such as the α-adrenergic-receptor inhibitor prazosin *(52)*, angiotensin-converting enzyme (ACE) inhibitors *(158)*, prostaglandin analogs *(24)*, NO donors *(159)*, and those with a more indirect vasodilatory action, i.e., ARIs *(33)*, antioxidants *(101,112–115)*, acetyl L-carnitine *(138,160)*, and evening primrose oil (EPO) *(161)*. Most of these agents also have important metabolic effects in addition to the vasodilatory capacity, so ascribing all of their therapeutic efficacy to a direct vascular action may be an over simplification. Suggestive fragmentary clinical evidence in support of nerve hypoxia in the development of DPN has been the finding of a reduction of endoneurial oxygen in the sural nerves of diabetic patients with far advanced polyneuropathy *(162)*, and the development of some abnormalities of neural conduction in nondiabetic hypoxic patients with chronic-obstructive airway disease *(163)*. Nondiabetic animals exposed to chronic hypoxia show some impairment of NCV and resistance to ischemic conduction block, abnormalities of which are reversible when the hypoxia is corrected *(164)*. Finally, experimentally induced reduction in caudal-nerve action potential in diabetic rats can be normalized by hyperbaric oxygenation, but NCV does not improve *(165)*. Thus, although hypoxia may play a role in the development of diabetic neuropathy, it probably is not the only factor. Indeed, unequivocal biochemical data supporting the presence of endoneurial hypoxia in EDN has not yet emerged.

Recently, the importance of the anatomical arrangement of the nerve vasculature has been highlighted in mediating both the diabetes-induced deficits of nerve blood flow as well as the effects of vasoactive therapeutic interventions. The nerve vascular supply comprises an intrinsic system consisting of microvessels that are situated longitudinally within the fascicular endoneurium and an extrinsic system composed of the larger nutritive arteries, arterioles, venules, and epineural vessels. The nerve has only a very limited capacity to autoregulate its vascular supply *(166)*: Perhaps only the epineural and perineural vessels are capable of autoregulation. This means that alterations in system pressure lead to passive fluctuations in perfusion in the nerve *(166)*, so assessments of nerve perfusion are best expressed as a "vascular conductance" that corrects for mean blood pressure *(158)*. Extensive anastomoses (both arteriovenous [AV] and arterioarterial) are formed between the two systems by the epi- and perineural vessels, which together with the low metabolic requirements of the nerve confer a resistance to ischemic insults *(167)*. Extensive perineurial AV anastomoses have recently been demonstrated in neuropathic diabetic subjects and have lead to speculation regarding the role of a "steal phenomenon" occurring in which the nutritive endoneurial capillary flow is impaired by the high shunt flow *(168)*. Conversely, whether this putatively increased shunt flow is a result of chronic endoneurial ischemia/sclerosis is unknown. Many successful therapeutic interventions have been shown to differentially regulate endoneurial nutritive and/or AV shunt flow.

A lack of standardization of techniques for the assessment of nerve blood flow in EDN may have contributed to the divergent interpretations of the direction of blood flow change. For example, although a reduction in nerve blood flow in EDN is generally demonstrated by techniques including laser Doppler flowmetry *(161)* and hydrogen clearance *(8)*, an increase in blood flow (or no change) has been reported using microsphere techniques *(30)*. All the generally used methods have some limitations that appear to adversely affect their utility. For example, laser flowmetry measures composite nerve blood flow, and in general measurements made using this technique have correlated well with hydrogen polarography techniques. A limitation of this technique, is however its inability to distinguish nutritive (capillary) from nonnutritive (large vessel and anastomotic) flow and its capacity to underestimate the former. As agents such as ARIs and acetyl-L-carntine (in contrast to EPO and prostaglandins analogs) may selectively increase endoneurial nutritive flow, without a measurable effect on large-vessel flow *(32,160)*, then these effects may not be detected using laser flowmetry. In common with laser flowmetry, hydrogen-clearance techniques require that the nerve is surgically exposed, a procedure that may alter resting nerve blood flow *(169)*. Microsphere techniques may be misleading because of increased trapping of microspheres in the diabetic vasculature leading to overestimates of nerve blood flow in diabetes, although they allow assessment of flow in unexposed nerve *(170)*. Therefore, in general, disagreement still exists over the best technique to use. The widely agreed success of vasodilatory therapy in preventing or ameliorating nerve dysfunction in EDN *(52,158,159)*, suggests that whatever the direction of blood-flow change, an increase in flow is beneficial to nerve function.

### *Altered Nitric Oxide Metabolism in Diabetic Neuropathy*

The emergence of the endothelium-derived relaxing factor NO as a potent mediator of vasodilatation, macrophage cytotoxicity, and neurotransmission *(17,18,171)* and its altered metabolism in diabetes *(22,23,109–111)*, leads to the speculation that it may be of critical importance to the pathogenesis of diabetic complications, including diabetic neuropathy. NO synthase, the enzyme catalyzing the conversion of L-arginine to citrulline and NO at the expense of NADPH *(171)* is critically situated in endothelial cells, vascular smooth muscle cells, and sympathetic ganglia. NOS is constitutively expressed in endothelial (eNOS) and neuronal (nNOS) cells at the mRNA and protein level, with gene-product activity critically dependent on posttranslational modification by calcium-calmodulin-dependent protein kinases and perhaps other kinases, including PKC *(17,171)*. Impaired synthesis of NO has been linked to polyol-pathway activation through an NADPH-mediated mechanism (via the redox hypothesis), and alterations in protein-kinase activation and calcium levels (via the osmotic hypothesis).

Metabolic competition for NADPH by AR and NOS has been proposed as a potential mechanism leading to NO depletion *(6,172)*. Aldose-reductase-mediated consumption of NADPH may not only directly impair the activity of NO synthetase activity, but may also lead to increased levels of superoxide radicals (that may chemically quench NO) *(18)* as NADPH is required for the production of reduced glutathione *(7)*. The diabetic endothelium is abnormally sensitive to damage mediated by both increased production of superoxide radicals, and to the increased formation of AGEs by glucose *(7)* and fructose that may also quench NO. PKC may also regulate NOS by direct phosphorylation *(173)*. However, the effect of PKC on NOS is controversial, as PKC activation has been reported to either increase *(173)* or decrease *(174)* NOS activity. Moreover, the putatively cell-specific bidirectional effects of hyperglycemia on DAG levels and PKC activation suggests that tissue-specific differences in these regulatory factors may determine the predominant response of NOS to hyperglycemia. Deficiency of the NOS substrate L-arginine in vivo appears not to be responsible for the reduced action of NO on the vasa nervorum, as a 6× increase in dietary L-arginine has been reported to have little effect on NCV deficits in diabetic rats after 1 mo *(159)*. L-arginine transport also does not appear to be impaired *(175)*.

Support for metabolic competition between NOS and AR and/or AR-mediated abnormalities in PKC is provided by the fact that ARIs not only restore osmolyte and redox balance in the nerve *(6)* but also improve nerve blood flow *(33)*. Aldose reductase protein is found within the endoneurium as well as the perineurium *(133)*, and presumably the sympathetic ganglia, which would thus make such metabolic interactions a possibility at any of these sites. In a 3-mo STZ-D rat model, ARI treatment has been reported to normalize endothelium-dependent relaxation *(172)* and the specific NOS inhibitor L-nitro-*N*-methyl arginine ester (L-NAME) was found to reverse the effects of an ARI in acute EDN, despite the ability of the ARI to significantly decrease nerve sorbitol and increase nerve MI in the L-NAME treated rats *(23)*. Despite becoming hypertensive, L-NAME had little acute effect on motor NCV in untreated diabetic animals *(23)* and short-term (3-wk) treatment of nondiabetic rats with L-NAME only insignificantly reduced NCV. In contrast to the vasculature, sciatic-nerve $Na^+$, $K^+$-ATPase activity was not measurably affected by this period of NO inhibition, suggesting that NO may not be the principal regulator of nerve $Na^+$, $K^+$-ATPase activity in the acute rat model. However, 3-mo treatment did slow nerve conduction and reduce $Na^+$-$K^+$-ATPase activity *(23)*. These data support a role for NO in mediating, at least partially, the beneficial effects of ARIs on nerve blood flow and nerve conduction in diabetic rats and possibly also in the chronic maintenance of nerve $Na^+$-$K^+$-ATPase.

Stimulation of NO synthesis is thought to mediate the therapeutic effects of many differing agents, including the ARIs *(23)*, EPO *(161)*, and acetyl L-carnitine *(160)*, as blockade of NO synthesis reverses many of their beneficial effects in EDN. Recently, chronic treatment of diabetic rats for up to 2 mo with the nitrovasodilator isosorbide dinitrate has been reported to prevent motor and sensory NCV deficits and correct reduced nutritive endoneurial blood flow, although nerve $Na^+$, $K^+$-ATPase activity was not measured *(159)*. The failure of L-NAME to block the beneficial effects of 1% dietary MI supplementation on NCV slowing despite the animals remaining hypertensive *(23)*, suggests that although MI may alter NO synthesis *(59)*, its effects on NCV slowing are mediated at least in part by other mechanisms.

In diabetes, NO deficiency may impair nerve blood flow from effects at sites within the nerve vasculature or remote from it, in for example, the sympathetic ganglia. In the endoneurial microvasculature, locally released NO together with locally derived prostacyclins may modulate regional blood flow. In diabetes, deficiencies of these vasodilatory agents may be compounded by elevated plasma levels of the immunoreactive vasoconstrictor endothelin *(20,21)*. Endothelium-dependent relaxation of smooth muscle has been shown to be impaired in both human *(176)* and experimentally induced diabetes *(177)*. The mechanisms underlying this deficit are unclear but may involve depletion of NO *(172,177,178)* or altered smooth-muscle sensitivity to NO *(179)*. Impaired endoneurial vasodilatory responses to acetyl choline *(177)* but preserved endothelial-independent vasodilatory responses to sodium nitroprusside, nitroglycerin, and other agents that directly release NO, implicate a defect or defects in either endoneurial NO synthesis or release as the cause of impaired vascular responses in diabetes. Impaired local synthesis of NO may alter basal vascular tone either by reduced

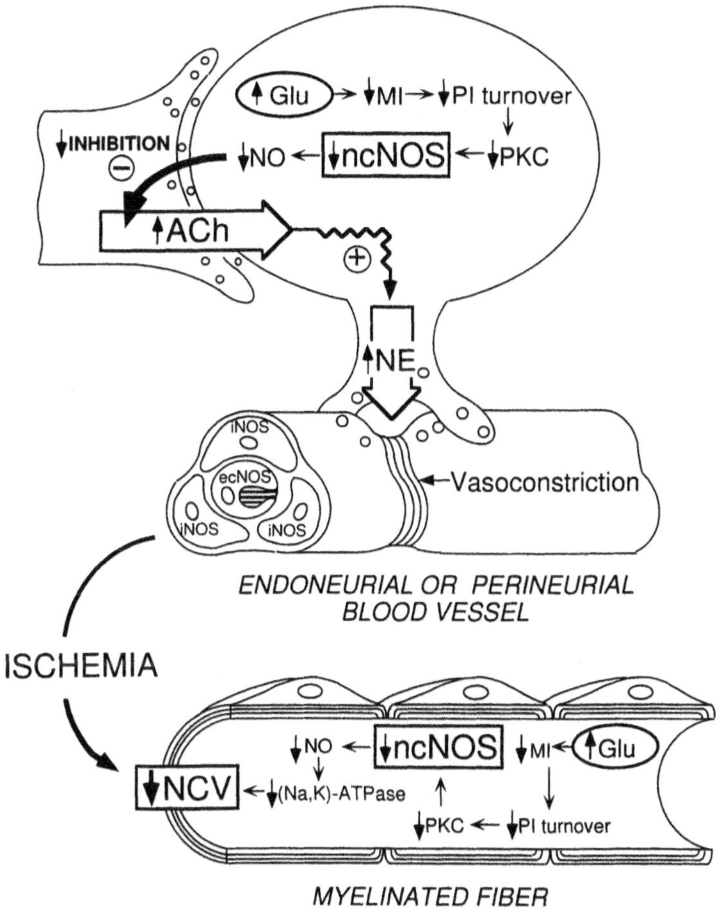


**Fig. 7.** Model for glucose (Glu)-induced inhibition of ncNOS in postganglionic sympathetic or myelinated peripheral somatic neurons resulting in slowing of nerve-conduction velocity (NCV) in acute experimental diabetes. In both postganglionic sympathetic neurons (top) and in myelinated peripheral somatic neurons (bottom) ncNOS is tonically regulated by PKC whose activity is altered in diabetes. In postganglionic sympathetic neurons, NO inhibits presynaptic release of acetylcholine (Ach) and decreases sympathetic tone. NO deficiency at this site may therefore lead to increased vasoconstricting sympathetic tone and reduced nerve blood flow. In large myelinated somatic neurons, NO regulates metabolic processes including $Na^+$,$K^+$-ATPase activity.

activation of soluble guanylate cyclase in vascular smooth muscle *(177)* or by decreased vascular $Na^+$-K-ATPase *(24)* activity potentially resulting in decreased blood flow in the endoneurium of peripheral nerves. Indeed it is apparent that the vascular $Na^+$, $K^+$-ATPase is exquisitely sensitive to changes in NO levels, and NOS inhibition potently decreases $Na^+$, $K^+$-ATPase activity that is associated with hypertension and enhanced vascular reactivity.

Like the prostanoids, NO may play an important role as a neurotransmitter with both central and peripheral effects *(180)*. In the sympathetic autonomic nervous system, NO may function as an inhibitory neurotransmitter, released by postsynaptic sympathetic neurons and thereby inhibiting the presynaptic release of acetylcholine, reducing sympathetic tone *(23,59)* (Fig. 7). Thus, redox perturbations, and alterations of signal-trans-

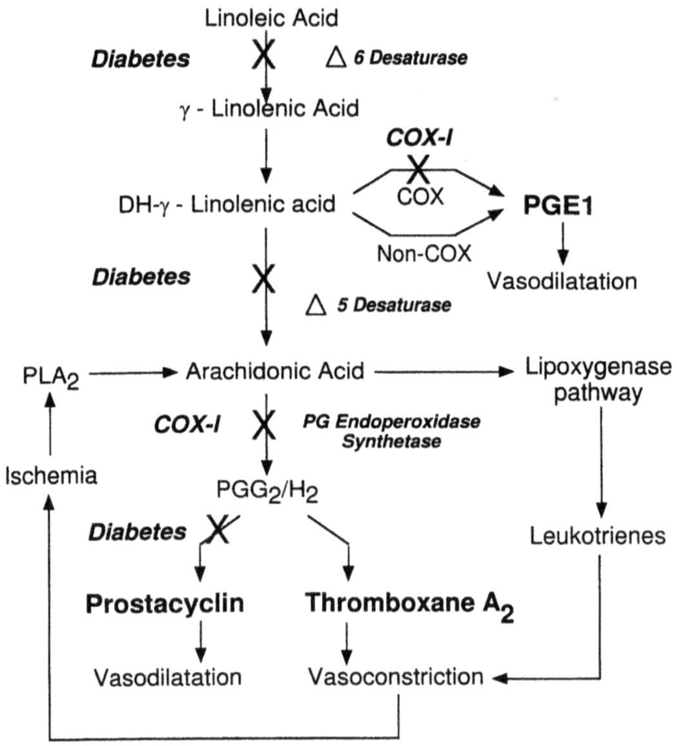


**Fig. 8.** Eicosanoid metabolism in diabetes. COX-I (cyclo-oxygenase inhibitor), $PLA_2$ (Phospholipase $A_2$).

duction pathways may impair nNOS activity in postsynaptic sympathetic neurons, thereby increasing sympathetic vascular tone *(6,59)* (Fig. 7). Acute STZ-D is a state of adrenergic hyperactivity *(181)*, which may be exacerbated by ganglionic NO deficiency. This may explain the observation that inhibition of basal sympathetic vascular tone by guanethidine, restores both nerve blood flow and nerve conduction to normal levels in acute experimental diabetes *(51)*.

Therefore, a decrease in the production of NO in diabetes resulting from sorbitol pathway-related osmolyte depletion or redox imbalance could contribute to NCV slowing by decreasing endoneurial blood flow. Alternatively, NO depletion may exert more distal effects on nerve function independently of nerve blood flow via direct effects on the nerve $Na^+$-$K^+$-ATPase activity.

## *Eicosanoids and Diabetic Neuropathy*

Alterations in fatty-acid metabolism, including the well-described block in the conversion of γ-linoleic acid to α-linolenic acid (Fig. 8), have been invoked (182–184) in the pathogenesis of diabetic neuropathy. Accumulation of long-chain fatty-acid esters in the nerve may perturb cellular metabolism and membrane function potentially by mechanism(s) involving alterations in nerve metabolites, PKC and/or $Na^+$-$K^+$-ATPase activity (Fig. 6). Reduced nerve prostacyclin (secondary to decreased availability of arachidonate *(105)* has been found in chronic (4-mo) experimental diabetes and prostaglandin E1-analog administration has been shown to restore NCV to normal in diabetic rats *(185)*. Depletion of PGE1 in diabetes *(182)*, which is synthesized by both COX-dependent and COX-independent *(183,184)* mechanisms (Fig. 8) could have critical effects on nerve function. It has direct effects on nerve blood flow *(185)*, nerve energy utilization, intracellular calcium mobilization, PKC activity *(183,186)*, and blockade of its synthesis is associated with a reduction in the nerve action-potential amplitude *(187)*. Nerve cAMP levels are reduced in EDN *(188)* and nerve prostacyclin levels, cAMP *(188)*, and $Na^+$-$K^+$-ATPase activity *(185)* correlate with each other and are corrected by prostaglandin E1 administration. Since prostacyclin levels are typically not depleted early in EDN *(105)*, they probably do not precipitate the early decrease in endoneurial blood flow that is observed. However, alterations in the metabolism of COX products probably cannot account for all the acute manifestations of EDN. For example, potent COX inhibition alone does not reproduce the degree of NCV slowing observed in the untreated STZ-D rat, as simultaneous NOS blockade is also required to achieve this *(189)*. Although COX inhibition results in a significant reduction in endoneurial capillary density *(190)*, COX products appear to also regulate nonnutritive flow such as that in the AV shunts *(189)*. COX inhibition with flurbiprofen in STZ-D rats has been reported to increase the total percentage of nutritive nerve blood flow, but decrease composite flow, a finding consistent with nutritive capillary flow diversion secondary to closure of AV shunts *(189)*. An alternative explanation is that COX inhibition may enhance arachidonic acid flux through the lipoxygenase pathway and augment vasoactive leukotriene production and thereby produce collateral vessel vasoconstriction *(191)* (Fig. 8).

The possible interactions between polyol-pathway activity, nerve-osmolyte composition, and redox balance and the secondary effects of these disturbances on prostanoid metabolism are potentially complex. Arachidonic acid, which can become rate-limiting for eicosanoid metabolism, is released from membrane phosphoinositides and is dependent upon cytoplasmic redox for synthesis and metabolism. Altered prostaglandin production and hypersensitivity in diabetes may predispose to either tissue hyperemia or ischemia depending upon the balance between vasoconstrictive or vasodilatory eicosanoids.

In diabetes, alterations in prostanoid metabolism may decrease nerve blood flow secondarily to effects on neurotransmission at the sympathetic ganglia or from local effects within the endoneurial vasculature. Eicosanoids appear to modulate autonomic tone as both PGE1 and PGE2 inhibit sympathetic neurotransmission, mainly by reducing the release of norepinephrine from adrenergic nerve terminals *(192,193)*. This may in part be modulated by regulation of neuronal $Na^+$, $K^+$-ATPase, as decreased activity increases norepinephrine overflow. Disinhibition of sympathetic neurotransmission would act in concert with NO depletion and lead to augmentation of vasoconstricting sympathetic tone. Within the endoneurial vasculature, microvascular tone is dependent on the opposing actions of prostacyclin, which is located within the endothelial cells, which together with NO elicits vasodilatation, and thromboxane $A_2$, which is found mainly in blood platelets but also in endothelium and produces vasoconstriction *(194)* (Fig. 8). Increases in vasoconstricting PGH2 *(195)*, (TX) $A_2$ *(194)*, PGF2a, and reduction in vasodilating prostacyclin have been described in isolated diabetic vascular tissue *(196)*. An increase in the thromboxane:prostacyclin ratio *(118)* may contribute to a reduction of blood flow and possibly $Na^+$-$K^+$-ATPase activity in diabetic nerve. Ischemia in the nerve may activate phospholipase $A_2$ *(197)*, which will disrupt membrane phospholipids and generate prostaglandins from activated arachidonic acid *(198)* (Fig. 8). A hypoxic insult may also be one of the triggers for the production of the superoxide radical via the breakdown of ATP and the generation of reducing equivalents such as NADPH in the xanthine–xanthine oxidase reaction *(105)*. The generation of lipid hydroperoxides by the action of free radicals may result in increased COX activity and a reduction in prostacyclin synthase activity, thus increasing the thromboxane:prostacyclin ratio with resultant vasoconstriction and platelet aggregation. Phospholipase activation may also generate leukotrienes, which may further compound the damage to the endothelial cell and are important regulators of AV shunt flow *(191)*. However, eicosanoids may also serve to limit the detrimental effects of ischemia by inhibiting superoxide anion production *(199)*. Thus, disruption of eicosanoid metabolism may lead to nerve blood flow deficits in diabetes by a complex array of mechanisms.

Correction of defects in eicosanoid metabolism may be the final common pathway by which a number of seemingly diverse therapeutic interventions correct nerve blood flow deficits, $Na^+$-$K^+$-ATPase activity and NCV slowing. Dietary MI supplementation and gamma-linolenic acid (GLA, from evening primrose oil) *(49,136,200)*, may be working at least partly by increasing eicosanoid production as both may increase arachidonic acid and their effects on nerve function can be blocked by COX inhibition (Stevens, unpublished observations refs. *189,190)*. A major component of the beneficial effects of ARIs may also be mediated by COX products, as decreased cAMP levels in STZ-D rat nerves are corrected by AR inhibition *(144)* and the beneficial effects of ARIs on MNCV slowing are also blocked by flurbiprofen *(189)*. Therefore, it seems likely that many therapeutic agents act through a variety of different interdependent pathways involving both the eicosanoids and NO. Recently, a functional synergism between subtherapeutic doses of different metabolic agents on nerve function has been demonstrated in the STZ-D rat model *(189)*, suggesting that even partial correction of deficits in some metabolic pathways may minimize deficits in others.

## DISRUPTION OF GROWTH FACTORS

Increasingly, alterations in the metabolism of nerve growth factors are implicated in the pathogenesis of both DPN as well as autonomic neuropathy. Growth factors can rescue the nervous system from damage *(201,202)*. The prototypic and perhaps best-studied neurotrophic agent is nerve growth factor (NGF) *(203)*. Targets of innervation regulate the final density of innervating neurons through the production of trophic factors that are required for neuronal survival. Nerve growth factor protein is found in target organs of sympathetic and neural-crest-derived dorsal-root ganglion sensory neurons in which levels of NGF mRNA parallel the density of innervation *(203)*. In the rat heart for example, high levels of NGF mRNA and protein are found in the densely innervated atria, but not in the more sparsely innervated ventricles, although regional ventricular differences have not been reported *(204)*.

During embryogenesis 50–70% of dorsal root ganglion neurons (mostly comprising nociceptive C-fibers with small cell bodies and unmyelinated axons) *(205)* are responsive to NGF. In the last 5 yr, the neurotrophin family *(206,207)* has been expanded to include three additional neurotrophic factors, namely brain-derived neurotrophin factor (BDNF), neurotrophin-3 (NT-3), and neurotrophin-4/5 (NT-4/5), which have approximately 50% amino acid sequence homology *(206)*. These neurotrophins bind to a family of tyrosine kinase receptors called Trk (trophomyson-related kinase) *(207)*, whose altered expression represents another possible means by which diabetes could impair neurotrophism. NGF binds to the high-affinity receptor Trk A, Trk B serves as the receptor for both BNDF and NT-4/5 and Trk C binds NT-3. There is documented "promiscuity" in the neurotrophin family in that factors can bind and activate more than one receptor, especially NT-3 *(208)*. In addition to the Trk receptors, a "low" affinity receptor for all the neurotrophins exists, termed p75, which is also the most abundant receptor *(209)*. The low-affinity receptor p75 receptor may modulate NGF sensitivity *(209,210)* and determine the survival requirement of mature sympathetic neurons to NGF *(211)*. p75 is upregulated by NGF *(212)*, axonal injury *(213)*, and collateral sprouting *(214)*, and is expressed in target fields during their innervation *(215)* suggesting that it may present neurotrophins to high-affinity receptors on the growing axons *(209)*. It may interact with TrkA to form the high-affinity receptor *(209)*. Schwann cells express NGF receptors during normal development with a dramatic decline in receptor number (25-fold) upon peripheral nervous system maturation *(216)*. The effects of diabetes and denervation on p75 gene expression are unknown. Trk B and C exist in truncated forms, devoid of the active kinase domain.

Like NGF, retrograde transport of neurotrophins from target organs to neuronal cell bodies is required for normal growth, maintenance, and regeneration of the peripheral nervous system, although an additional local action of NGF has been proposed *(217)*. In general, dorsal root ganglion neurons and primary sensory neurons derived from neural crest are responsive to NGF, BDNF, and NT-3. In contrast, however, cranial-nerve sensory ganglia respond to BDNF or NT-3, but not NGF. During chick development, approx 50% of the dorsal root ganglion neurons are NGF responsive, whereas 30–40% require BDNF. NT-3 promotes the survival of muscle afferents and may primarily support proprioceptive neurons. NT-3 may also regulate the survival of sympathetic ganglion neuronal precursors that transiently express TrkC *(218,219)*. Recently, the roles of neurotrophins have been explored using knockout mice models. Deletion of the high-affinity NGF receptor TrkA in mice results in extensive loss of sympathetic ganglionic neurons and small neural crest-derived sensory neurons (nocioceptive C neurons) *(220,221)*. NT-3 knockout animals are deficient in both type 1a sensory afferents and muscle spindles, whereas BDNF and NT-4/5 null mutants lack neural placode-derived sensory cranial ganglia *(221)*.

Increasingly, it is evident that the role of target-derived neurotrophins changes during development. In the embryo, for example, neurotrophins are required for neuron survival, whereas in the adult they define the neuronal phenotype and promote local regeneration *(206)*. An important function of the neurotrophins is to regulate the expression of phenotypic neuropeptides including substance P and calcitonin gene-related peptide (CGRP) in adult dorsal root ganglion neurons. After nerve injury in the adult, they promote local neurite sprouting and regeneration *(222)*. Thus blunting of these neurotrophic responses may contribute to the pathogenesis of nervous system diseases *(223)*. This may be especially true of diabetic neuropathy, in which persistent hyperglycemia may decrease neurotrophin synthesis by target organs or supporting cells, disrupt retrograde transport of neurotrophins to the neuronal cell body, alter neurotrophin signaling at the level of Trk receptors or at more downstream signaling cascades, or promote neuronal cell death *(224,225)*.

NGF remains the best studied of the neurotrophins and alterations of its actions in diabetes may be particularly important in small nerve fiber damage and autonomic dysfunction. Produced by target cells of sympathetic and neural-crest-derived sensory neurons, retrograde axonal transport is an important modulator of target-tissue NGF as, for example, total sympathetic denervation in adult rats produces high NGF protein levels in the heart *(226,227)*, without affecting tissue mRNA levels *(227,228)*. Retrograde transport of NGF from target organs to neuronal cell bodies is required for normal growth, maintenance, and regeneration of the peripheral nervous system. Loss of NGF leads to neuronal dysfunction and/or death depending on the developmental stage of the animal *(229)*. Ganglionic NGF is required for signal transduction, neurotransmitter synthesis, protein phosphorylation, methylation, and gene expression of ras-like proteins in sympathetic and sensory neurons *(229)*. Systemic administration of NGF to neonatal rats, promotes growth and sprouting of sympathetic neurons *(223)*. NGF increases its own neuronal receptor mRNA levels in a coordinated program of induced gene expression that includes upregulation of tyrosine hydroxylase (TH) mRNA and T$\alpha$1 $\alpha$-tubulin mRNA in sympathetic neurons *(222,230)*. T$\alpha$1 $\alpha$-tubulin mRNA increases after axotomy of sympathetic neurons *(230)* and decreases as reinnervation is achieved *(231)*. However, in the absence of successful reinnervation it remains elevated *(230)*. In adult rat sciatic nerve, NGF production is low as long as axonal contact is maintained *(231,232)*. With nerve transection, Schwann cells distal to the cut, including those ensheathing motor axons, dramatically increase their production of NGF *(233)* and NGF receptors *(234)*, which reach maximal levels at 5–7 d. Transection of selective ventral roots entering the sciatic nerve results in increased NGF-receptor expression by Schwann cells associated with degenerating motor neurons alone, but not intact sensory neurons *(235)*. In patients with diabetic neuropathy *(236)*, however, there is no change in p75 NGF-receptor expression in sural nerve biopsy specimens.

Evidence suggests that altered NGF metabolism may play a role in the pathogenesis of diabetic neuropathy. In diabetes, even small changes in endogenous NGF levels may be of pathophysiological significance as NGF-sensitive neurons are normally NGF starved as endogenous NGF levels are limited *(237)* and their NGF receptors are unsaturated *(238)*. Indeed, in diabetic autonomic neuropathy subjects, serum NGF levels are reduced *(239)* and it has been suggested that NGF autoantibodies may play a role in the development of autonomic neuropathy *(240)*. Decreased skin-axon reflexes, mediated by small sensory fibers, correlate with loss of NGF expression in keratinocytes in patients with early diabetic neuropathy *(241,242)*. Endogenous NGF levels are reduced in some sympathetically innervated target organs of diabetic rodents *(237)* including the sciatic nerve *(237)* and submandibular glands (the latter decreasing NGF in the superior cervical ganglion) *(243,244)*. However, in some target tissues, including the atria and ventricles, NGF content increases after the induction of diabetes, which may reflect impaired axonal transport or possibly increased regional synthesis *(237,245,246)*. NGF binds selectively to the terminal portions of sympathetic and neural crest-derived sensory neurons, and, after internalization, is transported by retrograde axonal flow to the cell bodies, a process that is altered in ST2-D rats *(245,246)*. During experimentally induced diabetes, retrograde axonal transport of NGF along the mesenteric nerves (that supply the alimentary tract) to the superior mesenteric ganglion is reduced by approx half *(246)* and these nerves can develop a distal diabetic axonopathy. In a similar fashion, NGF transport is decreased in diabetic somatic sensory neurons *(247)*. Alterations in NGF transport are only a part of a more widespread transport dysfunction in diabetes that includes proteins, glycoproteins, and neurotransmitters *(246)*. Thus impaired axonal transport, particularly the retrograde flow of neurotrophins, may play a role in the pathogenesis of diabetic neuropathy.

Limited evidence suggests that NGF treatment may be effective in the management of sensory neuropathies. In experimental diabetes, NGF treatment protects against the development of diabetic sensory neuropathy *(248,249)* and ameliorates diabetes-induced decreases in neuropeptide levels in vivo *(250)* and in vitro *(251)*. NGF-treated diabetic rodents retain the ability to respond to noxious thermal stimuli and express normal neuropeptide levels *(249)*. Treatment with 4-methylcatechol, which stimulates endogenous NGF synthesis, also ameliorates neuropathy in streptozocin-treated rodents *(252)*. A preliminary clinical trial in man suggests that NGF may be effective in the treatment of diabetic neuropathy although its use it limited by side effects *(205)*.

When compared to NGF, much less is known about the expression of the other neurotrophin family members in the diabetic state. A recent study has reported a 30–50% decrease in NT-3 and NT-4/5 gene expression in nerves from rodents with experimental diabetes, whereas BDNF was undetectable *(253)*. Levels of NT-3 are decreased in the leg muscles from diabetic rodents and its administration is reported to increase the NCV of sensory nerves *(254)*. Therefore evidence is accumulating of a broad alteration of neurotrophin metabolism in diabetes, which may contribute to the development of diabetic neuropathy.

Another family of growth factors, thought to be important in the pathogenesis and potentially the treatment of diabetic neuropathy *(255)* are the insulin-like growth factors (IGFs). IGF-I and IGF-II are polypeptides essential for normal fetal, neonatal, and pubertal growth *(256)*. IGFs are abundant during fetal development *(257)*, but postnatal IGF expression rapidly decreases *(258)*. In adult rats, the brain and spinal cord contain the highest concentrations of IGF-II mRNAs *(259)*. Gial, but not neuronal cells express IGF-II mRNAs *(260)*, unlike IGF I, which is expressed by both *(260)*. Both IGF I and II increase the number of cells with neurites and the length of neurites in cultured human neuroblastoma cells *(261)* and cultured spinal-cord motor neurons *(262)* as well as act as mitogens for the former. IGF receptors are found on the shafts and terminals of axons *(262,263)*. Six IGFBPs regulate the action of the IGFs *(264,265)* and serve as possible targets for disruption by diabetes. IGFBP II preferentially binds IGF-II and is the predominant IGFBP in the CNS and CSF *(266)*. IGFBP3, which binds both IGF-I and II is the principal form found in the circulation *(267)*. Sites of production of IGFBPs include the neurons and glia *(265,268)*.

IGFs share many important neurotrophic properties with NGF. IGFs have neurotrophic actions in sensory *(267)*, sympathetic *(267,269)*, and motor neurons *(267)*, all of which are affected by diabetes *(270)*. IGFs are presently the only known neurotrophic factors, found in nerve and muscle, capable of supporting both sensory- and motor-nerve regeneration in adult animals *(270,271)*. Local production of IGFs and their binding proteins may stimulate nerve-fiber regeneration. IGF-I and II mRNAs are increased in denervated nerve *(272)*, peaking 6 d after crush, and are downregulated after the axons have regenerated *(272)*. *In situ* hybridization demonstrates that IGF mRNAs are increased in the nerve distal but not proximal to the crush or in the ganglia *(273)*. Neurons may have a trophic-factor requirement that is directly proportional to the length of their axons *(267)*. Local infusion of IGF-I increases the distance of regeneration of sensory axons in lesioned rat sciatic nerve *(274)* and IGF-II stimulates motor-axon regeneration in crushed sciatic nerve *(275)* and increases the rate of sensory axon regeneration *(276)*, which can be decreased by anti-IGF antiserum, implicating a role for endogenous IGF in spontaneous regeneration. Local production of IGF is probably important in stimulating regeneration as IGFBPs would tend to block more distant effects *(267)*.

IGF expression and/or action appears to be altered in diabetes in both rodents and humans. For example, Schwann cells from genetically diabetic rodents express lowered amounts of IGF-I, IGF-IR, and NGF *(277)*. In streptozotocin-treated rats, there is a decrease in serum IGF-I levels *(277–279)* and a reduction in IGF-I mRNA in sciatic nerve, liver, kidney, lung, and heart *(277,280–283)*. Treatment of ST2-D rats with IGF-I protects against the development of diabetic neuropathy and restores normal nerve function *(224,270)*. Studies in humans are currently planned to explore the utility of IGF-I as a treatment for diabetic peripheral neuropathy. Since successful axonal maintenance, regeneration, and reformation of axon-Schwann cell contacts is likely dependent on local synthesis of growth factors and growth-factor receptors, disruption of these processes in diabetes is becoming a key research area in the search for a treatment in humans.

## SUMMARY

In summary, diabetic neuropathy is a result of complex yet interdependent deficits at the molecular, biochemical, and microvascular level, reflecting the detrimental effects of persistent hyperglycemia. Many of these deficits appear related to activation of the AR pathway that may result in altered metabolism of intracellular nonionic osmolytes and adenine-nucleotide-linked chemical reactions. These proceed to involve cellular fuel metabolism, redox potential, signal transduction, and neurotrophism in a profound way. Since complication-prone diabetic tissues are necessarily complex and heterogeneous, the effects of hyperglycemia most likely vary from cell to cell, and differentially effect different vascular beds in complex and diverse ways. Critically, the consequences of these diverse and tissue-specific molecular, metabolic, and physiological perturbations are just beginning to be understood and appreciated. The interdependence of many pathogenetic pathways factors suggests that selective intervention aimed at a key early defect may be therapeutically beneficial. Indeed, recent clinical trials with potent inhibitors of the initial inciting event, metabolism of glucose through AR, in concert with tight glycemic control appear to offer the best opportunity to treat or possibly prevent the diabetic neuropathy.

## REFERENCES

1. Greene DA, Lattimer SA, Sima AAF. Sorbitol, phosphoinositides and sodium-potassium-ATPase in the pathogenesis of diabetic complications. N Engl J Med 1990;316:599.
2. DCCT Research Group. The effect of intensive treatment of diabetes on the development and progression of long-term complications in insulin-dependent diabetes mellitus. N Engl J Med 1993;329:977–986.
3. Pirart J. Diabetes mellitus and its degenerative complications: a prospective study of 4,400 patients observed between 1947 and 1973. Diabetes Care 1978;1:168–188, 252–263.
4. Young MJ, Boulton AJM, Macleod AF, Williams DRR, Sonksen PH. A multicentre study of the prevalence of diabetic peripheral neuropathy in the United Kingdom hospital clinic population. Diabetologia 1993;36:150–154.
5. The DCCT Research Group. The effect of intensive diabetes therapy on the development and progression of neuropathy. Ann Intern Med 1995;122:561–568.

6. Greene DA, Sima AAF, Stevens MJ, Feldman EL, Lattimer SA. Complications: neuropathy, pathogenetic considerations. Diabetes Care 1992;15:1902–1925.
7. Dvornik D. Hyperglycemia in the pathogenesis of diabetic complications. In: Porte D, ed. Aldose Reductase Inhibition. An Approach to the Prevention of Diabetic Complications. Biomedical Information, New York, pp. 69–151.
8. Tuck RR, Schmelzer JD, Low PA. Endoneurial blood flow and oxygen tension in the sciatic nerves of rats with experimental diabetic neuropathy. Brain 1984;107:935–950.
9. Marano CW, Matchinsky FM. Biochemical aspects of diabetes mellitus in microscopic layers of the cornea and retina. Diabetes Metab Rev 1989;5:1–15.
10. Suarez G, Rajaram R, Bhuyan KC, Oronsky AL, Gold JA. Administration of an aldose reductase inhibitor induces a decrease of collagen fluorescence in diabetic rats. J Clin Invest 1988;82:624–627.
11. Nakamura J, Del Monte DA, Shewach D, Lattimer SA, Greene DA. Inhibition of phosphatidylinositol synthase by glucose in human retinal pigment epithelial cells. Am J Physiol 1992;262:E417–E426.
12. Stevens MJ, Lattimer SA, Kamijo M, VanHuysen C, Sima AAF, Greene DA. Osmotically induced nerve taurine depletion and the compatible osmolyte hypothesis in experimental diabetic neuropathy in the rat. Diabetologia 1993;36:608–614.
13. Dyck PJ, Karnes JL, O'Brien P, Okazaki H, Lois A, Engelstad J. The spatial distribution of fiber loss in diabetic polyneuropathy suggests ischemia. Ann Neurol 1986;19:440–449.
14. Vracko RA. Comparison of the microvascular lesions in diabetic mellitus with those of normal aging. J Am Geriatr Soc 1982;30:201–205.
15. Lowe GDO, Lowe JM, Drummond MM, et al. Blood viscosity in young male diabetics with or without retinopathy. Diabetologia 1980;18:359–363.
16. Bauersachs RM, Shaw SJ, Ziedler A, Meiselman HJ. Red blood cell aggregation and blood viscosity in poorly controlled type 2 diabetes mellitus. Clin Hemorheol 1989;9:935.
17. Moncada S, Palmer RMJ, Higgs EA. Nitric oxide: physiology, patho-physiology and pharmacology. Pharmacol Rev 1991;43:109–142.
18. Gryglewski RJ, Palmer RMJ, Moncada S. Superoxide anion is involved in the breakdown of endothelium-derived vascular relaxing factor. Nature 1986;320:454–458.
19. Ward KK, Low PA, Schmelzer JD, Zochodne DW. Prostacyclin and nora-drenaline in peripheral nerve of chronic experimental diabetic in rats. Brain 1989;112:197–208.
20. Takahashi K, Ghatei MA, Lam H-C, O-Halloran DJ, Bloom SR. Elevated plasma endothelin levels in patients with diabetes mellitus. Diabetologia 1990;33:306–310.
21. Takeda Y, Miyamori I, Yoneda T, Takeda R. Production of endothelin-1 from the mesenteric arteries of streptozotocin-induced diabetic rats. Life Sci 1991;48:2553–2556.
22. Greene DA, Sima AAF, Stevens MJ, Feldman EL, Killen PD, Henry DN, Thomas T, Dananberg J, Lattimer SA. Aldose reductase inhibitors: an approach to the treatment of diabetic nerve damage. Diabetes Metab Rev 1993;9:189–217.
23. Stevens MJ, Dananberg J, Feldman EL, Lattimer, SA, Kamijo M, Thomas TP, Shindo H, Sima AAF, Green DA. The linked roles of nitric oxide, aldose reductase and ($NA^+$,$K^+$)-ATPase in the slowing of nerve conduction in the streptozotocin diabetic rat. J Clin Invest 1994;94:853–859.
24. Gupta S, Sussman I, McArthur CS, Tornheim K, Cohen RA, Ruderman NB. Endothelium-dependent inhibition of Na/K-ATPase activity in rabbit aorta by hyperglycemia. J Clin Invest 1992;90:727–732.
25. Sima AAF, Bril V, Nathaniel V, McEwen TA, Brown M, Lattimer SA, Greene DA. Regeneration and repair of myelinated fibers in sural nerve biopsies from patients with diabetic neuropathy treated with an ARI. N Engl J Med 1988;319:548–555.
26. Greene Arezzo J, Brown M, Zenarestat Study Group. Dose-related effects of the aldose reductase inhibitor Zenarestat on nerve sorbitol levels, nerve conduction velocity and nerve fiber density in human diabetic neuropathy. Diabetes 1996;45:A9.
27. Sima AAF, Prashar A, Zhang W-X, Chakrabarti S, Greene DA. Preventative effect of long-term aldose reductase inhibition (Ponalrestat) on nerve conduction and sural nerve structure in the spontaneously diabetic bio-breeding rat. J Clin Invest 1990;85:1410–1420.
28. Tomlinson DR, Sidenius P, Larsen JR. Slow component-a of axonal transport, nerve myo-inositol and aldose reductase inhibition in streptozotocin-diabetic rats. Diabetes 1986;34:398–402.
29. Mayer JH, Tomlinson DR. The influence of aldose reductase inhibition and nerve myoinositol on axonal transport and nerve conduction velocity in rats with experimental Diabetes. J Physiol (London) 1983;340:25P–26P.

30. Williamson JR, Ostrow E, Eades D, Chang K, Allison W, Kilo C, Sherman WR. Glucose-induced microvascular functional changes in nondiabetic rats are stereospecific and are prevented by an aldose reductase inhibitor. J Clin Invest 1990;85:1167–1172.
31. Greene DA, Lattimer SA. Action of sorbinil in diabetic peripheral nerve. Relationship of polyol (sorbitol) pathway inhibition to a myo-inositol-mediated defect in sodium-potassium ATPase activity. Diabetes 1984;33:712–716.
32. Cameron NE, Cotter MA, Dines KC, Maxfield EK, Carey F, Mirrlees DJ. Aldose reductase inhibition, nerve perfusion, oxygenation and function in streptozotocin-diabetic rats: dose-response considerations and independence from a myo-inositol mechanism. Diabetologia 1994;37:651–663.
33. Yasuda H, Masanobu S, Yamashita M, Teradam M, Hatanaka I, Huitian Z, Shigeta Y. Effect of prostaglandin E, analogue TFC612 on diabetic neuropathy in streptozotocin-induced diabetic rats; comparison with aldose reductase inhibitor ONO2235. Diabetes 1989;38:832–838.
34. Burg MB, Kador PF. Sorbitol, osmoregulation, and the complications of diabetes. J Clin Invest 1988;81:635–640.
35. Moriyama T, Garcia-Perez A, Burg MB. Factors affecting the ratio of different organic osmolytes in renal medullary cells. Am J Physiol 1990;259:F847–F858.
36. Moriyama T, Garcia-Perez A, Burg MB. Osmotic regulation of aldose reductase protein synthesis in renal medullary cells. J Biol Chem 1989;264:16,810–16,814.
37. Moo Kwon H, Yamauchi A, Uchida S, Robey R, Garcia-Perez A, Burg MB, Handler JS. Renal Na-myo-inositol cotransporter mRNA expression in *Xenopus oocytes*: regulation by hypertonicity. Am J Physiol 1991;260:F258–F263.
38. Uchida S, Kwon HM, Preston AS, Handler JS. Taurine behaves as an osmolyte in MDCK cells: protection by polarized, regulated transport of taurine. J Clin Invest 1991;88:656–662.
39. Henry DN, Del Monte M, Greene DA, Killen PD. Aldose reductase gene regulation in cultured human retinal pigment epithelial cells. J Clin Invest 1993;92:617–623.
40. Stevens MJ, Henry DN, Thomas TP, Killen PD, Greene DA. Aldose reductase gene expression and osmotic dysregulation in cultured human retinal pigment epithelial cells. Am J Physiol: Endocrinol Metab 1993;265:E428–E438.
41. Hosaka Y, Stevens MJ, Porcellati FA, Larkin D, Masterson J, Killein P, Greene DA. Glucose decreases human Na-dependent myo-inositol transporter mRNA levels in cultured human retinal pigment epithelial cells. Diabetes 1996;45:A1017.
42. Stevens M, Masterson J, Hosaka Y, Larkin D. Glucose induces down-regulation of the human taurine transporter by both osmotic and metabolic mechanisms. Diabetes 1996;45:A765.
43. Jackson PS, Strange K. Volume-sensitive anion channels mediate swelling-activated inositol and taurine efflux. Am J Physiol 1993;265:C1489–C1500.
44. Huxtable RJ. From heart to hypothesis: a mechanism for the calcium modulatory effects actions of taurine. In: Huxtable RJ, Franconi F, Giotti A, eds. The Biology of Taurine: Methods and Mechanisms. Plenum, New York, 1987, pp. 371–388.
45. Malone JI, Lowitt S, Cook WR. Nonosmotic diabetic cataracts. Ped Res 1990;27:293–296.
46. Dent MT, Tebbs SE, Gonzales AM, Ward JD, Wilson RM. Neutrophil aldose reductase activity and its association with established diabetic microvascular complications. Diab Med 1991;8:439–442.
47. Vinores SA, Campochiaro PA, Williams EH, May EE, Green R, Sorenson RL. Aldose reductase expression in human diabetic retina and retinal pigment epithelium. Diabetes 1988;37:1658–1664.
48. Greene DA, Lattimer SA. Impaired energy utilization and Na-K-ATPase in diabetic peripheral nerve. Am J Physiol 1984;246:E311–E318.
49. Greene DA, DeJesus PV, Winegrad AI. Effects of insulin and dietary myo-inositol on impaired motor nerve conduction velocity in acute streptozotocin diabetes. J Clin Invest 1975;55:1326–1336.
50. Finegold D, Lattimer S, Nolle S, Bernstein M, Greene DA. Polyol pathway activity and myo-inositol metabolism. Diabetes 1983;32:988–992.
51. Cameron NE, Cotter MA, Low PA. Nerve blood flow in early experimental diabetes in rats: relation to conduction deficits. Am J Physiol 1991;261:E1–E8.
52. Cameron NE, Cotter MA, Ferguson K, Robertson S, Radcliffe MA. Effects of chronic alpha-adrenergic receptor blockade on peripheral nerve conduction, hypoxic resistance, polyols, Na/K-ATPase activity, and vascular supply in STZ-D rats. Diabetes 1991;40:1652–1658.
53. Tomlinson DR, Mayer JH. Reversal of deficits in axonal transport and nerve conduction velocity by treatment of streptozotocin diabetic rats with myo-inositol. Exp Neurol 1985;89:420–427.

54. Kim J, Rushovich EA, Thomas TA, Ueda T, Agranoff BW, Greene DA. Diminished specific activity of cytosolic protein kinase C in sciatic nerve of streptozotocin-diabetic rats, and its correction by dietary myo-inositol. Diabetes 1991;40:1545–1554.
55. Stevens M, Van Huysen C, Beyer L, Thomas T, Yorek M. Amelioration of nerve blood flow deficits by myo-inositol in streptozotocin-diabetic rats. Diabetes 1996;45:A775.
56. Greene DA, Chakrabarti S, Lattimer SA, Sima AAF. Role of sorbitol accumulation and myoinositol depletion in paranodal swelling of large myelinated nerve fibers in the insulin-deficient spontaneously diabetic biobreeding rat. J Clin Invest 1987;79:1479–1485.
57. Zhu X, Eichberg J. 1,2-diacylglycerol content and its arachidonyl-containing molecular species are reduced in sciatic nerve from streptozotocin-induced diabetic rats. J Neurochem 1990;55:1087–1090.
58. Kim J, Kyriazi H, Greene DA. Normalization of Na,K-ATPase activity in isolated membrane fraction from sciatic nerves of streptozotocin-induced diabetic rats by dietary myo-inositol supplementation in vivo or protein kinase C agonists in vitro. Diabetes 1990;40:558–567.
59. Shindo H, Thomas TP, Larkin DD, Karihaloo AK, Stevens MJ, Greene DA. Modulation of nitric oxide-dependent cyclic-GMP by ambient glucose, myo-inositol and protein kinase C in cultured SH-SY5Y human neuroblastoma cells. J Clin Invest 1996;97:736–745.
60. Karmazyn M, Horrobin DF, Manku MS, Karmali RA, Morgan RO, Ally AI. Myo-inositol in physiological concentrations stimulates production of prostaglandin-like material. Prostaglandins 1977;4:967–974.
61. Yorek MA, Wiese TJ, Davidson EP, Dunlap JA, Stefani MR, Conner CE, Lattimer SA, Kamijo M, Greene DA, Sima AA. Reduced motor nerve conduction velocity and $Na(^{+})$-$K(^{+})$-ATPase activity in rats maintained on L-fucose diet. Reversal by myo-inositol supplementation. Diabetes 1993;42:1401–1406.
62. Malone JI, Benford SA, Malone J Jr. Taurine prevents galactose-induced cataracts. J Diabetes Comp 1993;1:44–48.
63. Trachtman H, Futterweit S, Bienkowski RS. Taurine prevents glucose-induced lipid peroxidation and increased collagen production in cultured rat mesangial cells. Biochem. Biophys Res Comm 1993;191:759–765.
64. Wright CE, Tallan HH, Kin YY, Gaull GE. Taurine: biological update. Ann Rev Biochem 1986;55:427–453.
65. Halliwell B, Gutteridge JMC. The antioxidants of human extracellular fluids. Arch Biochem Biophys 1990;280:1–8.
66. Lombardini JB. Effects of taurine on protein phosphorylation in mammalian tissues. In: Lombardini JB, Schaffer SW, Azuma J, eds. Advances in Experimental and Cell Biology. Taurine: Nutritional Value and Mechanisms of Action. Plenum, New York, 315, 1992, pp. 309–318.
67. Li Y-P, Lombardini JB. Inhibition by taurine of the phosphorylation of specific synaptosomal proteins in the rat cortex: effects of taurine on the stimulation of calcium uptake in the mitochondria and inhibition of phosphoinositide turnover. Brain Res 1991;553:89–96.
68. Whitton PS, Nicholson RA, Strong HC. Effect of taurine on calcium accumulation in resting and repolarized insect synaptosomes. J Neurochem 1988;50:1743–1746.
69. Davidson AN, Kaczmarek LN. Taurine-a possible neurotransmitter? Nature 1971;234:107–108.
70. Lerma J, Herranz AS, Herreras O, Munoz D, Solis JM, del Rio RM, Delgado JMR. Gamma-aminobutyric acid increases the in vivo extracellular taurine in the rat hippocampus. J Neurochem 1985;44:983–986.
71. Aruoma OI, Halliwell B, Hoey BM, Butler J. The antioxidant action of taurine, hypotaurine and their metabolic precursors. Biochem J 1988;256:251–255.
72. Fukuda K, Hirai Y, Yoshida H, Hakajima T, Usii T. Free amino acid content of lymphocytes and granulocytes compared. Clin Chem 1982;28:1758–1761.
73. Yeh LA, Ashton MA. The increase in lipid peroxidation in diabetic rat lens can be reversed by oral sorbinil. Metabolism 1990;39:619–622.
74. Trachtman H, Futterweit S, Prenner J, Hanon S. Antioxidants reverse the antiproliferative effect of high glucose and advanced glycosylation end products in cultured rat mesangial cells. Biochem Biophys Res Comm 1994;199:346–352.
75. Curcio F, Ceriello A. Decreased cultured endothelial cell proliferation in high glucose medium is reversed by antioxidants: new insights on the pathophysiological mechanisms of diabetic vascular complications. In vitro Cell Dev Biol 1992;28A:787–790.

76. Kunisaki M, Bursell S-V, Umeda F, Nawata H, King GL. Normalization of diacylglycerol-protein kinase C activation by vitamin E in aorta of diabetic rats and cultured rat smooth muscle cells exposed to elevated glucose levels. Diabetes 1994;43:1372–1377.
77. Shiba T, Inoguchi T, Sportsman JR, Heath WF, Bursell S, King GL. Correlation of diacylglycerol level and protein kinase C activity in rat retina to retinal circulation. Am J Physiol 1993;265:E783–E793.
78. Sellstrom A, Sjoberg L-B, Hamberger A. Neuronal and glial systems for gamma aminobutyric acid metabolism. J Neurochem 1975;25:393–398.
79. Sanchez-Olea R, Moran J, Schousboe A, Pasantes-Morales H. Changes in taurine transport evoked by hyperosmolarity in cultured astrocytes. J Neurosci Res 1992;32:86–92.
80. Altshular D, Turco JJL, Rusch J, Cepko C. Taurine promotes the differentiation of a vertebrate retinal cell type in vitro. Development 1993;119:1317–1328.
81. Oja SS, Kontro P, Neuromodulatory and trophic actions of taurine. In: Pasantes Morales H, Martin DL, Shain W, del Rio M, eds. Taurine: Functional Neurochemistry, Physiology and Cardiology. Wiley-Liss, 1990, pp. 1–20.
82. Taber KH, Thalman RH. Response of rat hippocampal neurons to taurine. Soc Neurosci Abstr 1983;9:414.
83. Oberley LW. Free radicals and Diabetes. Free Radic Biol Med 1988;5:113–124.
84. Hunt JV, Dean RT, Wolff SP. Hydroxyl radical production and autoxidative glycosylation: glucose autoxidation as the source of protein damage in the experimental glycation model of diabetes mellitus and aging. Biochem J 1988;256:205–212.
85. Baynes JW. Role of oxidative stress in development of complications of diabetes. Diabetes 1991;40:405–412.
86. Wolff SP. Diabetes mellitus and free radicals. Br Med Bull 1993;49:642–652.
87. Cameron NE, Cotter MA, Archibald V, Dines KC, Maxfield EK. Anti-oxidant and pro-oxidant effects on nerve conduction velocity and endoneurial blood flow and oxygen tensions in non-diabetic and streptozotocin-diabetic rats. Diabetologia 1994;37:449–459.
88. Karpen CW, Pritachard KA Jr, Arnold JH, Cornwell DG, Panganamala RV. Restoration of the prostacyclin-thromboxane A2 balance in the diabetic rat: influence of vitamin E. Diabetes 1982;31:947–951.
89. Sato Y, Hotta N, Sakamoto N, Matsuoka S, Ohishi N, Yagi K. Lipid peroxide level in plasma of diabetic patients. Biochem Med 1979;21:104–107.
90. Karpen CW, Cataland S, O'Dorisio TM, Panganamala RV. Interrelation of platelet vitamin E and thromboxane synthesis in type I diabetes mellitus. Diabetes 1994;33:239–243.
91. Karpen CW, Cataland S, O'Dorisio TM, Panganamala RV. Production of 12-hydroxyeicosatetraenoic acid and vitamin E status in platelets from type I human diabetic subjects. Diabetes 1985;34:526–531.
92. Franconi F, Bennardini F, Mattana A, Miceli M, Ciuti M, Mian M, Gironi A, Anichini R, Seghieri G. Plasma and platelet taurine are reduced in subjects with insulin-dependent diabetes mellitus: effects of taurine supplementation. Am J Clin Nutr 1995;61:1115–1119.
93. Luzi L, Castellino P, Simonson DC, Petrides AS, De Fronzo RA. Leucine metabolism in IDDM. Role of insulin and substrate availability. Diabetes 1990;39:38–48.
94. McLennan S, Yue SK, Fisher E, Capogreco C, Heffernan S, Ross GR, Turtle JR. Deficiency of ascorbic acid in experimental diabetes: relationship with collagen and polyol pathway activities. Diabetes 1988;37:359–361.
95. Morel DW, Chisolm GM. Antioxidant treatment of diabetic rats inhibits lipoprotein oxidation and cytotoxicity. J Lipid Res 1989;30:1827–1834.
96. Godin DV, Wohaieb SA, Ganrett ME, Goumeniouk AD. Antioxidant enzyme alterations in experimental and clinical diabetes. Mol Cell Biochem 1988;84:223–231.
97. Wohaieb SA, Godin DV. Alterations in free radical tissue-defense mechanisms in streptozotocin-induced diabetes in the rat. Diabetes 1987;36:1014–1018.
98. Wolff SP. The potential role of oxidative stress in diabetes and its complications: novel implications for theory and therapy. In: Crabbe MJC, ed. Diabetic Complications: Scientific and Clinical Aspects. Churchill-Livingstone, New York, 1982, pp. 167–220.
99. Fondelli C, Signorini AM, Borgogni L, Gragnoli G. Tolrestat and superoxide anion production in type 2 diabetic patients. Diabetologia 1993;36(Suppl. 1):A203.
100. Low PA, Nickander KK. Oxygen free radical effects in sciatic nerve in experimental diabetes. Diabetes 1991;40:873–877.

101. Bravenboer B, Kapelle AC, Hamers FPT, van Buren T, Erkelens DW, Gispen WH. Potential use of glutathione for the prevention and treatment of diabetic neuropathy in the streptozotocin-induced diabetic rat. Diabetologia 1992;35:813–817.
102. McCord JM. Oxygen free radicals in postischemic tissue injury. N Engl J Med 1985;312:159–163.
103. Rechthand E, Smith QR, Latker CH, Rapoport SI. Altered blood-nerve barrier to small molecules in experimental diabetes mellitus. J Neuropath Exp Neurol 1987;46:302–314.
104. Ohi T, Poduslo JF, Dyck PJ. Increased endoneurial albumin in diabetic neuropathy. Neurology 1985;35:1790–1791.
105. Ward KK, Low PA, Schmelzer JD, Zochodne DW. Prostacyclin and noradrenaline in peripheral nerve of chronic experimental diabetic in rats. Brain 1989;112:197–208.
106. Crouch R, Kimsey G, Priest DG, Sarda A, Buse MG. Effect of streptozotocin on erthrocyte and retinal superoxide dismutase. Diabetologia 1978;15:53–57.
107. Kaji H, Kurasak M, Ito K. Increased lipoperoxide value and glutathione peroxidase activity in blood plasma of type 2 (non-insulin dependent) diabetic women. Klin Wochenschr 1985;63:765–768.
108. Moncada S, Gryglewski RJ, Bunting S, Vane JR. A lipid peroxide inhibits the enzyme in blood vessel microsomes that generates from prostaglandin endoperoxides the substance (prostaglandin X) which prevents platelet aggregation. Prostaglandin 1976;12:715–737.
109. Hattori Y, Kawasaki H, Kazuhiro A, Kanno M. Superoxide dismutase recovers altered endothelium-dependent relaxation in diabetic rat aorta. Am J Physiol 1991;261:H1086–H1094.
110. Langenstroer P, Pieper GM. Regulation of spontaneous EDRF release in diabetic rat aorta by oxygen free radicals. Am J Physiol 1992;263:H257–H265.
111. Tesfamarian B, Cohen RA. Free radicals mediate endothelial cell dysfunction caused by elevated glucose. Am J Physiol 1992;263:H321–H326.
112. Cameron NE, Cotter MA, Maxfield EK. Antioxidant treatment prevents the development of peripheral nerve dysfunction in streptozotocin-diabetic rats. Diabetologia 1993;36:299–304.
113. Sagara M, Satoh J, Wada R, Yagihashi S, Takahashi K, Fukuzawa M, Muto G, Muto Y, Toyota T. Inhibition of development of peripheral neuropathy in streptozotocin-induced diabetic rats with N-acetylcysteine. Diabetologia 1996;39:263–269.
114. Nagamatsu M, Nickander KK, Schmelzer JD, Raya A, Wittrock DA, Tritschler H, Low PA. Lipoic acid improves nerve blood flow, reduces oxidative stress, and improves distal nerve conduction in experimental diabetic neuropathy. Diabetes Care 1995;18:1160–7.
115. Cotter MA, Love A, Watt MJ, Cameron NE, Dines KC. Effects of natural free radical scavengers on peripheral nerve and neurovascular function in diabetic rats. Diabetologia 1995;38:1285–1294.
116. Cameron NE, Cotter MA, Dines K, Love A. Effects of aminoguanidine on peripheral nerve function and polyol pathway metabolites in streptozotocin-diabetic rats. Diabetologia 1992;35:946–950.
117. Kihara M, Schmelzer JD, Pouslo JF, Curran FF, Nickander KK, Low PA. Aminoguanidine effect on nerve blood flow, vascular permeability, electrophysiology, and oxygen free radicals. Proc Natl Acad Sci USA 1991;88:6107–6111.
118. Brownlee M. Glycation products and the pathogenesis of diabetic complications. Diabetes Care 1992;15:1835–1843.
119. Odetti PR, Borgoglio A, De Pascale A, Rolandi R, Adezati L. Prevention of Diabetes-increased aging effect on rat collagen-linked fluorescence by aminoguanidine and rutin. Diabetes 1990;39:796–801.
120. Wautier JL, Zoukourian C, Chappey O, Wautier MP, Guillausseau PJ, Cao R, Hori O, Stern D, Schmidt AM. Receptor-mediated endothelial cell dysfunction in diabetic vasculopathy. Soluble receptor for advanced glycation end products blocks hyperpermeability in diabetic rats. J Clin Invest 1996;97:238–243.
121. Haitoglou CS, Tsilibary EC, Brownlee M, Charonis AS. Altered cellular interactions between endothelial cells and nonenzymatically glucosylated laminin/type IV collagen. J Biol Chem 1992;267:12,404–12,407.
122. Szwergold BS, Kappler E, Brown TR. Identification of fructose 3-phosphate in the lens of diabetic rats. Science 1990;247:451–454.
123. Williamson JR, Arrigoni-Martelli E. The roles of glucose-induced metabolic hypoxia and imbalances in carnitine metabolism in mediating diabetes induced vascular dysfunction. Int J Clin Pharm Res 1992;12:247–252.
124. Williamson JR, Chang K, Frangos M, Hasan KS, Ido Y, Kawamura T, Nyengaard JR, Maria Van Den Enden, Kiloc, Tilton RG. Hyperglcemic "pseudohypoxia" and diabetic complications. Diabetes 1993;42:801–813.

125. Thomas TP, Porcellati F, Kato K, Stevens MJ, Sherman WR, Greene DA. Effects of glucose on sorbitol pathway activation, cellular redox and metabolism of myo-inositol, phosphoinositide and diacylglyerol in cultured human retinal pigment epithelial cells. J Clin Invest 1994;93:2718–2724.
126. Thomas TP, Feldman EL, Nakamura J, Kato K, Lien M, Stevens MJ, Greene DA. Ambient glucose and aldose reductase-induced myo-inositol depletion modulate basal and carbachol-stimulated inositol phospholipid metabolism and diacylglycerol accumulation in human retinal pigment epithelial cells in culture. Proc Natl Acad Sci USA 1993;90:9712.
127. De La Rubia G, Oliver FJ, Inoguchi T, King GL. Induction of resistance of endothelin-1's biochemical actions by elevated glucose levels in retinal pericytes. Diabetes 1992;41:1533.
128. Ludwigson MA, Sorenson RL. Immunohistochemical localization of aldose reductase; 1. enzyme purification and antibody preparation-localization in peripheral nerve, artery and testis. Diabetes 1980;29:438–449.
129. Lee T-S, Slatsman KA, Ohashi H, King GL. Activation of protein kinase C by elevation of glucose concentration: proposal for a mechanism in the development of diabetic vascular complications. Proc Natl Acad Sci USA 1989;86:5141–5145.
130. Craven PA, DeRubertis FR. Protein kinase C is activated in glomeruli from streptozotocin diabetic rats: possible mediation by glucose. J Clin Invest 1989;83:1667–1675.
131. Akagi Y, Yajima PF, Kador PF, Kuwabara T, Kinoshita JH. Localization of aldose reductase in the human eye. Diabetes 1984;33:562.
132. Ludwigson MA, Sorenson RL. Immunohistochemical localization of aldose reductase; 2. In rat eye and kidney. Diabetes 1980;29:450–459.
133. Chakrabarti S, Sima AAF, Nakajima T, Yagihashi S, Greene DA. Aldose reductase in the BB rat: isolation, immunological identification and localization in the retina and peripheral nerve. Diabetologia 1987;30:244–251.
134. Leach KL, Ruff VA, Wright TM, Pessin MS, Raben DM. Dissociation of protein kinase C activation and sn-1,2-diacylglycerol formation. Comparison of phosphatidylinositol- and phosphatidylcholine-derived diglycerides in thrombin-stimulated fibroblasts. J Biol Chem 1991;266:3215–3221.
135. Tomlinson DR, Robinson JP, Compton A, Keen P. Essential fatty acid treatment—effects on nerve conduction, polyol pathway and axonal transport in streptozotocin diabetic rats. Diabetologia 1989;32:655–659.
136. Cameron NE, Cotter MA, Robertson S. Effects of essential fatty acid dietary supplementation on peripheral nerve and skeletal muscle function and capillarisation in streptozotocin diabetic rats. Diabetes 1991;40:532–539.
137. Ishii H, Jirousek MR, Koya D, Takagi C, Xia P, Clermont A, Bursell SE, Kern TS, Ballas LM, Heath WF, Stramm LE, Feener EP, King GL. Amelioration of vascular dysfunctions in diabetic rats by an oral PKC beta inhibitor. Science 1996;272:728–731.
138. Stevens MJ, Lattimer SA, Feldman EL, Helton ED, Millington DS, Sima AAF, Greene DA. Acetyl-l-carnitine deficiency as a cause of altered nerve myo-inositol content, Na,K-ATPase activity and motor conduction velocity in the streptozotocin-diabetic rat. Metabolism 1996;45:865–872.
139. Pop-busui R, Van Huysen C, Beyer L, Towns R, Greene DA, Stevens M. Dissociation of nerve blood flow and nerve conduction velocity by acetyl-L-carntine treatment in streptozotocin diabetes. Diabetes 1996;45:A12.
140. Jones DP, Miller LA, Dowling C, Chesney RW. Regulation of taurine transporter activity in LLC-PK1 cells: role of protein synthesis and protein kinase C activation. J Am Soc Nephrol 1991;2:1021–1029.
141. Karihaloo A, Kato K, Greene DA, Thomas T. Coordinated regulation of Na-dependent myo-inositol uptake and efflux by protein kinases in retinal pigment epithelial cells. Implications for glucose-induced diabetic complications. Diabetes 1996;45:190A.
142. Greene DA, Winegrad AI. Effects of acute experimental diabetes on composite energy metabolism in peripheral nerve axons and Schwann cells. Diabetes 1981;30:967–974.
143. Brismar T, Sima AAF, Greene DA. Reversible and irreversible nodal dysfunction in diabetic neuropathy. Ann Neurol 1987;21:504–507.
144. Shindo H, Tawata M, Onaya T. Cyclic adenosine 3′,5′-monophosphate enhances sodium, potassium-adenosine triphosphatase activity in the sciatic nerve of streptozotocin-induced diabetic rats. Endocrinology 1993;132:510–516.
145. Xia P, Kramer RMN, King GL. Identification of the mechanism for the inhibition of Na,K-adenosine triphosphatase by hyperglycemia involving activation of protein kinase C and cytosolic phospholipase A2. J Clin Invest 1995;96:733–740.

146. Powell HC, Garrett RS, Kador PF, Mizisin AP. Fine-structural localization of aldose reductase and ouabain-sensitive, K-dependent p-nitro-phenylphosphatase in rat peripheral nerve. Acta Neuropathol 1991;81:529–539.
147. Fink DJ, Datta S, Mata M. Isoform specific reduction in Na,K-ATPase catalytic (a) subunits in the nerve of rats with streptozotocin-induced Diabetes. J Neurochem 1994;63:1782–1786.
148. Borghini I, Geering K, Gjinovci A, Woilheim CB, Pralong WF. In vivo phosphorylation of the Na,K-ATPase a subunit in sciatic nerves of control and diabetic rats: effects of protein kinase modulators. Proc Natl Acad Sci 1994;91:6211–6215.
149. Landdown D, Ritchie JM. The binding of titrated ouabain to mammalian non-myelinated nerve fibres. J Physiol 1970;207:529–537.
150. Cantley LC. Structure and mechanism of the Na,K-ATPase. Curr Top Bioenerg 1981;11:201–237.
151. Shull GE, Greeb J, Lingrel JB. Molecular cloning of three distinct forms of the Na,K-ATPase a-subunit from rat Brain. Biochemistry 1986;25:8125–8132.
152. Bertorello AM, Aperia A, Ivar Walaas S, Nairn AC, Greengard P. Phosphorylation of the catalytic subunit of $Na^+,K^+$-ATPase inhibits the activity of the enzyme. Proc Natl Acad Sci USA 1991;88:11,359–11,362.
153. McDonough AA, Geering K, Farley RA. The sodium pump needs its B subunit. FASEB J 1990;4:1598–1605.
154. Urayama O, Shutt H, Sweadner KJ. Identification of three isozyme proteins of the catalytic subunit of the Na,K-ATPase in rat Brain. J Biol Chem 1989;264:8271–8280.
155. Lattimer SA, Sima AAF, Greene DA. In vitro correction of impaired $Na^+$-$K^+$-ATPase in diabetic nerve by protein kinase C agonists. Am J Physiol 1989;256:E264–E269.
156. Hermenegildo C, Felipo V, Minana MD, Grisola S. Inhibition of protein kinase C restores Na/K-ATPase activity in the sciatic nerve of diabetic mice. J Neurochem 1992;58:1246–1249.
157. Tilton RG, Pugliese G, Eades DM, Privince MA, Sherman WR, Kilo C, Williamson JR. Prevention of hemodynamic and vascular albumin filtration changes in diabetic rats by ARIs. Diabetes 1989;38:1258–1270.
158. Cameron NE, Cotter MA, Robertson S. Rapid reversal of a motor nerve conduction deficit in streptozotocin-diabetic rats by the angiotensin converting enzyme inhibitor lisinopril. Acta Diabetol 1993;30:46–48.
159. Cameron NE, Cotter MA. Effects of chronic treatment with a nitric oxide donor on nerve conduction abnormalities and endoneurial blood flow in streptozotocin-diabetic rats. Eur J Clin Invest 1995;25:19–24.
160. Cotter MA, Cameron NE, Keegan A, Dines KC. Effects of acetyl- and proprionyl-L-carnitine on peripheral nerve function and vascular supply in experimental diabetes. Metabolism 1995;44:1209–1214.
161. Stevens EJ, Lockett MJ, Carrington AL, Tomlinson DR. Essential fatty acid treatment prevents nerve ischemia and associated conduction anomalies in rats with experimental diabetes mellitus. Diabetologia 1993;36:111–117.
162. Newrick PG, Wilson AJ, Jakubowski J, Boulton AJM, Ward JD. Sural nerve oxygen tension in diabetes. Br Med J 1986;293:1053–1054.
163. Appenzeller O, Parks RD, MacGee J. Peripheral neuropathy in chronic disease of the respiratory tract. Am J Med 1968;44:873–880.
164. Low PA, Schmelzer JD, Ward KK. Experimental hypoxic neuropathy: relavence to diabetic neuropathy. Am J Physiol 1986b;250:E94–E98.
165. Low PA, Schmelzer JD, Ward KK, Curran GL, Poduslo JF. Effect of hyperbaric oxygenation on normal and chronic streptozotocin diabetic peripheral nerves. Exp Neurol 1988;99:201–212.
166. Takeuchi M, Low PA. Dynamic peripheral nerve metabolic and blood pressure responses to exsanguination. Am J Physiol 1987;253:E349–E353.
167. Adams WE. The blood supply of nerves. II. The effects of exclusion of its regional sources of supply on the sciatic nerve of the rabbit. J Anat 1943;77:243–250.
168. Tesfaye S, Harris N, Jakubowski JJ, Mody C, Wilson RM, Renme IG, Ward JD. Impaired blood flow and arterio-venous shunting in human diabetic neuropathy: a novel technique of nerve physiology and fluorescein angiography. Diabetologia 1993;36:1266–1274.
169. Kinoshita Y, Monafo WW. Effect of surgical trauma on regional blood flow in rat sciatic nerve. Exp Neurol 1994;125:296–301.
170. Ido Y, McHowat J, Chang KC, Arrigoni-Martelli E, Orfalian Z, Kilo C, Corr PB, Williamson JR.

Neural dysfunction and metabolic imbalances in diabetic rats: prevention by acetyl-l-carnitine. Diabetes 1994;43:1469–1477.
171. Moncada S, Palmer RMJ, Higgs EA. Biosynthesis of nitric oxide from L-arginine: a pathway for the regulation of cell function and communication. Biochem Pharmacol 1989;38:1709–1715.
172. Cameron NE, Cotter MA. Impaired contraction and relaxation in aorta from streptozotocin-diabetic rats: role of polyol pathway. Diabetologia 1992;35:1011–1019.
173. Nakane ML, Mitchel L, Forstermann U, Murad F. Phosphorylation by calcium calmodulin-dependent protein kinase II and protein kinase C modulates the activity of nitric oxide synthetase. Biochem Biophys Res Comun 1991;180:1396–1402.
174. Bredt DS, Ferris CD, Snyder SH. Nitric oxide synthetase regulatory sites. J Biol Chem 1992;267:10,976–10,981.
175. Sobrevia L, Jay MT, Morgan DML, Yudilevich DL, Mann GE. Arginine transport is elevated in human umbilical vein endothelial cells isolated from insulin-treated diabetic pregnancies and in normal cells cultured in hyperglycemic media. J Physiol 1995;475:67P.
176. Saenz de Tejada I, Goldstein I, Azadzoi K, Krane RJ, Cohen RA. Impaired neurogenic and endothelium-mediated relaxation of the penile smooth muscle from diabetic men with impotence. N Engl J Med 1989;320:1025–1030.
177. Kamata K, Miyata N, Kasuya Y. Impairment of endothelium-dependent relaxation and changes in levels of cyclic GMP in aorta from streptozotocin-induced diabetic rats. Br J Pharmacol 1989;97:614–618.
178. Vallence P, Collier J, Moncada S. Effects of endothelium-derived nitric oxide on peripheral arterial tone in man. Lancet ii 1989;997–1000.
179. Calver A, Collier J, Vallance P. Inhibition and stimulation of nitric oxide synthesis in the human forearm arterial bed of patients with insulin-dependent diabetes. J Clin Invest 1992;90:2548–2554.
180. Bult H, Boeckxstaens GE, Pelckmans PA, Jordaens FH, Van Maercke YM, Herman AG. Nitric oxide as an inhibitory non-adrenergic non-cholinergic neurotransmitter. Nature 1990a;345:346–347.
181. Felton SY, Peterson RG, Shea PA, Besch HR, Felton DL. Effects of streptozotocin diabetes on the noradrenergic innervation of the rat heart: a longitudinal histofluorescence and neurochemical study. Brain Res Bull 1982;8:593–607.
182. Sima AAF, Ristic H, Merry A, Kamijo M, Lattimer SA, Stevens MJ, Greene DA. The primary preventive and secondary interventionary effects of acetyl-L-carnitine on diabetic neuropathy in the BB/W-rat. J Clin Invest 1996;97:1900–1907.
183. Horrobin DF. The roles of essential fatty acids in the development of diabetic neuropathy and other complications of diabetes melitus. Prostaglandins Leukot Essent Fatty Acids 1988;31:181–197.
184. Nugteren DH, Vonkeman H, Van Dorp DA. Non-enzymatic conversion of all-cis 8,11,14-eicosatrienoic acid into prostaglandin E1. RECUEIL 1967;86:1237–1245.
185. Sonobe M, Yasuda H, Hisanaga T, Maeda K, Yamashita M, Kawabata T, Kikkawa R, Taniguchi Y, Shigeta Y. Amelioration of nerve Na/K-ATPase activity independently of myo-inositol level by PGE1 analogue OP-1206 a-CD in streptozotocin-induced diabetic rats. Diabetes 1991;40:726.
186. Yamashita T, Tsuda T, Hamamori Y, Takai Y. Possible involvement of cyclic AMP and calcium ion in PGE1-induced elevation of C-myc mRNA levels in Swiss 3T3 fibroblasts. J Biol Chem 1986;261:16,878–16,882.
187. Horrobin DF, Durand LG, Manku MS. Prostaglandin E1 modifies nerve conduction and interfers with local anaesthetic action. Prostaglandins 1977;14:103–108.
188. Shindo H, Tawata M, Aida K, Onaya T. The role of cyclic adenosine 3′, 5′ -monophosphate and polyol metabolism in diabetic neuropathy. J Clin Endocrinol Metab 1992;74:393–398.
189. Cameron NE, Cotter MA, Hohman TC. Interactions between essential fatty acid, prostanoid, polyol pathway and nitric oxide mechanisms in the neurovascular deficit of diabetic rats. Diabetologia 1996;39:172–182.
190. Cameron NE, Cotter MA, Dines KC, Roberston S, Cox D. The effects of evening primrose oil on nerve function and capillarization in streptozotocin-diabetic rats: modulation by the cyclo-oxygenase inhibitor flurbiprofen. Br J Pharmacol 1993;109:972–979.
191. Brune K, Aehringhaus U, Peskar BA. Pharmacological control of leukotriene and prostaglandin production from mouse peritoneal macrophages. Agents Actions 1984;14:729–734.
192. Hedqvist P, Wennmalm A. Comparison of the effects of prostaglandins E1, E2 and F2 alpha on the sympathetically stimulated rabbit heart. Acta Physiol Scand 1971;83:156–162.
193. Wennmalm A, Hedqvist P. Inhibition by prostaglandin E1 of parasympathetic neurotransmission in the rabbit heart. Life Sci 1971;10:465–470.

194. Subbiah MTR, Deitemeyer D. Altered synthesis of prostaglandins in platelet and aorta from spontaneously diabetic Wistar rats. Biochem Med 1980;23:231–235.
195. Shimizu K, Muramatsu M, Kakegawa Y, Asano H, Toki Y, Miyazaki Y, Okumura K, Hashimoto H, Ito T. Role of prostaglandin H2 as an endothelium-derived contracting factor in diabetic state. Diabetes 1993;42:1246–1252.
196. Harrison HE, Reece AH, Johnson M. Decreased vascular prostacyclin in experimental Diabetes. Life Sci 1978;23:354–356.
197. Bazan NG. Effects of ischemia and electroconvulsive shock on free fatty acid pool in the brain. Biochimica Biophysica Acta 1970;218:1–10.
198. Wolfe LS. Eicosanoids, prostaglandins, thromboxanes, leukotrienes, and other derivatives of carbon-2 unsaturated fatty acids. J Neurochem 1982;38:1–14.
199. Simpson PJ, Mickelson J, Fantone JC, Gallagher KP, Lucchesi BR. Reduction of experimental canine infarct size with prostaglandin E1: inhibition of neutrophil migration and activation. J Pharmacol Exp Therapeut 1988;244:619–624.
200. Houtsmiller AJ, van Hal-Ferwerda J, Zahn KJ, Henkes HE. Favourable influences of linoleic acid on the progression of diabetic micro- and microangiopathy in adult onset diabetes mellitus. Prog Lipid Res 1982;20:377–386.
201. McMahon SB, Priestley JV. Peripheral neuropathies and neurotrophic factors: animal models and clinical perspectives. Curr Opinion Neurobiol 1995;5:616–624.
202. Davies AM. The neurotrophic hypothesis: where does it stand? Philos Trans Royal Soc London, Series B: Biol Sci 1996;351:389–394.
203. Levi-Montaicini R, Calissano P. Nerve growth factor as a paradigm for other polypeptide growth factors. Trends Neurosci 1986;9:473–477.
204. Korsching S, Thoenen H. Nerve growth factor in sympathetic ganglia and corresponding target organs of the rat: correlation with the density of sympathetic innervation. Proc Natl Acad Sci USA 1983a;80:3513–3516.
205. Anand P. Nerve growth factor regulates nociception in human health and disease. Br J Anaesth 1995;75:201–208.
206. Lindsay RM. Role of neurotrophins and trk receptors in the development and maintenance of sensory neurons: an overview. Philos Trans Royal Soc London, Series B: Biol Sci 1996;351:365–373.
207. Bothwell M. Functional interactions of neurotrophins and neurotrophin receptors. Ann Rev Neurosci 1995;18:223–253.
208. Chalazonitis A. Neurotrophin-3 as an essential signal for the developing nervous system. Mol Neurobiol 1996;12:39–53.
209. Chao MV. The p75 neurotrophin receptor. J Neurobiol 1994;25:1373–1385.
210. Davies A, Lee K-F, Jaenisach R. The p75-deficient trigeminal sensory neurons have an altered response to NGF but not to other neurotrophins. Neuron 1993;11:1–20.
211. Lee K-F, Davies AM, Jaenisch R. p75-deficient embryonic dorsal root sensory and neonatal sympathetic neurons display a decreased sensitivity to NGF. Development 1994;120:1027–1033.
212. Doherty P, Seaton P, Flanigan TP, Walsh FS. Factors controlling the expression of the NGF receptor in PC12 cells. Neurosci Lett 1988;92:222–227.
213. Taniuchi M, Clark HB, Johnson EM. Induction of nerve growth factor receptor in Schwann cells after axotomy. Proc Natl Acad Sci USA 1986;83:4094–4098.
214. Diamond J, Holmes M, Coughlin M. Endogenous NGF and nerve impulses regulate the collateral sprouting of sensory axons in the skin of the adult rat. J Neurosci 1992;12:1454–1466.
215. Wyatt S, Shooter EM, Davies AM. Expression of the NGF receptor gene in sensory neurons and their cutaneous targets prior to and during innervation. Neuron 1990;4:421–427.
216. Yan O, Johnson EM. A quantitative study of the developmental expression of nerve growth factor (NGF) receptor in rats. Dev Biol 1987;121:139–148.
217. Campenot RB. Compartmented culture analysis of nerve growth. In: Stevenson B, Paul D, Gallin W, eds. Cell-Cell Interactions: A Practical Approach. IRL Press, Oxford, 1992, pp. 275–298.
218. Birren SJ, LoL, Anderson DJ. Sympathetic neuroblasts undergo a developmental switch in trophic dependence. Development 1993;119:597–610.
219. DiCicco-Bloom E, Friedman WJ, Black IB. NT-3 stimulates sympathetic neuroblast proliferation by promoting precursor survival. Neuron 1993;11:1101–1111.
220. Smeyne RJ, Klein R, Schnapp A, Long LK, Bryant S, Lewin A, Lira SA, Barbacid M. Severe sensory and sympathetic neuropathies in mice carrying a disrupted Trk/NGF receptor gene. Nature 1994;368:256–249.

221. Barbacid M. The Trk family of neurotrophin receptors. J Neurobiol 1994;25:1386–1403.
222. Thoenen H, Angeletti PU, Levi-Montalcici R, Kettler R. Selective induction by nerve growth factor of tyrosine hydroxylase and dopamine hydroxylase in the rat superior cervical ganglion. Proc Natl Acad Sci USA 1971;68:1598–1602.
223. Levi-Montalcini R, Booker B. Excessive growth of the sympathetic ganglia evoked by a protein isolated from mouse salivary glands. Proc Natl Acad Sci USA 1960;42:373–384.
224. Brewster WJ, Fernyhough P, Diemel LT, Mohiuddin L, Tomlinson DR. Diabetic neuropathy, nerve growth factor and other neurotrophic factors. Trends Neurosci 1994;17:321–325.
225. Yagihashi S. Pathology and pathogenetic mechanisms of diabetic neuropathy. Diabetes Metab Rev 1995;11:193–225.
226. Whittemore SR, Larkfors L, Ebendal T, Holets VR, Ericsson A, Persson H. Increased b-nerve growth factor messenger RNA and protein levels in neonatal rat hippocampus following specific cholinergic lesions. J Neurosci 1987;7:244–251.
227. Korsching S, Thoenen H. Treatment with 6-hydroxydopamine and colchicine decreases nerve growth factor levels in the sympathetic ganglia and increases them in the corresponding tissues. J Neurosci 1985a;5:1058–1061.
228. Clegg DO, Large TH, Bodary SC, Reichardt LF. Regulation of nerve growth factor mRNA levels in developing rat heart venticle is not altered by sympathectomy. Dev Biol 1989;134:30–37.
229. Gorin PD, Johnson EM Jr. Effects of long-term nerve growth factor deprivation on the nervous system of the adult rat: an experimental autoimmune approach. Brain Res 1980;198:27–42.
230. Mathew TC, Miller FD. Increased expression of Tal a-tubulin mRNA during collateral and NGF-induced sprouting of sympathetic neurons. Dev Biol 1990;141:84–92.
231. Johnson EM, Taniuchi M, DiStefano PA. Expression and possible function of nerve growth factor receptors on Schwann Cells. Trends Neurosci 1988;111:299–304.
232. Bosch EP, Zhong W, Lim R. Axonal signals regulate expression of glia maturation factor-α in Schwann cells: an immunohistochemical study of injured sciatic nerves and cultured Schwann cells. J Neurosci 1989;9:3690–3698.
233. Heumann R, Korsching S, Bandtlow C, Thoenen H. Changes of nerve growth factor synthesis in non-neuronal cells in response to sciatic nerve transection. J Cell Biol 1987;104:1623–1631.
234. Taniuchi M, Clark HB, Johnson EM. Induction of nerve growth factor receptor in Schwann cells after axotomy. Proc Natl Acad Sci USA 1986;83:4094–4098.
235. Taniuchi M, Clark HB, Schweitzer JB, Johnson EJ. Expression of nerve growth factor receptors by Schwann cells of axotomized peripheral nerves: ultrastructural location, suppression by axonal contact, and binding properties. J Neurosci 1988;8:664–681.
236. Bradley JL, Thomas PK, King RHM, Muddle JR, Ward JD, Tesfaye S, Boulton AJM, Tsigos C, Young RJ. Myelinated nerve fibre regeneration in diabetic sensory polyneuropathy: correlation with type of diabetes. Acta Neuropathologica 1995;90:403–410.
237. Hellweg R, Hartung H-D. Endogenous levels of nerve growth factor (NGF) are altered in experimental diabetes mellitus: a possible role for NGF in the pathogenesis of diabetic neuropathy. J Neurosci Res 1990;26:258–267.
238. Thoenen H, Bandtlow C, Heumann R. The physiological function of nerve growth factor in the central nervous system: comparison with the periphery. Rev Physiol Biochem Pharmacol 1987;109:145–178.
239. Faradji V, Sotelo J. Low serum levels of nerve growth factor in diabetic neuropathy. Acta Neurol Scand 1990;81:402–406.
240. Zanone MM, Banga JP, Peakman M, Edmonds M, Watkins PJ. An investigation of antibodies to nerve growth factor in diabetic autonomic neuropathy. Diabetic Med 1994;11:378–383.
241. Anand P, Terenghi G, Warner G, Kopelman P, Williams-Chestnut RE, Sinicropi DV. The role of endogenous nerve growth factor in human diabetic neuropathy. Nature Med 1996;2:703–707.
242. Anand P. Neurotrophins and peripheral neuropathy. Philos Trans Royal Soc London. Series B: Biol Sci 1996;351:449–454.
243. Kasayama S, Oka T. Impaired production of nerve growth factor in the submandibular gland of diabetic mice. Am J Physiol 1989;257:E400–E404.
244. Ordonez G, Fernandez A, Perez R, Sotelo J. Low contents of nerve growth factor in serum and submaxillary gland of diabetic mice: a possible etiological element of diabetic neuropathy. J Neurol Sci 1994;121:163–166.
245. Hellweg R, Raivich G, Hartung H-D, Hock C, Kreutzberg GW. Axonal transport of endogenous

nerve growth factor (NGF) and NGF receptor in experimental diabetic neuropathy. Exp Neurol 1994;130:24–30.
246. Tomlinson DR, Mayer JH. Defects of axonal transport in diabetes mellitus-a possible contribution to the aetiology of diabetic neuropathy. J Aut Pharmacol 1984;4:59–72.
247. Jakobsen J, Brimijoin S, Skau K, Sidepius P, Wells D. Retrograde axonal transport of transmitter enzymes, fucose-labeled protein, and nerve growth factor in streptozotocin-diabetic rats. Diabetes 1981;30:797–803.
248. Fernyhough P, Diemel LT, Hardy J, Brewster WJ, Mohiuddin L, Tomlinson DR. Human recombinant nerve growth factor replaces deficient neurotrophic support in the diabetic rat. Eur J Neurosc 1995;7:1107–1110.
249. Apfel SC, Arezzo JC, Brownlee M, Federoff H, Kessler JA. Nerve growth factor administration protects against experimental diabetic sensory neuropathy. Brain Res 1994;634:7–12.
250. Schmidt Y, Unger JW, Bartke J, Reiter R. Effect of nerve growth factor on peptide neurons in dorsal root ganglia after taxol or cisplatin treatment and in diabetic (db/db) mice. Exp Neurol 1995;132:16–23.
251. Sango K, Verdes JM, Hikawa N, Horie H, Tanaka S, Inoue S, Sotelo JR, Takenaka T. Nerve growth factor (NGF) restores depletions of calcitonin gene-related peptide and substance P in sensory neurons from diabetic mice in vitro. J Neurol Sci 1994;126:1–5.
252. Hanaoka Y, Ohi T, Furukawa S, Furukawa Y, Hayashi K, Matsukura S. The therapeutic effects of 4-methylcatechol, a stimulator of endogenous nerve growth factor synthesis, on experimental diabetic neuropathy in rats. J Neuro Sci 1994;122:28–32.
253. Rodriguez-Pena A, Botana M, Gonzalez M, Requejo F. Expression of neurotrophins and their receptors in sciatic nerve of experimentally diabetic rats. Neurosci Lett 1995;200:37–40.
254. Tomlinson DR, Fernyhough P, Diemel LT. Neurotrophins and peripheral neuropathy. Philos Trans Royal Soc London. Series B. Biol Sci 1996;351:455–462.
255. Ishii DN. Implication of insulin-like growth factors in the pathogenesis of diabetic neuropathy. Brain Res Rev 1995;20:47–67.
256. Daughaday WH, Rotwein P. Insulin-like growth factor I and II. Peptide, messenger ribonucleic acid and gene structures, serum, and tissue concentrations. Endocr Rev 1989;10:68–91.
257. Stylianopoulou F, Herbert J, Soares MB, Efstratiadis A. Expression of the insulin-like growth factor II gene in the choroid plexus and the leptomeninges of the adult rat central nervous system. Proc Nat Acad Sci USA 1988;85:141–145.
258. Van Evercooren AB, Olichon-Berthe C. Expression of IGF-I and insulin receptor genes in the rat central nervous system: a developmental, regional, and cellular analysis. J Neurosci Res 1991;28:244–253.
259. Soares MB, Ishii DN, Efstratiadis A. Development and tissue-specific expression of a family of transcripts related to insulin-like growth factor II mRNA. Nucl Acids Res 1985;13:1119–1134.
260. Rotwein P, Burgess SK, Milbrandt JD, Krausse JE. Differential expression of insulin-like growth factor genes in rat central nervus system. Proc Natl Acad Sci USA 1988;85:265–269.
261. Caroni P, Grandes P. Nerve sprouting in innervated adult skeletal muscle induced by exposure to elevated levels of insulin-like growth factors. J Cell Biol 1990;vol 110:1307–1317.
262. Boyd FT Jr, Clarke DW, Muther TF, Raizada MK. Insulin receptors and insulin modulation of norepinephrine uptake in neuronal cultures from rat brain. J Biol Chem 1985;260:15,880–15,884.
263. Martin JL, Baxter RC. Insulin-like growth factor binding protein from the human plasma. Purification and characterization. J Biol Chem 1986;261:8754–8760.
264. Ocrant I, Fay CT, Parmelee JT. Characterization of insulin-like growth factor binding proteins produced in the rat central nervous system. Endocrinology 1990;127:1260–1267.
265. Tseng LY-H, Brown AL, Yang YW-H, Romanus JA, Orlowski CC, Taylor T, Rechler MM. The fetal rat binding protein for insulin-like growth factors is expressed in the choroid plexus and cerebrospinal fluid of adult rats. Molec Endocr 1989;3:1559–1568.
266. Ishii DN, Glazner GW, Pu S-F. Role of insulin-like growth factors in peripheral nerve regeneration. Pharmacol Ther 1994;62:125–144.
267. Lamson G, Pham H, Oh Y, Ocrant I, Schwander J. Expression of the BRL-3A insulin-like growth factor binding protein (rBP-30) in the rat central nervous system. Endocrinology 1989;123:1100–1102.
268. Zackenfels K, Oppenheim RW, Rohrer H. Evidence for an important role of IGF-I and IGF-II for the early development of chick sympathetic neurons. Neuron 1995;14:731–741.
269. Ishii DN. Implication of insulin-like growth factors in the pathogenesis of diabetic neuropathy. Brain Res Rev 1995;20:47–67.

270. Houenou LJ, Li L, Lo AC, Yan O, Oppenheim RW. Naturally occurring and axotomy-induced motorneuron death and its prevention by neurotrophic agents: a comparison between chick and mouse. In: Van Pelt J, Corner MA, Uylings HBM, Lopes da Silva FH, eds. Progress in Brain Research. Amsterdam, Elsevier, New York, 1994, pp. 217–226.
271. Glazner GW, Wright WG, Ishii DN. Kinetics of insulin-like growth factor (IGF) mRNA changes in rat nerve and muscle during IGF-dependent nerve regeneration. Soc Neurosci Abstr 1993b;19:253.
272. Pu S-F, Ishii DN. Distribution of insulin-like growth factor mRNAs in rat nerve and muscle during nerve regeneration by in situ hybridization. Soc Neurosci Abstr 1993;19:253.
273. Kanje M, Skottner A, Sjoberg J, Lundborg G. Insulin-like growth factor I (IGF-I) stimulates regeneration of the rat sciatic nerve. Brain Res 1989;486:396–398.
274. Near S, Whalen LR, Miller JA, Ishii DN. Insulin-like growth factor II stimulates motor nerve regeneration. Proc Natl Acad Sci USA 1992;89:11,716–11,720.
275. Glazner GW, Lupien S, Miller JA, Ishii DN. Insulin-like growth factor II increased the rate of sciatic nerve regeneration in rats. Neuroscience 1993a;54:791–797.
276. Yang H, Scheff AJ, Schalch DS. Effects of streptozotocin-induced diabetes mellitus on growth and hepatic insulin-like growth factor I gene expression in the rat. Metabolism 1990;39:295–301.
277. Ekstrom AR, Kanje M, Skottner A. Nerve regeneration and serum levels of insulin-like growth factor-I in rats with streptozotocin-induced insulin deficiency. Brain Res 1989;496:141–147.
278. Graubert MD, Goldstein S, Phillips LS. Nutrition and somatomedin: XXVII. Total and free IGF-I and IGF binding proteins in rats with streptozocin-induced diabetes. Diabetes 1991;40:959–965.
279. Bornfeldt KE, Arnqvist HJ, Enberg B, Mathews LS, Norstedt G. Regulation of insulin-like growth factor-I and growth hormone receptor gene expression by Diabetes and nutritional state in rat tissues. J Endocrinol 1989;122:651–656.
280. Luo J, Murphy LJ. Differential expression of insulin-like growth factor-I and insulin-like growth factor binding protein-1 in the diabetic rat. Mol Cell Biochem 1991;103:41–50.
281. Ishii DN, Guertin DM, Whalen LR. Reduced insulin-like growth factor-I mRNA content in liver, adrenal glands and spinal cord of diabetic rats. Diabetologia 1994;37:1073–1081.
282. Wuarin L, Guertin DM, Ishii DN. Early reduction in insulin-like growth factor gene expression in diabetic nerve. Exp Neurol 1994;130:106–114.
283. Ishii DN, Lupien SB. Insulin-like growth factors protect against diabetic neuropathy: effects on sensory nerve regeneration in rats. J Neurosci Res 1995;40:138–144.

# 3 Clinical Features of Diabetic Polyneuropathy

*Solomon Tesfaye,* MD, MRCP, *and*
*John D. Ward,* MD, FRCP

*CONTENTS*



## INTRODUCTION

Diabetic polyneuropathy is one of the most common complications of the diabetic state. There are now a number of both clinic-*(1,2)* and population-based studies *(3,4)* that have surprisingly similar prevalence rates for diabetic polyneuropathy, affecting approximately 30% of all diabetic people. The EURODIAB IDDM Complications Study, which involved the examination of 3250 type I patients, from 16 European countries, found a prevalence rate of 28% for diabetic peripheral neuropathy *(1)*. The study reported significant correlations with age, duration of diabetes, quality of metabolic control, height, the presence of background and proliferative retinopathy, microalbuminuria, severe ketoacidosis, elevated diastolic blood pressure, and other cardiovascular risk factors. Other recent population-based studies also report similar prevalence rates of neuropathy in type II diabetic patients *(4)*. Well-established correlates of diabetic neuropathy include increasing age, increasing duration of diabetes, poor glycemic control, retinopathy, and albuminuria *(1)*. Less well-established correlates of diabetic neuropathy include increasing height, hypertension, and cardiovascular risk factors *(1,4)*. The differing clinical presentations of the several neuropathic syndromes in diabetes suggest varied etiological factors.

The clinical consequences of diabetic neuropathy are also varied. Some may have minor complaints such as tingling in one or two toes; others may be affected with the devastating complications such as "the numb diabetic foot," or severe painful neuropathy that does not respond to drug therapy. Moreover, diabetic neuropathy is a major contributor to male impotence and other autonomic symptoms that are thankfully rare *(5,6)*.

From: *Contemporary Endocrinology: Clinical Management of Diabetic Neuropathy*
Edited by: A. Veves © Humana Press Inc., Totowa, NJ

**Table 1**
**The Varied Presentations of the Neuropathic Syndromes Associated with Diabetes (J D Ward)**

| |
|---|
| Chronic insidious sensory neuropathy |
| Acute painful neuropathy |
| Proximal motor neuropathy |
| Diffuse symmetrical motor neuropathy |
| The neuropathic foot |
| Pressure neuropathy |
| Focal vascular neuropathy |
| Neuropathy present at diagnosis |
| Treatment induced neuropathy |
| Hypoglycemic neuropathy |

Diabetic peripheral neuropathy presents in a similar way to neuropathies of other causes, and thus the physician needs to carefully exclude other common causes before attributing the neuropathy to diabetes. Absence of other complications of diabetes, rapid weight loss, excessive alcohol intake, and other atypical features in either the history or clinical examination should alert the physician to search for other causes of neuropathy.

## CLINICAL CLASSIFICATION OF DIABETIC NEUROPATHIES

Although clinical classification of the various syndromes of diabetic neuropathies are often difficult because of the very considerable overlap in the mixture of clinical features, attempts at classification stimulate thought as to the etiology of the various syndromes and also assist in the planning of management strategy for the patient. Watkins and Edmonds *(7)* have recently suggested a classification for diabetic neuropathies that clearly separates them into three distinct groups. These include:

1. Progressive neuropathies that are associated with increasing duration of diabetes and with other diabetic complications. These are predominantly sensory, and autonomic involvement is common. The onset is gradual and there is no recovery.
2. Reversible neuropathies that have rapid onset, often occurring at the presentation of diabetes itself, and which are not related to diabetes duration or other complications of diabetes. There is spontaneous recovery of these acute neuropathies.
3. Pressure palsies that occur more frequently in the diabetic state, but are not specific to diabetes only. There is no association with duration of diabetes or other complications of diabetes.

An alternative way of classifying diabetic neuropathies takes into account the various distinct clinical presentations to the physician. One such classification proposed by Ward *(5)* is depicted in Table 1. This practical approach to the classification of diabetic neuropathies is useful in characterizing the various syndromes and hence enabling the clinician to have workable, crude definitions, and in planning treatment.

Low and Suarez *(8)* have recently suggested a modified form of classification of the diabetic neuropathies originally proposed by Bruyn and Garland *(9)*. This classification principally considers whether the presentation was symmetrical or asymmetrical as

Table 2
Classification of Diabetic Neuropathy

| |
|---|
| **Symmetrical neuropathies** |
| 1. Distal sensory and sensorimotor neuropathy |
| 2. Large-fiber type of diabetic neuropathy |
| 3. Small-fiber type of diabetic neuropathy |
| 4. Distal small-fiber neuropathy |
| 5. Insulin neuropathy |
| 6. Chronic inflammatory demyelinating polyradiculoneuropathy (CIDP) |
| **Asymmetrical neuropathies** |
| 1. Mononeuropathy |
| 2. Mononeuropathy multiplex |
| 3. Radiculopathies |
| 4. Lumbar plexopathy or radiculoplexopathy |
| 5. Chronic inflammatory demyelinating polyradiculoneuropathy |

Adapted from Low and Suarez *(8)*.

shown in Table 2. It is important to appreciate that the separation into symmetrical and asymmetrical neuropathies, although useful in identifying distinct entities, is an oversimplification of the truth as there is a great overlapping of the syndromes.

## SYMMETRICAL NEUROPATHIES

### *Chronic Distal Symmetrical Neuropathy*

This is the most common neuropathic syndrome. It is a diffuse symmetrical disorder, affecting principally the feet in a stocking distribution, involvement of the hands in a glove pattern being rare. There is a length-related pattern of sensory loss, with sensory symptoms starting in the toes and then extending to involve the feet and legs. When there is upper-limb involvement, there is a similar progression proximally starting in the fingers. There is a close association with autonomic neuropathy, which is often subclinical and can only be detected by autonomic function tests. As the disease advances, it becomes a sensorimotor neuropathy; however, significant motor involvement is rare in most cases, early in the course of the disease.

### *Symptoms*

The patient describes a progressive build-up of unpleasant sensory symptoms including tingling (parasthesia); burning pain; shooting pains down the legs; lancinating pains; contact pain often with daytime clothes and bedclothes (allodynia); pain on walking often described as "walking barefoot on marbles," or "walking barefoot on hot sand," sensations of heat or cold in the feet; persistent achy feeling in the feet; cramp-like sensations in the legs; and various grades of numbness in the feet. The feet and legs are principally affected with these symptoms, similar symptoms being rare in the upper limbs. This has prompted a speculation that the standing position, with all its effects on the peripheral vascular system, may have an etiological role in the development of peripheral neuropathy *(10)*. Alternatively, some have suggested that the longer nerve fibers may be affected, resulting in distal neuropathy, particularly as epidemiological studies have recently shown the association between height and prevalence of diabetic neuropathy *(1,11)*. This suggests a distal axonopathy of the "dying-back" type in which neurons with the longest axons are unable to support the more distal parts, possibly because of impairment of axonal transport.

Autonomic symptoms are rare, but subclinical autonomic neuropathy is commonly found in patients with chronic distal symmetrical neuropathy *(12)*. Depressive symptoms are also not uncommon, particularly in those who have painful neuropathy that is complicated with loss of sleep, unemployment, and limitation in exercise tolerance *(13–15)*. Diabetic neuropathic pain is characteristically more severe at night, and often prevents sleep *(14,15)*. Occasionally, severe pain can extend above the feet and may involve the whole of the legs, and when this is the case there is upper-limb involvement also. The presence of neuropathic pain is usually unrelated to the severity of nerve dysfunction or pathology *(16)*. Despite pain being the prominent feature in these subjects, however recent sural nerve biopsy studies have shown axonal degeneration affecting fibers of all sizes *(16)*. Assessment of severity of neuropathic symptoms is discussed in Chapter 9.

Some patients may never have had any symptoms at all, and their first presentation may be with a foot ulcer *(17)*. Moreover, in some patients with painful neuropathy, progressive degeneration of nerve fibers may lead to foot numbness, the so called "painful, painless" leg *(18)*. The numb foot is at risk of developing mechanical and thermal injuries, and patients must therefore be warned about these *(17,18)*. With severe large-fiber involvement, patients may have unsteadiness on walking because of sensory ataxia.

### *Signs*

On clinical examination, the most common presenting abnormality is a reduction or absence of vibration sense in the toes. As the disease progresses there is sensory loss in a "stocking" and sometimes in a "glove" distribution involving all modalities. When there is severe sensory loss, proprioception may also be impaired, so as to cause positive Romberg's sign. Tendon reflexes at the level of the ankle and occasionally in the knees are usually reduced or absent. Muscle strength is usually normal, although mild weakness may be found in toe extensors. With progressive disease, there is significant generalized muscular wasting, particularly in the small muscles of the hands and feet, occasionally leading to clawing. This leads to elevated pressure points at the metatarsal heads that are prone to callus formation and recurrent foot ulceration *(17)*.

Upper-limb involvement is uncommon, and occurs usually in patients with advanced disease in the feet and legs. The fine movements of fingers would then be affected, and there is difficulty in handling small objects. However, wasting of dorsal interossei is usually caused by entrapment of the ulnar nerve at the elbow. Entrapment of the median nerve causing carpel tunnel syndrome is more commonly found in diabetes than in the general population, and results in a reduction of the muscle bulk in the thenar eminence.

Bedside cardiovascular autonomic function tests (changes in blood pressure and heart rate from the lying position to standing), are frequently abnormal in patients with peripheral neuropathy. Autonomic neuropathy affecting the feet can also cause a reduction in sweating and consequently dry skin that is likely to crack easily, predisposing the patient to the risk of infection *(17)*. The purely neuropathic foot is also warm because of arterio/venous shunting *(19)*, which causes the distension of foot veins that fail to collapse even when the foot is elevated. The oxygen tension of the blood in these veins is typically raised *(20)*. The increasing blood flow brought about by autonomic neuropathy can sometimes result in neuropathic edema, which is resistant to treatment with diuretics.

With severe peripheral neuropathy, there could be complete anesthesia below the knees, with marked loss of proprioception. Tendon reflexes are usually absent. The patient is disabled with marked unsteadiness on walking, because of sensory ataxia. This is more evident in the dark or with the eyes closed (positive Romberg's test). Measurement of body sway has shown posture instability that correlates with the severity of neuropathy *(21)*. There may rarely be an associated bilateral foot drop, and the patient is disabled with marked unsteadiness on walking and adopts a typical stamping gait.

The more serious consequence of advanced diabetic peripheral neuropathy is the development of diabetic foot ulceration and deformities (clawing of feet with high arch as a consequence of wasting of the small muscles of the feet, which leads to prominent metatarsal heads). Rarely, patients with long-standing diabetes with both somatic and autonomic neuropathy, may develop Charcot arthropathy. The feet should therefore be carefully examined for the presence of neuropathic foot ulcers that are usually located over the metatarsal heads but are also commonly encountered over the toes (occasionally hidden between toes) and sometimes over the heels or the malleoli. Neuropathy causing loss of pain and temperature sensation coupled with elevated pressure points is the usual initiating factor for diabetic foot ulceration. Other contributing factors include limited joint mobility, autonomic neuropathy (skin dryness and fissuring caused by anhidrosis; arteriovenous shunting causing impaired nutritive capillary blood flow), and peripheral vascular disease.

### *Small-Fiber Neuropathy*

Some authorities have advocated the existence of small-fiber neuropathy as a distinct entity *(22)*. A prominent feature of this syndrome is neuropathic pain that may be disabling, even though physical signs of neurological damage are relatively not severe. Occasionally patients with small-fiber neuropathy also have foot ulceration, and not all patients also have pain. The syndrome tends to develop within a few years of diabetes as a relatively early complication.

The pain is described as burning, deep, and aching. The sensation of pins and needles (parasthesia) is also often experienced. Contact hypersensitivity may be present. On clinical examination there is little evidence of objective signs of nerve damage, apart from a reduction in pinprick and temperature sensation, which are reduced in a "stocking" and "glove" distribution. There is relative sparing of vibration and position sense (because of relative sparing of the large diameter A β fibers). Muscle strength is usually normal and reflexes are also usually normal. Autonomic function tests are frequently abnormal and affected male patients usually have erectile dysfunction.

Electrophysiological tests support small-fiber dysfunction. Sural sensory conduction velocity may be normal, although the amplitude may be reduced. Motor nerves appear to be less affected. Controversy still exists as to whether small-fiber neuropathy is a distinct entity or an earlier manifestation of chronic sensory motor neuropathy *(22–24)*. Said et al.'s *(22)* morphometric study reported that there is small-fiber degeneration initially. Veves et al. *(25)* found a varying degree of early small-fiber involvement in all diabetic polyneuropathies that was confirmed by detailed sensory and autonomic function tests. If this is the case, the syndrome of small-fiber neuropathy may simply represent an early process that is not detected unless pain is a prominent feature.

### *Natural History of Chronic Distal Symmetrical Neuropathy*

The natural history of chronic distal symmetrical neuropathy is still poorly understood *(26)*. This is to a large extent the result of inadequate knowledge regarding the etiopathogenesis of distal symmetrical neuropathy although several different mechanisms have been suggested *(6,27–29)*. Boulton et al. *(30)* reported that neuropathic symptoms remain or get worse over a 5-yr period in patients with chronic distal symmetrical neuropathy. In contrast, a more recent study reported improvements in painful symptoms over 3.5 yr *(31)*. In this study, 50 diabetic patients with chronic painful sensory motor neuropathy were studied prospectively to clarify the natural history of diabetic peripheral neuropathy, in particular the role of small-fiber damage. Neuropathic pain was assessed using a visual analog scale, and small-fiber function by thermal limen, heat pain threshold, and weighted pinprick threshold. At follow-up 3.5 yr later one third of the patients had died or were lost to follow-up. Despite this major drawback, there was symptomatic improvement in painful neuropathy in the majority of the remaining patients. Despite this symptomatic improvement, small-fiber function as measured by the above tests deteriorated significantly. The study concluded that although neuropathic pain tends to improve with time, and may resolve completely, small-fiber function continues to deteriorate, indicating that the above neurophysiological measures do not predict the evolution of painful neuropathic symptoms.

In the natural history of chronic distal symmetrical neuropathy, controversy still exists as to what sensory modality or modalities are affected initially. Zeigler et al. *(32)* performed detailed neurophysiological tests including thermal discrimination thresholds, pain perception thresholds to heat and cold stimuli, vibration perception thresholds, and nerve conduction studies on 30 asymptomatic patients with type I diabetes of long duration, and an age-matched group of 30 type I patients with painful neuropathy. The study found that in the diabetic group as a whole, the most frequent abnormality was an elevated threshold for thermal sensation in the feet *(32)*. Not surprisingly, nerve dysfunction was more severe in the lower limbs, particularly when painful symptoms had developed.

There is also a great deal of controversy as to whether the clinical features, neurophysiological parameters, and morphometric findings are distinctly different in subjects with painful and painless diabetic neuropathy associated with foot ulceration. Young et al. *(33)* found that electrophysiological tests were appreciably worse in patients with foot ulceration than in patients with painful neuropathy, whereas patients with painful neuropathy had a higher ratio of autonomic (small-fiber) abnormality to electrophysiologic (large-fiber) abnormality. They concluded that in chronic distal symmetrical neuropathy, the relationship between large-fiber and small-fiber damage is not uniform, and that there may be different etiological influences on large- and small-fiber neuropathy in diabetic subjects, with the predominant type of fiber damage determining the form of the presenting clinical syndrome *(33)*. Support for this assertion is provided by the study of Tsigos et al. *(34)*, who also suggested that painful and painless neuropathies represent two distinct clinical entities with little overlap. In contrast, Veves et al. *(35)* found that painful symptoms were frequent in diabetic neuropathy, irrespective of the presence or absence of foot ulceration, and that these symptoms can occur at any stage of the disease. This study concluded that there is a spectrum of neuropathic syndromes from the painful to the patients with foot ulceration, and that much overlap exists *(35)*. In the authors' experience, painful symptoms are often similarly present in patients with and without foot ulceration, suggesting that painless and painful neuropathy represent extreme forms of the same syndrome. Thus, the presence or absence of symptoms cannot predict foot ulceration, and the painful-painless foot with ulceration as described by Ward *(18)*, is often observed in the diabetic foot clinic. However, vibration perception threshold is often higher in patients with foot ulceration, and indeed elevated levels predict foot ulceration *(36)*.

## ACUTE PAINFUL NEUROPATHIES

These syndromes are relatively uncommon and are characterised by relatively sudden onset of pain in the feet and legs and sometimes thighs. The pain is usually severe and distressing. Painful neuropathies present in the context of poor glycaemic control or rapid improvements in metabolic control.

### *Acute Painful Neuropathy of Poor Glycaemic Control*

This may occur in the context of poor glycemic control and is often not related to the presence of other chronic diabetic complications. There is often marked weight loss *(37)*. Ellenberg coined the description of this condition as "neuropathic cachexia" *(38)*. Patients typically develop persistent burning pain associated with allodynia (discomfort produced by tactile stimuli), and there is nocturnal exacerbation of symptoms. The pain is likened to walking on burning sand. There is also a subjective feeling of the feet being swollen. The pain is most marked in the feet, but it often affects the whole of the lower extremities. Patients also describe intermittent bouts of stabbing pain that shoot up the legs from the feet ("peak pain"), superimposed on the background burning pain. Not surprisingly, these disabling symptoms often lead to depression. In contrast to the severe pain, sensory loss is often mild and sometimes absent. There are usually no motor signs, although ankle jerks are lost in some. Nerve conduction studies are also usually normal or mildly abnormal. Temperature discrimination threshold is affected more commonly than vibration perception threshold *(39)*. There is complete resolution of symptoms within 10 mo, and weight gain is usual with continued improvement in glycemic control with the use of insulin.

### *Acute Painful Neuropathy of Rapid Glycaemic Control (Insulin Neuritis)*

The natural history of acute painful neuropathies is an almost guaranteed improvement *(37)* in contrast to chronic distal symmetrical neuropathy *(30,31)*. The term "insulin neuritis" was first used to describe the syndrome of acute painful neuropathy of rapid glycemic control, by Caravati *(40)*. The term is a misnomer as the condition can follow rapid improvement in glycemic control with oral antidiabetic agents, and "neuritis" implies an inflammatory process for which there is no evidence. It is therefore recommended that the term "acute painful neuropathy of rapid glycemic control" be used to describe this condition. The patient presents with burning pain, parasthesia, allodynia, often with a nocturnal exacerbation of symptoms; and depression may be a feature. There is no associated weight loss, unlike acute painful neuropathy of poor glycemic control. Sensory loss is often mild or absent, and there are no motor signs. There is little or no abnormality on nerve-conduction studies, but there is impaired exercise-induced conduction velocity increment *(41)*. There is complete resolution of symptoms within 10 mo. Sural nerve biopsy has shown changes of chronic neuropathy with active regeneration *(42)*, whereas degeneration of both myelinated and unmyelinated fibers was found in acute painful neuropathy of poor glycemic control *(37)*. A recent study looking into the epineurial vessels of sural nerves in patients with acute painful neuropathy of rapid glycemic control demonstrated marked arterio/venous abnormality including the presence of proliferating new vessels, similar to those found in the retina *(43)*. The study suggested that the presence of this fine network of epineural vessels may lead to a "steal" effect rendering the endoneurium ischemic, and this process was also thought to be important in the genesis of neuropathic pain *(43)*. These findings were also supported by studies in experimental diabetes that demonstrated that insulin administration led to acute endoneurial hypoxia, by increasing nerve arterio-venous flow, and reducing the nutritive flow of normal nerves *(44)*.

## ASYMMETRICAL NEUROPATHIES

The diabetic state can also affect single nerves (diabetic mononeuropathy), multiple nerves (diabetic mononeuropathy multiplex), or groups of nerve roots. These focal neuropathies have a relatively rapid onset, and complete recovery is usual in most cases. This contrasts with chronic distal symmetrical neuropathy, in which most sufferers report no improvement in symptoms 5 yr after onset *(30)*. A vascular etiology has been suggested by virtue of the rapid onset of symptoms and the focal nature of the neuropathic syndromes *(45)*. Asymmetrical neuropathies tend to predominantly affect older patients *(46,47)*, and are more common in men. Unlike chronic distal symmetrical neuropathies, they are often unrelated to the presence of other diabetic complications. A careful history should be taken to identify any associated symptoms that might point to another cause for the neuropathy. Investigations should also be carried out to exclude other possible causes of neuropathy in those patients.

### *Mononeuropathies*

By far the most common mononeuropathy other than "entrapment/pressure," neuropathy is the third cranial nerve palsy. The patient presents with pain in the orbit, or sometimes with a frontal headache *(45,48)*. There is typically ptosis and ophthalmoplegia, although the pupil is usually spared *(49,50)*. Recovery occurs usually over 3 mo. The clinical onset and time-scale for recovery, and the focal nature of the lesions on the third cranial nerve, on postmortem studies suggested an ischemic etiology *(45,51)*. It is important to exclude any other cause of third cranial nerve palsy (aneurysm or tumor) by CT or MR scanning, where the diagnosis is in doubt.

Fourth, sixth, and seventh cranial nerve palsies have also been described in diabetic subjects, but the association is not as strong as that with third cranial nerve palsy. Phrenic nerve involvement in association with diabetes has also been described, although the possibility of a pressure lesion could not be excluded *(52)*.

### *Pressure (Entrapment) Neuropathies*

A number of nerves are vulnerable to pressure damage in diabetes. In the Rochester Diabetic Neuropathy Study, which was a population-based epidemiological study, Dyck et al. *(53)*, found electrophysiological evidence of median nerve lesions at the wrist in approx 30% of diabetic subjects, although the typical symptoms of carpel tunnel syndrome occurred in less than 10%. The patient typically has pain and paresthesia in the hands that sometimes radiate to the forearm and are particularly marked at night. In severe cases, clinical examination may reveal a reduction in sensation in the median territory in the hands, and wasting of the muscle bulk in the thenar eminence. The clinical diagnosis is easily confirmed by median-nerve conduction studies and treatment involves surgical decompression at the carpel tunnel in the wrist. There is generally good response to surgery, although painful symptoms appear to relapse more commonly than in the nondiabetic population *(54)*.

The ulnar nerve is also vulnerable to pressure damage at the elbow in the ulnar groove. This results in wasting of the dorsal interossei, particularly the first dorsal interossius. This is easily confirmed by ulnar electrophysiological studies that localize the lesion to the elbow. Rarely, the patients may present with wrist drop because of radial nerve palsy after prolonged sitting (with pressure over the radial nerve in the back of the arms) while unconscious during hypoglycemia or asleep after an alcohol binge. In the lower limbs, the common peroneal (lateral popliteal) is the most commonly affected nerve. The compression is at the level of the head of the fibula and causes foot drop. Unfortunately, complete recovery is unusual. The lateral cutaneous nerve of the thigh is occasionally also affected with entrapment neuropathy in diabetes.

### *Truncal Radiculopathies*

Diabetic truncal radiculopathies are characterized by acute onset pain in a dermatomal distribution over the thorax or the abdomen *(55)*. The pain is usually asymmetrical, and can cause local bulging of the muscle *(56)*. There may be patchy sensory loss and other causes of nerve root compression should be excluded. Some patients presenting with abdominal pain have undergone unnecessary investigations such as barium enema, colonoscopy, and even laparotomy, when the diagnosis could easily have been made by careful clinical history and examination. Recovery is usually the rule within several mo, although symptoms can sometimes persist for a few yr.

### *Proximal Motor Neuropathy (Femoral Neuropathy, Amyotrophy, Plexopathy)*

This syndrome of progressive asymmetrical proximal leg weakness and atrophy was first described by Garland *(57)*, who coined the term diabetic amyotrophy. The patient presents with severe pain that is felt deep in the thigh, but can sometimes be of burning quality and extend below the knee. The pain is usually continuous and often causes insomnia and depression *(58)*. Both type I and type II patients over the age of 50 are affected *(57,59,60)*. There is an associated weight loss that can sometimes be very severe, and can raise the possibility of an occult malignancy. On examination, there is profound wasting of the quadriceps with marked weakness in these muscle groups, although hip flexors and hip abductors can also be affected *(61)*. Thigh adductors, glutei, and hamstring muscles may also be involved. The knee jerk is usually reduced or absent. The profound weakness can lead to difficulty getting out of a low chair or climbing stairs. Sensory loss is unusual, and if present, indicates a coexistent distal sensory neuropathy.

It is important to carefully exclude other causes of quadriceps wasting such as nerve root and cauda equina lesions, and the possibility of occult malignancy causing proximal myopathy syndromes such as polymyocytis. An erythrocyte sedimentation rate

(ESR), an X-ray of the lumbar/sacral spine, a chest X-ray, and ultrasound of the abdomen may be required. Electrophysiological studies may demonstrate increased femoral-nerve latency and active denervation of affected muscles. Occasionally more detailed investigation with MR imaging may be required. Cerbrospinal fluid protein has been reported to be raised.

The cause of diabetic proximal motor neuropathy is not known. It tends to occur within the background of diabetic distal symmetrical neuropathy *(62)*. Some have suggested that the combination of focal features superimposed on diffuse peripheral neuropathy may suggest vascular damage to the femoral nerve roots as a cause of this condition.

Coppack and Watkins *(58)* have reported that pain usually starts to settle after approx 3 mo, and usually settles by 1 yr, whereas the knee jerk is restored in 50% of the patients after 2 yr. Recurrence on the other side is a rare event. Management is largely symptomatic and supportive. Patients should be encouraged and reassured that this condition is likely to resolve. There is still controversy as to whether the use of insulin therapy influences the natural history of this syndrome *(58)*. Accompanying pain and depression should be adequately treated (*see* Chapters 9 and 10). Extension exercises aimed at strengthening the quadriceps may also be of some value.

## REFERENCES


1. Tesfaye S, Stephens L, Stephenson J, Fuller J, Platter ME, Ionescu-Tirgoviste C, Ward JD. The prevalence of diabetic neuropathy and its relation to glycaemic control and potential risk factors: the EURODIAB IDDM Complications Study. Diabetologia 1996;39:1377–1384.
2. Young MJ, Boulton AJM, Macleod AF, Williams DRR, Sonksen PH. A multicentre study of the prevalence of diabetic peripheral neuropathy in the United Kingdom hospital clinic population. Diabetologia 1993;36:150–154.
3. Maser RE, Steenkiste AR, Dorman JS et al. Epidemiological correlates of diabetic neuropathy. Report from Pittsburgh Epidemiology of Diabetes Complications Study. Diabetes 1989;38:1456–1461.
4. Ziegler D. Diagnosis, staging and epidemiology of diabetic peripheral neuropathy. Diab Nutr Metab 1994;7:342–348.
5. Ward JD. Clinical features of diabetic neuropathies. In: Ward JD, Goto Y, eds. Diabetic Neuropathy. 1990, pp. 281–296.
6. Ward JD, Tesfaye S. Pathogenesis of diabetic neuropathy. In: Pickup J, Williams G, eds. Textbook of Diabetes vol. 2. Oxford, UK,1997, pp. 49.1–49.19.
7. Watkins PJ, Edmonds ME. Clinical features of diabetic neuropathy. In: Pickup J, Williams G, eds Textbook of Diabetes vol. 2. Oxford, UK, 1997, pp. 50.1–50.20.
8. Low PA, Suarez GA. Diabetic neuropathies. In: Bailliere's Clinical Neurology. Oxford, UK, 1995, pp. 401–425.
9. Bruyn GW, Garland H. Neuropathies of endocrine origin. In: Vinken PJ, Bruyn GW, eds. Handbook of Clinical Neurology, vol 8. North-Holland Publishing Co., Amsterdam, 1970, p. 29.
10. Ward JD. The Claude Bernard Lecture, Vienna, 1996.
11. Sosenko JM, Gadia MT, Fournier AM, O'Connell MT, Aguiar MC, Skyler JS. Body stature as a risk factor for diabetic sensory neuropathy. Am J Med 1986;80:1031–1034.
12. Ewing DJ, Borsey DQ, Bellavere F, Clarke BF. Cardiac autonomic neuropathy in diabetes: comparison of measures of R-R interval variation. Diabetologia 1981;21:18–24.
13. Tesfaye S, Watt J, Benbow SJ, Pang KA, Miles J, MacFarlane IA. Electrical spinal cord stimulation for painful diabetic peripheral neuropathy. Lancet 1996;348:1696–1701.
14. Tesfaye S, Price D. Therapeutic approaches in diabetic neuropathy and neuropathic pain. In: Boulton AJM, ed. Diabetic Neuropathy. 1997, pp. 159–181.
15. Watkins PJ. Pain and diabetic neuropathy. Br Med J 1984;288:168, 169.
16. Britland ST, Young RJ, Sharma AK, Clarke BF. Association of painful and painless diabetic polyneuropathy with different patterns of nerve fiber degeneration and regeneration. Diabetes 1990;39:898–907.
17. Boulton AJM. Foot problems in patients with diabetes mellitus. In: Pickup J, Williams G, eds. Textbook of Diabetes vol 2. Oxford, UK, 1997, pp. 58.1–58.20.

18. Ward JD. The diabetic leg. Diabetologia 1982;22:141–147.
19. Ward JD, Simms JM, Knight G, Boulton AJM, Sandler DA. Venous distension in the diabetic neuropathic foot (physical sign of arterio-venous shunting). J Roy Soc Med 1983;76:1011–1014.
20. Boulton AJM, Scarpello JHB, Ward JD. Venous oxygenation in the diabetic neuropathic foot: evidence of arterial venous shunting? Diabetologia 1982;22:6–8.
21. Ojala JM, Matikaien E, Groop L. Body sway in diabetic neuropathy. J Neurol 1985;232 (Suppl.):188.
22. Said G, Slama G, Selva J. Progressive centripital degeneration of axons in small-fiber type diabetic polyneuropathy. A clinical and pathological study. Brain 1983;106:791.
23. Harati Y. Diabetic peripheral neuropathies. Ann Intern Med 1987;107:546.
24. Vinik AI, Holland MT, LeBeau JM, Liuzzi FJ, Stansberry KB, Colen LB. Diabetic neuropathies. Diabetes Care 1992;15:1926–1975.
25. Veves A, Young MJ, Manes C, Boulton AJ. Differences in peripheral and autonomic nerve function measurements in painful and painless neuropathy: a clinical study. Diabetes Care 1994;17:1200–1202.
26. Boulton AJM. What causes neuropathic pain? J Diab Comp 1992;6:58–63.
27. Harati Y. Diabetes and the nervous system. Endoc Metab Clin North Am 1996;25:325–359.
28. Tesfaye S, Malik R, Ward JD. Vascular factors in diabetic neuropathy. Diabetologia 1994;37:847–854.
29. Tesfaye S, Harris N, Jakubowski J, Mody C, Wilson RM, Rennie IG, Ward JD. Impaired blood flow and arterio-venous shunting in human diabetic neuropathy: a novel technique of nerve photography and fluorescein angiography. Diabetologia 36:1266–1274.
30. Boulton AJM, Armstrong WD, Scarpello JHB, Ward JD. The natural history of painful diabetic neuropathy-a 4 year study. Postgrad Med J 1983;59:556–559.
31. Benbow SJ, Chan AW, Bowsher D, McFarlane IA, Williams G. A prospective study of painful symptoms, small fiber function and peripheral vascular disease in chronic painful diabetic neuropathy. Diabetic Med 1994;11:17–21.
32. Ziegler D, Mayer P, Wiefels K, Gries FA. Assessment of small and large fiber function in long-term type 1 (insulin-dependent) diabetic patients with and without painful neuropathy. Pain 1988;34:1–10.
33. Young RJ, Zhou YQ, Rodriguez E, Prescott RJ, Ewing DJ, Clarke BF. Variable relationship between peripheral somatic and autonomic neuropathy in patients with different syndromes of diabetic polyneuropathy. Diabetes 1986;35:192–197.
34. Tsigos C, White A, Young RJ. Discrimination between painful and painless diabetic neuropathy based on testing of large somatic nerve and sympathetic nerve function. Diabetic Med 1992;9:359–365.
35. Veves A, Manes C, Murray HJ, Young MJ, Boulton AJM. Painful neuropathy and foot ulceration in diabetic patients. Diabetes Care 1993;vol: 1187–1189.
36. Young MJ, Manes C, Boulton AJM. Vibration perception threshold predicts foot ulceration: a prospective study (Abstract). Diabetic Med 1992;9 (Suppl. 2):542.
37. Archer AG, Watkins PJ, Thomas PJ, Sharma AK, Payan J. The natural history of acute painful neuropathy in diabetes mellitus. J Neurol Neurosurg Psychiatr 1983;46:491–496.
38. Ellenberg M. Diabetic neuropathic cachexia. Diabetes 1974;23:418–423.
39. Guy RJC, Clark CA, Malcolm PN, Watkins PJ. Evaluation of thermal and vibration sensation in diabetic neuropathy. Diabetologia 1985;28:131.
40. Caravati CM. Insulin neuritis: a case report. Va Med Mon 1933;59:745, 746.
41. Tesfaye S, Harris N, Wilson RM, Ward JD. Exercise induced conduction velocity increment: a marker of impaired nerve blood flow in diabetic neuropathy. Diabetologia 1992;35:155–159.
42. Llewelyn JG, Thomas PK, Fonseca V, King RHM, Dandona P. Acute painful diabetic neuropathy precipitated by strict glycaemic control. Acta Neuropathol (Berl) 1986;72:157–163.
43. Tesfaye S, Malik R, Harris N, Jakubowski J, Mody C, Rennie IG, Ward JD. Arteriovenous shunting and proliferating new vessels in acute painful neuropathy of rapid glycaemic control (insulin neuritis). Diabetologia 1996;39:329–335.
44. Kihara M, Zollman PJ, Smithson IL, Lagerlund TD, Low PA. Hypoxic effect of endogenous insulin on normal and diabetic peripheral nerve. Am J Physiol 1994;266:E980–E985.
45. Asbury AK. Aldredge H, Hershberg R, Fisher CM. Oculomotor palsy in diabetes mellitus: a clinico-pathological study. Brain 1970;93:555–557.
46. Clements RS, Bell DSH. Diagnostic, pathogenic and therapeutic aspects of diabetic neuropathy. Special Topics Endocrinol Metab 1982;3:1–43.
47. Matikainen E, Juntunen J. Diabetic neuropathy: epidemiological, pathogenetic, and clinical aspects with special emphasis on type 2 diabetes mellitus. Acta Endocrinol Suppl 1984;262:89–94.
48. Zorilla E, Kozak GP. Ophthalmoplegia in diabetes mellitus. Ann Intern Med 1967;67:968–976.

49. Goldstein JE, Cogan DG. Diabetic ophthalmoplegia with special reference to the pupil. Arch Ophthalmol 1960;64:592–600.
50. Leslie RDG, Ellis C. Clinical course following diabetic ocular palsy. Postgrad Med J 1978;54:791, 792.
51. Dreyfuss PM, Hakim S, Adams RD. Diabetic ophthalmoplegia. Arch Neurol Psychiatry 1957;77:337–349.
52. White JES, Bullock RF, Hudgson P, Home PD, Gibson GJ. Phrenic neuropathy in association with diabetes. Diabet Med 1992;9:954–956.
53. Dyck PJ, Kratz KM, Karnes JL, Suarez GA, Low PA, Pineda AA, Windebank AJ, Karnes JL, O'Brien PC. The prevalence by staged severity of various types of diabetic neuropathy, retinopathy, and nephropathy in a population-based cohort: the Rochester Diabetic Neuropathy Study. Neurology 1993;43:817–824.
54. Clayburgh RH, Beckenbaugh RD, Dobyns JH. Carpal tunnel release in patients with diffuse peripheral neuropathy. J Hand Surg 1987;12A:380–383.
55. Ellenberg M. Diabetic truncal mononeuropathy—a new clinical syndrome. Diabetes Care 1978;1:10–13.
56. Boulton AJM, Angus E, Ayyar DR, Weiss R. Diabetic thoracic polyradiculopathy presenting as abdominal swelling. BMJ 1984;289:798, 799.
57. Garland H. Diabetic amyotrophy. BMJ 1955;2:1287–1290.
58. Coppack SW, Watkins PJ. The natural history of femoral neuropathy. QJ Med 1991;79:307–313.
59. Casey EB, Harrison MJG. Diabetic amyotrophy: a follow-up study. Br Med J 1972;1:656.
60. Garland H, Taverner D. Diabetic myelopathy. Br Med J 1953;1:1405.
61. Subramony SH, Willbourn AJ. Diabetic proximal neuropathy. Clinical and electromyographic studies. J Neurol Sci 1982;53:293–304.
62. Bastron JA, Thomas JE. Diabetic polyradiculoneuropathy: clinical and electromyographic findings in 105 patients. Mayo Clinic Proc 1981;56:725–732.

# 4 Diagnosis of Diabetic Neuropathy

*Aristidis Veves, MD*

***Contents***



## INTRODUCTION

The diagnosis and staging of severity of the diabetic neuropathy plays an important role not only for following up patients in a daily clinical practice, but also for the conduction of research that studies the etiopathogenesis of the disease and the development of new therapeutic modalities.

According to the recommendations of the San Antonio Consensus Statement, the diagnosis of the Diabetic Neuropathy should be based on the clinical symptoms, the clinical signs, quantitative sensory testing, electrophysiological measurements and, in rare occasions, on sural nerve biopsies *(1)*. However, as is discussed in this chapter, not all these methods are necessary for the daily clinical practice.

## CLINICAL SYMPTOMS

As discussed in the previous chapter, the most common symptoms of the peripheral diabetic neuropathy are numbness, tingling sensation often described by the patient as pins and needles, lancinating pain, deep aching pain, burning pain, and muscular cramps. They usually involve the feet and legs and present first or get worse during the night.

The staging of the severity of the symptoms of diabetic neuropathy is not an easy task because the reaction to an unpleasant stimulus is strongly influenced by previous simi-

From: *Contemporary Endocrinology: Clinical Management of Diabetic Neuropathy*
Edited by: A. Veves © Humana Press Inc., Totowa, NJ

lar experiences and the personality of the patient. For a stoic person, a seriously painful symptom can be described as a mild or disturbing pain, whereas to others, mild painful symptoms can seem unbearable. It is helpful that before detailed questions about specific symptoms are being made, the patient should be allowed to describe in their own words any possible neuropathic symptoms.

Over the last decade, a variety of methods have been developed in an effort to quantify pain in various conditions and many of these have also been employed for the evaluation of diabetic neuropathic symptoms. The McGill Pain Questionnaire consists of three types of descriptive words: sensory, affective, and evaluative, which are used by the patient in order to characterize the properties of the painful symptoms and also contains an intensity scale that is used to quantify the pain *(2)*. The application of this method in diabetic neuropathy has been limited but, one study found it sufficiently sensitive for detecting differences among different pain relieving methods *(3)*. Another method that was employed in early studies is the graphic scale of pain that can quantify the intensity of pain but cannot discriminate the various symptoms *(4,5)*. Additional details about these methods are given in Chapter 9.

Most of the currently used techniques are based on methods developed by PJ Dyck and his colleagues at the Mayo Clinic. They first developed the Neuropathy Symptom Score (NSS) which consisted of 17 symptoms of muscle weakness and sensory disturbances in the head, torso, and upper and lower limbs *(6)*. The NSS was later expanded to a true or false questionnaire that included a few hundred questions about motor, sensory, and autonomic neuropathic symptoms and was named Neuropathy Symptom Profile (NSP) *(7)*. The main advantage of the NSP is that it can detect and quantify the severity of peripheral neuropathy, but it carries the disadvantage of being cumbersome and time consuming, limiting its use for clinical trials.

A simplified Neuropathy Symptom Score, which is based on the original NSS, has been extensively used for epidemiological or intervention clinical trials and can also be easily used for daily clinical practice *(8,9,10)*. In this simplified NSS, the patients are asked for the existence of the following typical symptoms of diabetic neuropathy in their feet and legs: muscular cramps, numbness, pins and needles, abnormal cold or hot sensations, lancinating pain, deep aching pain, burning pain, and irritation in their feet and legs caused by the bedclothes at night. Each symptom is scored as 0 if it is absent, 1 if it is present, and 2 if there is nocturnal exacerbation. The total sum from all the symptoms represents the Neuropathy Symptom Score.

The main disadvantage of all methods trying to assess the severity of neuropathic symptoms is their poor reproducibility, mainly related to the fact that both the intensity of the symptoms and the response of the patient to the painful stimuli vary with time *(11)*. Therefore, although neuropathic symptoms are very useful in diagnosing diabetic neuropathy, they are of little help in designing longitudinal studies that examine the natural history of the disease or access the efficacy of various therapeutic modalities.

## CLINICAL SIGNS

The quantification of the clinical signs was also pioneered at the Mayo Clinic by Dyck et al. who first described the Neuropathy Disability Score (Mayo NDS) *(6,7)*. According to this method, the severity of each neurologic deficit was scored using a scale from 0–4, with 0 indicating no deficit and 4 the most severe. The total score was based on the evaluation of muscular weakness, including the face, torso and extremities, the reflexes of upper and lower extremities, the sensation to pain, touch, and vibration, and joint position at the index finger and great toe. The main advantage of this technique is that it is reproducible and can give a very detailed and accurate picture of the severity of the neuropathy *(11)*. However, this applies only if it is performed by well-trained neurologists who can accurately evaluate muscular weakness and grade the severity of the sensory deficit rendering it a very useful research tool with a limited role in the daily clinical practice.

A modified NDS that can be performed by a nonspecialist but still provide valuable information was first described by Young et al. *(12)*. According to this technique the NDS is the sum of the sensory and reflex deficit score. For the evaluation of the sensory score, the sensations of pain, touch, cold, and vibration at both legs are tested. The pain perception is examined with a pin, the touch perception with a cotton wool, the cold perception with a tuning fork immersed in icy water, and the vibration with a tuning fork of 128-Hz frequency. Each sensory deficit is graded according to the level up to which the sensation is found to be impaired as follows: (0) no abnormality, (1) impaired sensation up to the base of the toes, (2) up to midfoot, (3) ankle, (4) midleg, and (5) knee. The average of both feet for each modality is calculated and the sum of all four deficits represents the sensory score. For the evaluation of the reflex score, the knee and ankle reflexes are examined and scored as following: normal 0, elicited with reinforcement 1, and absent 2. The sum total of all four reflexes and the sensory score represented the NDS (maximum 28). A score from 1 to 5 is considered to be indicative of mild neuropathy, 6–16 moderate, and 17–28 severe. Comparing to the previous method, the modified NDS has the advantage of being simpler and therefore can be used in conducting large clinical or epidemiological trials in which more than one center are involved or can be part of the clinical routine practice.

More recently, Feldman et al. proposed a new, two-step program for the diagnosis and staging of diabetic neuropathy on an outpatient basis *(13)*. The first step consists of the Michigan Neuropathy Screening Instrument (MNSI) which consists of 15 "yes or no" questions for symptoms related to sensation, general asthenia, and peripheral vascular disease. In addition, a brief clinical examination, involving inspection of the foot, semiquantitative assessment of the vibration sensation, and examination of the ankle reflexes, is performed. Patients with an abnormal MNSI score are then refereed for the second part of the examination, the Michigan Diabetic Neuropathy Score (MNDS) that includes a clinical neurological examination, involving vibration perception threshold measurements, pain, light touch, and a 10-g monofilament, and nerve electrophysiological assessments. All these measurements are scored and according to the total scored neuropathy is characterized as absent, mild, moderate, or severe.

## QUANTITATIVE SENSORY TESTING

The development of the quantitative sensory testing over the last two decades has been an important step in diagnosing and quantifying peripheral nerve damage. Its main advantage is that it can quantitatively measure the minimal stimulus perceived by the patient, something impossible during clinical examination in which a sensation can be described as present, reduced, or absent. Its main disadvantage is that it does not exclusively evaluate the function of the peripheral nerve system but the integrity of the whole

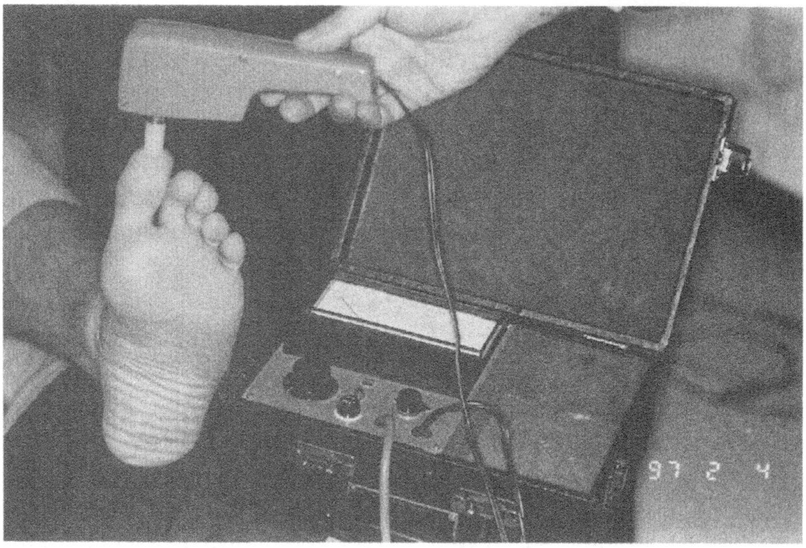


**Fig. 1.** Assessment of the vibration perception threshold by a Biothesiometer. The most important thing is to standardize the pressure applied on the skin and this can be achieved by keeping the stylus in vertical position so that the only pressure applied on the skin is that from the weight of the unit. The vibration of the stylus can be increased from 0 to 50 V by a switch in the main unit.

nerve pathway up to the higher brain centers. Thus, the full cooperation and concentration of the patient is required if reliable results are to be obtained, hence the term psychophysical testing *(1)*.

A number of different methods have been described, but in this chapter, the main emphasis will be given on two simple techniques that are simple, cost-effective, and can be easily used in daily clinical practice by nonspecialists.

### *Vibration Perception Threshold*

The sense of vibration is transmitted through the large myelinated (A–β) fibers. In healthy subjects, the vibration threshold is higher in the lower extremities when compared to other parts of the body *(14)*. The vibration perception threshold increases significantly with age and tables with age-related upper normal values are required for the correct interpretation of the obtained results *(15,16)*. Other factors that can influence the thresholds are the height and skin temperature *(16,17)*.

The most commonly employed device to evaluate the vibration perception threshold (VPT) is the biothesiometer (Bio-Medical Instrument Company, Newbury, OH) (Fig. 1). It consists of a hand-held unit with a tractor that vibrates proportionally to the applied voltage, which can be increased from 0 to 50 V using a control switch. The VPT is usually measured at the great toe and/or the medial malleolus, whereas the tractor is kept in vertical position and in firm contact with the skin. As the vibration perception depends on the applied pressure, it is important that during testing the vibrating stylus is kept vertical and that no additional pressure is applied so that the pressure to the skin is stable and is determined only by the weight of the unit. The Vibrameter and the Vibratron II are alternative devices that can be used for the assessment of the vibration thresholds.

The coefficient of variation of VPT measurements is 25–50%, not unsatisfactory for a psychophysical quantitative sensory testing technique *(18)*. Nevertheless, as considerable variability exists in measurements of two symmetrical parts of the body in both healthy subjects and diabetic patients, more than one site should be tested, even for screening purposes *(19,20)*.

Despite the above limitations, the Biothesiometer is an inexpensive, portable device requiring 2–3 min for each patient and can be operated with minimal training by doctors, nurses, or other paramedical staff. VPT measurements can be used for both the diagnosis of diabetic neuropathy and for screening large numbers of patients in order to identify the ones at risk for foot ulceration. A large prospective study has already shown that VPT is a very effective predictor of the risk for foot ulceration in diabetes and that patients with a threshold more than 25 V should be considered at high risk and receive preventive treatment *(21)*.

### *Semmes-Weinstein Monofilaments*

The Semmes-Weinstein monofilaments test the function of the myelinated sensory fibers that are responsible for the pressure sensation. Sets of three or six monofilaments with progressively increasing diameter are available for clinical use. When force is applied on a filament until is buckles, it always applies the same pressure on the skin and the amount of pressure depends only on the diameter of this particular filament (Fig. 2). Therefore, by quantifying the minimum pressure perceived by the patient it is possible to diagnose and stage the severity of the diabetic neuropathy *(22)*. Moreover, as this is a very easy technique, it is ideal for screening purposes. Patients who are unable to feel a pressure of 10 g are at high risk for foot ulceration and candidates for preventive treatment *(23,24)*.

The main advantages of the Semmes-Weinstein monofilaments are that they are inexpensive, very easy to use for medical or paramedical staff, and not time consuming. A pen-like device with a 5.07 monofilament exists, making it easy to be carried by the examiner and be used at different places such as the practice office or at the bedside dur-

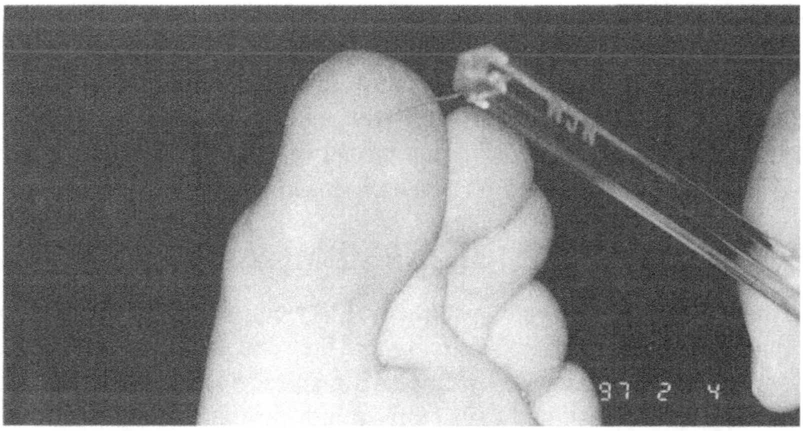


**Fig. 2.** The 5.07 Semmes-Weinstein monofilament. When the filaments is flexed it applies a constant pressure of 10 g on the tested area. A number of monofilaments are available with different diameter applying different amount of pressure on the skin. Failure to feel a pressure of 10 g or less is indicative of high risk for foot ulceration.

ing a brief clinical examination. All the above make this technique the most applicable in clinical practice and can be easily incorporated in the standard annual review visit, which should be performed on every diabetic patient.

### *Other Techniques*

A number of quantitative sensory testing techniques have been developed over the last years and have been used for the conduction of clinical studies. However, as none of them have been widely accepted for clinical practice, a detailed description of these methods would be beyond the scope of this chapter.

#### Warm and Cold Perception Thresholds

The sensation of warm and cold is served by small myelinated and unmyelinated fibers and is usually the first nerve function to be affected in diabetic patients *(25)*. Various methods have been proposed for the evaluation of the warm and cold thresholds but they are all hampered by the same problems, namely poor reproducibility, high intersubject and interobserver variation, time consuming, and requiring expensive equipment *(26,27)*. As a result of this, their use is restricted to research purposes in major institutions.

#### Current Perception Thresholds

This technique uses constant current delivered through the skin by a specifically designed device, the Neurometer (Neurotron, Baltimore, MD). Three frequencies can be measured (5, 250, and 2000 Hz) and previous studies have suggested a certain neuroselectivity with the 5 and 250 Hz frequencies mainly stimulating the small fibers and the 2000 Hz the large fibers *(28,29,30)*. The ability to test the function of both small and large fibers with the same device would obviously make the Neurometer an appealing alternative to currently employed methods. However, further studies that will examine the issues of neuroselectivity and reproducibility in more details are required before this technique gains general approval as first choice method *(31)*.

#### Computer-Assisted Sensory Examination (CASE)

The computer-assisted sensory examination (CASE), pioneered at the Mayo Clinic by Dyck and colleagues, is a computerized device that can evaluate the touch-pressure, vibration, and warm-cold perceptions using forced-choice testing *(32)*. Its main advantage is that it can offer reliable quantitative evaluation of all the above-mentioned sensations but as it requires expensive equipment installed in permanent facilities and well-trained staff, it is mainly used for research purposes.

## ELECTROPHYSIOLOGICAL MEASUREMENTS

The two main electrophysiological studies widely employed for the diagnosis of diabetic neuropathy are the conduction velocity and the sensory action potential. Both tests are noninvasive and are conducted by employing surface electrodes that do not expose the patient to any serious risk and cause only minor discomfort, related to the stimulation of the nerve by high-voltage electrical current. The nerve conduction velocity measures the function of the largest nerve fibers, which are also the fastest in conducting a stimulus, whereas the sensory action potential evaluates the number of the functioning fibers and is reduced in cases where there is fiber loss *(33,34)*.

In diabetic neuropathy, the sural nerve sensory amplitude is the first measurement to be affected and is followed by the conduction velocities of the sural and peroneal nerves, whereas in later stages, the nerves of the upper extremities may be involved *(35,36)*. The most commonly tested nerves are the median and ulnar (both sensory and motor) in the upper extremities and the peroneal (motor only) and sural (sensory only) in the lower extremity. Other electrophysiological measurements, which are used less frequently, are the compound muscle action potentials, F-Wave latency, and needle electromyography.

Factors that influence the electrophysiological measurements are the age, the skin temperature, the blood flow, and the glycemic control. Provided that age-related tables are used and the other factors are controlled, electrophysiology can provide very reliable results with coefficient variations ranging 4–7% for the conduction velocities and 10–15% for the sensory amplitudes *(37)*. This significant improvement in comparison to the quantitative sensory testing is related to the fact that electrophysiology provides objective measurements of the function of the peripheral nerves that do not require the collaboration of the patient. The above properties have established electrophysiological measurements as primary end-points in clinical trials of new therapeutic modalities *(1)*. However, despite all these advantages, the use of electrophysiology in clinical practice is limited by the fact that it requires expensive equipment and properly trained staff.

## SURAL NERVE BIOPSIES

This is an invasive technique that is mainly used for the conduction of research projects under the auspices of major clinical centers. There is no place for sural nerve biopsies in daily clinical practice, with the very rare exception of patients in whom the cause of peripheral neuropathy cannot be determined by any other method.

Both whole-nerve and fascicular-nerve biopsies can be employed. The myelinated fiber density is the most reliable single morphometric parameter for the evaluation of the severity of diabetic neuropathy, whereas other reliable indexes include the size of the myelinated fibers and the existence of axonal atrophy *(39)*. Another alternative is the index of pathology that was proposed by Dyck et al. and accommodates both the loss of myelinated fibers and the existence of abnormal teased fibers in one measurement *(40)*.

## COMPARISON AND RELATIONSHIP OF THE DIFFERENT METHODS USED FOR THE DIAGNOSIS AND STAGING OF DIABETIC NEUROPATHY

The histologic changes in sural nerve biopsies are the gold standard against which the efficacy of every other method employed in the diagnosis of diabetic neuropathy is compared. As nerve biopsies cannot be performed on a routine basis, extensive research has been conducted over the past decade examining the relationship of all the previously described noninvasive techniques and the morphometric measurements.

### *Assessments of the Neuropathic Symptoms*

No clinically significant correlations have been found by most of the studies between neuropathic symptoms and objective measurements of neuropathic severity, although

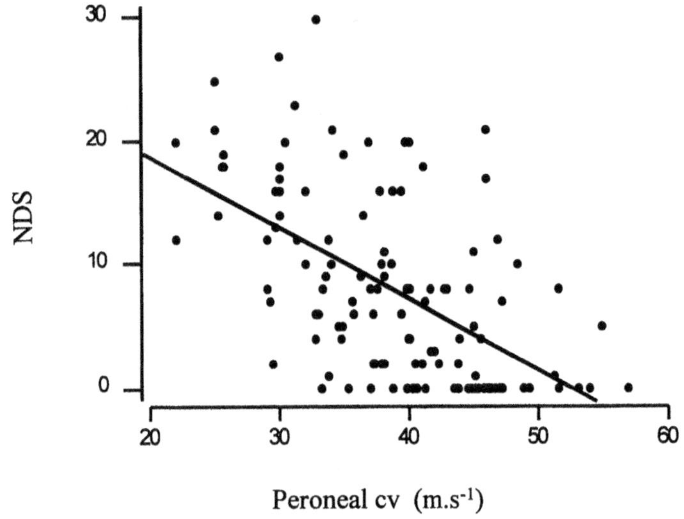


**Fig. 3.** A satisfactory relationship was found between the modified neuropathy, disability score (NDS), and the peroneal motor conduction velocity, coefficient correlation $r = -0.58$ (data from ref. *30*).

small but statistically significant correlations have been reported *(41–43)*. The two main reasons for this significant lack of correlation are the poor reproducibility of the employed techniques and that symptoms may be absent even in the most severe cases of neuropathy *(44)*.

### *Assessments of Clinical Signs*

In contrast with the clinical symptoms, satisfactory correlations have been obtained between measurements of clinical signs, using the previously described techniques, and objective measurements of diabetic neuropathy. In the few studies that employed sural nerve biopsies, significant relationships were reported between morphometric measurements and both the original Mayo Neuropathy Disability Score (NDS) and the modified NDS *(40,45)*.

Larger studies that have correlated the results of different NDS and electrophysiological measurements have also shown positive results. The regression between the modified NDS and peroneal motor nerve conduction velocity in a large number of diabetic patients with or without neuropathy is shown in Fig. 3 *(30)*. The correlation coefficient between the different NDS and the vibration perception threshold and nerve conduction velocities, as reported in two separate studies, are shown in Table 1 *(13,30)*. In brief, all NDS methods showed similar, and very satisfactory, relationships with VPT and nerve conduction velocities, indicating that a proper clinical examination can yield valuable information about the severity of diabetic neuropathy.

### *Quantitative Sensory Testing*

Initial studies of patients with moderate-to-severe neuropathy showed statistically significant correlations between quantitative sensory testing that included vibration perception threshold, warm discrimination thresholds, and myelinated fiber density of sural nerve biopsies *(46)*. However, these findings could not be reproduced in a subsequent

Table 1

| | *Modified NDS* | *Michigan NDS* | *Mayo NDS* |
|---|---|---|---|
| Vibration perception threshold (VPT) | 0.68 | 0.61 | 0.60 |
| Nerve conduction velocities | −0.58 | −0.59 | −0.66 |

The correlation coefficient between the three most commonly used Neuropathy Disability Scores (NDS), vibration perception threshold, and nerve conduction velocities measurements. The data in the first column (modified NDS) was derived from 122 diabetic patients *(30)* and in the second and third columns (Michigan and Mayo NDS) from 56 patients *(13)*.

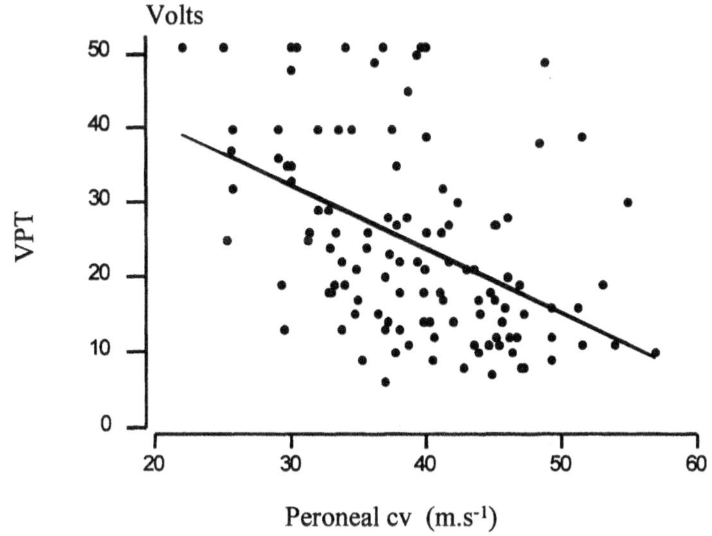


**Fig. 4.** Satisfactory correlation was found between peroneal motor conduction velocity and vibration perception threshold (VPT), $r = -0.50$ (data from ref. *30*).

study that included patients with mild neuropathy, indicating that in the early stages of the disease these techniques alone are not sufficient to quantify the severity of the diabetic neuropathy *(41)*.

Despite the above shortcomings, quantitative sensory testing has been shown to provide satisfactory correlations with electrophysiological measurements. As shown in Fig. 4, a significant correlation was found between vibration perception thresholds and the peroneal nerve conduction velocities in a large number of diabetic patients *(30)*. Similar results have been reported in other studies *(13,42)*.

### *Electrophysiologic Measurements*

As mentioned previously, electrophysiologic measurements provide objective results with a very satisfactory reliability and reproducibility. It is therefore no surprise that these measurements have been found to give the best correlations with the histopathologic nerve changes. In healthy subjects, the nerve conduction velocity of a particular nerve can be successfully estimated by the diameter of the largest fibers, but in diabetic

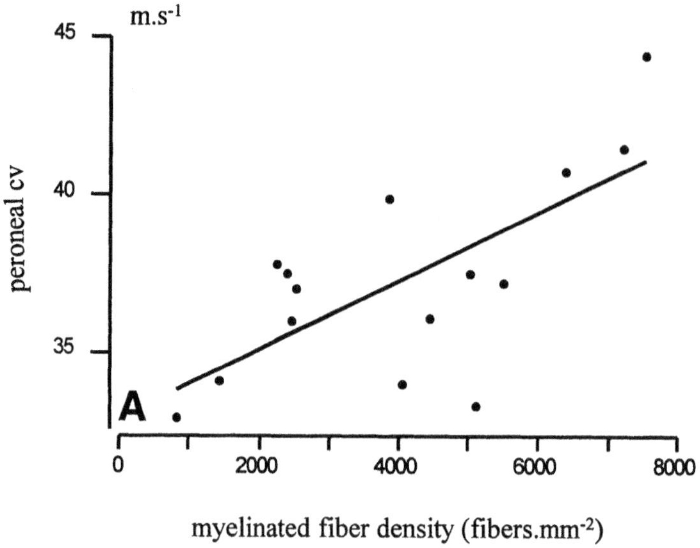


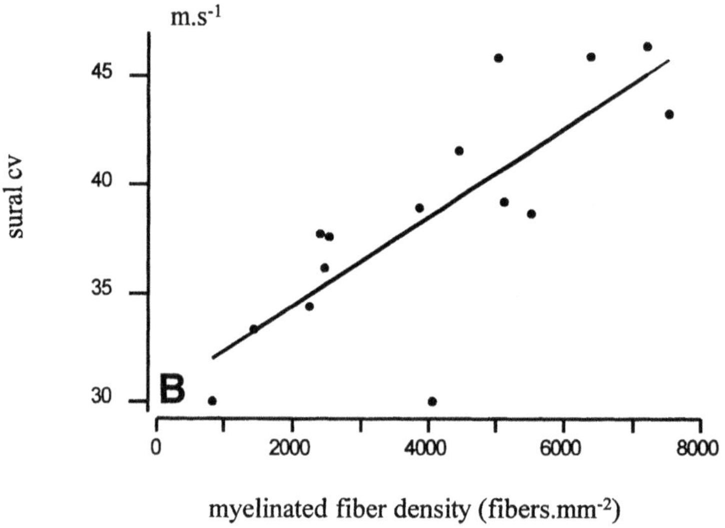


**Fig. 5.** The relationship between myelinated fiber density (MFD) in sural nerve biopsies and electrophysiological measurements in diabetic patients with mild diabetic neuropathy: Significant correlation was found between MFD and peroneal nerve conduction velocity, $r = 0.58$ (**A**), sural nerve conduction velocity, $r = 0.84$ (**B**), and sural sensory amplitude, $r = 0.74$ (**C**) (data from ref. *41*).

*(Figure continues on page 71)*

patients the actual velocity is usually 20–30% less than the expected one from such estimations *(47)*. This finding is related to functional changes in the nerve and is probably related to the nerve conduction velocity increments that follow the improvement of the glycemic control *(48)*.

Most of the electrophysiological changes are related to nerve structural damage and numerous studies have shown satisfactory correlations between these two measurements in mild, moderate, or severe neuropathy *(34,40,41,47)*. In Fig. 5, the regression

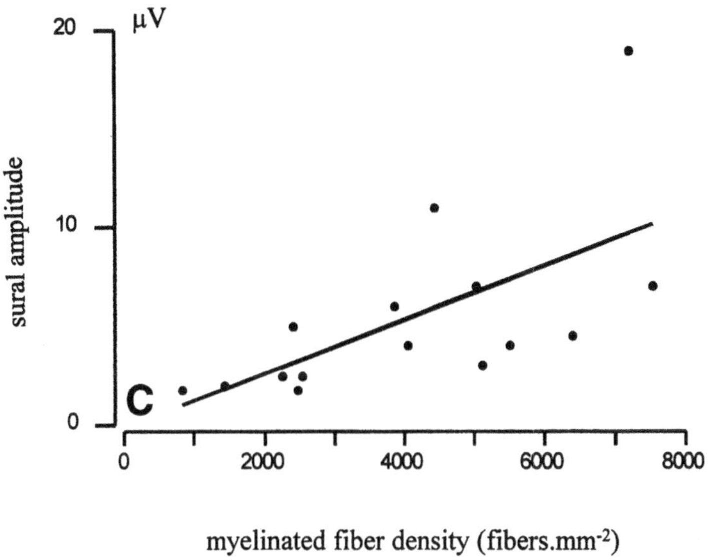


between myelinated fiber density of sural nerve biopsies and the peroneal motor conduction velocity, the sensory nerve conduction velocity and the sural sensory potential of patients with mild neuropathy is shown. The very close relationship between electrophysiologic and morphometric findings has prompted the use of electrophysiological measurements as surrogate methods for sural nerve biopsies in most of the clinical research studies.

## CRITERIA FOR THE DIAGNOSIS OF DIABETIC NEUROPATHY

There is no single set of criteria that is universally applicable for every case in which the diagnosis of the diabetic neuropathy is required. Instead, different criteria are applied in different situations, more simple criteria for daily clinical practice, simple but more standardized criteria for the conduction of large epidemiological studies, and more detailed criteria, sometimes including sural nerve biopsies, for studies in well-organized teaching hospitals which, as part of their mission, examine the pathogenesis of the disease or evaluate new medications. However, there is one rule that applies for all situations, namely that the diagnosis of diabetic neuropathy should be made only when abnormalities in two or more groups of tests are present and should never be based on abnormalities found in one test alone.

In routine clinical practice, where access to sophisticated equipment is limited, the diagnosis can be based on abnormalities of the clinical symptoms, signs, and quantitative sensory testing (vibration perception thresholds and/or Semmes-Weinstein monofilaments). Regarding the symptoms, the patients should be specifically asked for the existence of symptoms related to diabetic neuropathy such as numbness and/or painful symptoms in the lower extremities. The clinical signs should include the examination of the ankle and knee reflexes and the sensation of pain, touch, vibration, and cold sensation examined. The modified Neuropathy Symptom Score (NSS) and Neuropathy Disability Score (NDS), which require minimal additional time and allow a more structural examination, can be of particular help in following the progression of the disease. The assessment of the vibration perception threshold and/or the use of Semmes-Weinstein monofilaments will finally enable the physician not only in the diagnosis but also in identifying patients at risk of ulceration. The above tests require minimal and very inexpensive equipment and can be performed by every physician caring for diabetic patients without any specific training in 10–15 min. Therefore, they can easily be part of the annual check-up that should be performed on every patient, either in a hospital setting or in a primary-care practice.

In case a more detailed examination is required, most commonly related to research projects using algorithms such the one proposed by Dyck, a modification of this algorithm suggested by the San Antonio Consensus Statement or the Michigan algorithm proposed by Feldman can be used *(49,1,13)*. The inclusion of electrophysiological measurements in these algorithms allows a more detailed classification of the diabetic neuropathy and the detection of subclinical neuropathy. Thus, according to the San Antonio Consensus Statement, patients can be broadly classified into two categories: Class I in which both clinical symptoms and signs are absent and in Class II in which *either* symptoms or signs or both are present *(1)*. Each of these is then subdivided to classes A, B, and C according to the presence of abnormalities in quantitative sensory testing, electrophysiological measurements, and autonomic function testing.

It should again be emphasized that these algorithms are primarily useful for clinical research and not necessarily for use in daily clinical practice. Therefore, the practicing physician does not need to depend on them, but should be confident to make the diagnosis using the previously described methods.

## DIFFERENTIAL DIAGNOSIS

As there is no pathognomonic test for the diabetic neuropathy, its diagnosis can be made with confidence only when other possible causes have been excluded. Nevertheless, it should be kept in mind that in the great majority of diabetic patients with neurological findings, the underlying condition is diabetes. Findings that should alert the physician to the possibility of a neuropathy of another etiology would be an acute establishment of the neuropathy, asymmetrical neurological findings in the lower extremities, involvement of the central nervous system, and the existence of another systemic disease, e.g., malignancy or history of inherited neurological diseases in the family. Common causes for neuropathy with similar presentation to diabetic neuropathy include tabes dorsalis, B12 deficiency, leprosy, uremia, hypothyroidism, and diseases of the spinal column. If another cause for the neuropathy is suspected, further investigations under the supervision of a specialist may be required.

## CONCLUSIONS

The diagnosis of diabetic neuropathy is based on clinical symptoms, clinical signs, semiquantitative sensory testing, electrophysiological measurements, and in very rare cases, sural nerve biopsy. In clinical practice, abnormalities in two of the first three groups of tests, namely symptoms, signs, and quantitative sensory testing, are adequate to establish the diagnosis. What is more important, the use of vibration perception threshold measurements or Semmes-Weinstein monofilaments can identify patients at risk of foot ulceration and lead to preventive care. Various algorithms are also available for a more detailed examination of the peripheral nervous system and can help in the diagnosis of subclinical neuropathy and the staging of the severity of the disease. As discussed previously, these are usually employed for the conduction of clinical research.

## REFERENCES

1. Consensus Statement Report and Recommendations of the San Antonio Conference on Diabetic Neuropathy. Diabetes 1988;37:1000–1004.
2. Melzack R. The McGill Pain Questionnaire, major properties and scoring methods. Pain 1974;1:277–299.
3. Masson EA, Hunt L, Gem JM, Boulton AJM. A novel approach to the diagnosis and assessment of symptomatic diabetic neuropathy. Pain 1989;38:25–28.
4. Scott J, Huskisson EC. Graphic representation of pain. Pain 1976;2:175–184.
5. Boulton AJM, Scarpello JHB, Armstrong WD, Ward JD. The natural history of painful diabetic neuropathy—a 4-year study. Postgrad Med J 1983;59:16–19.
6. Dyck PJ, Sherman WR, Hallcher LM, Service J, O'Brian PC, Grina LC, Palumbo PJ, Swanson CJ. Human diabetic endoneurial sorbitol, fructose, and myo-inositol related to sural nerve morphometry. Ann Neurol 1980;8:590–596.
7. Dyck PJ, Karnes J, O'Brien PC, Swanson CJ. Neuropathy symptom profile in health, motor neuron disease, diabetic neuropathy, and amyloidosis. Neurology 1986;36:1300–1308.
8. Tesfaye S, Stevens L, Stephenson J, Fuller JH, Plater M, Ionescu-Tirgoviste C, Nuber A, Pozza G, Ward JD. The prevalence of diabetic peripheral neuropathy and its relation to glycemic control and potential risk factors: the Eurodiab IDDM complication study. Diabetologia 1996;39:1377–1384.
9. Veves A, Uccioli L, Manes C, Van Acker K, Komninou H, Philippides P, Katsilambros N, De Leeuw I, Menzinger G, Boulton AJM. Comparisons of risk factors for foot problems in diabetic patients attending teaching hospitals outpatient clinics in four different European states. Diabetic Med 1994;11:709–713.
10. Veves A, Donaghue VM, Sarnow MR, Giurini JM, Campbell DR, LoGerfo FW. The impact of reversal of hypoxia by revascularization in the peripheral nerve function of diabetic patients. Diabetologia 1996;39:344–348.
11. Dyck PJ, Kratz KM, Lehman KA, Karnes JL, Melton LJ, O'Brian PC, Litchy WJ, Windebank AJ, Smith BE, Low PA, Service FJ, Rizza RA, Zimmerman BR. The Rochester diabetic neuropathy study: design, criteria for types of neuropathy, selection bias, and reproducibility of neuropathic tests. Neurology 1991;41:799–807.
12. Young RJ, Zhou YQ, Rodriguez E, Prescott RJ, Ewing DJ, Clarke BF. Variable relationship between peripheral somatic and autonomic neuropathy in patients with different syndromes of diabetic polyneuropathy. Diabetes 1986;35:192–197.
13. Feldman EL, Srevens MJ, Thomas PK, Brown MB, Canal N, Greene DA. A practical two-step quantitative clinical and electrophysiological assessment for the diagnosis and staging of diabetic neuropathy. Diabetes Care 1994;17:1281–1289.
14. Steiness IB. Vibratory perception in normal subjects. A biothesiometer study. Acta Med Scandloose 1957;158:327–335.
15. Bloom S, Till S, Sonksen, Smith S. Use of a biothesiometer to measure individual vibration thresholds and their variation in 519 non-diabetic subjects. Brit Med J 1984;288:1783–1785.
16. Wiles PG, Pearce SM, Rice PJS, Mitchell JMO. Vibration Perception Threshold: influence of age, height, sex, and smoking and calculation of accurate centile values. Diabetic Med 1991;8:157–161.
17. Tegner R. The effect of skin temperature on vibratory sensitivity in polyneuropathy. J Neurol Neurosurg Psychiatry 1985;48:176–178.
18. Valensi P, Attali JR, Gagnat S. Reproducibility of parameters for assessment of diabetic neuropathy. The French Group for Research and Study of Diabetic Neuropathy. Diabetic Med 1993;10:933–939.
19. Williams G, Gill JS, Aber V, Mather HM. Variability in vibration perception threshold among sites: a potential source of error in biothesiometry. Brit Med J 1988;286:233–235.
20. Donaghue VM, Giurini JM, Rosenblum BI, Weissman PN, Veves A. Variability in function measurements of three sensory foot nerves in neuropathic diabetic patients. Diabet Res Clin Pract 1995;29:37–42.
21. Young MJ, Breddy JL, Veves A, Boulton AJM. The prediction of diabetic foot ulceration using vibration thresholds: a prospective study. Diabetes Care 1994;17:557–560.

22. Sosenko JM, Kato M, Soto R, Bild DE. Comparison of quantitative sensory-threshold measures for their association with foot ulceration in diabetic patients. Diabetes Care 1990;13:1057–1061.
23. Birke JA, Sims DS. Plantar sensory threshold in ulcerative foot. Leprosy Rev 1986;57:261–267.
24. Kumar S, Fernando DJS, Veves A, Knowles EA, Young MJ, Boulton AJM. Semmes-Weinstein monofilaments: a simple, effective and inexpensive screening device for identifying diabetic patients at risk of foot ulceration. Diabetes Res Clin Pract 1991;13:63–68.
25. Ziegler D, Mayer P, Wiefels K, Gries FA. Assessment of small and large fiber function in long-term type 1 (insulin-dependent) diabetic patients with and without painful neuropathy. Pain 1988;34:1–10.
26. Jamal GA, Weir AI, Hansen S, Ballantyne JP. An improved automated method for the measurement of thermal thresholds. 2. Patients with peripheral neuropathy. J Neurol Neurosurg Psychiatry 1985;48:361–366.
27. Bertelsmann FW, Heimans JJ, Weber EJM, Van der Veen EA, Schouten JA. Thermal discrimination threshold in normal subjects and in patients with diabetic neuropathy. J Neurol Neurosurg Psychiatry 1985;48:686–690.
28. Masson EA, Veves A, Fernando D, Boulton AJM. Current perception thresholds: a new, quick, and reproducible method for the assessment of peripheral neuropathy in diabetes mellitus. Diabetologia 1989;32:724–728.
29. Pitei DL, Watkins PJ, Stevens MJ, Edmonds ME. The value of neurometer is assessing diabetic neuropathy by measurement of the current perception threshold. Diabetic Med 1994;11:872–876.
30. Veves A, Young MJ, Manes C, Boulton AJM. Differences in peripheral and autonomic nerve function measurements in painful and painless neuropathy: a clinical study. Diabetes Care 1994;17:1200–1203.
31. Vinik AI, Suwanwalaikorn S, Stansberry KB, Holland MT, McNitt PM, Colen LE. Quantitative measurement of cutaneous perception in diabetic neuropathy. Muscle Nerve 1995;18:574–584.
32. Dyck PJ, Karnes J, O'Brian PC. Detection Thresholds of cutaneous sensation. In: Dyck PJ, Thomas PK, Asbury AK, Winegrad AI, Porte D, eds. Diabetic Neuropathy. WB Saunders, Philadelphia, 1987, pp. 107–121.
33. Kimura J. Nerve conduction studies and electromyography. In: Dyck PJ, Thomas PK, Lambert EH, Bunge R, eds. Peripheral Neuropathy. Saunders, Philadelphia, 1984, pp. 919–966.
34. Behse F, Buchthal F. Sensory action potentials and biopsy of the sural nerve in neuropathy. Brain 1978;101:473–493.
35. Baba M. Diabetic nerve function: its electrophysiological evaluation. In: Ward JD, Goto Y, eds. Diabetic Neuropathy. Wiley, Chichester, UK, 1991, pp. 269–280.
36. Daube JR. Electrophysiologic testing in diabetic neuropathy. In: Dyck PJ, Thomas PK, Asbury AK, Winegrad AI, Porte D, eds. Diabetic Neuropathy. Saunders, Philadelphia, 1987, pp. 162–176.
37. Daube JR. Electrophysiologic testing in diabetic neuropathy. In: Dyck PJ, Thomas PK, Asbury AK, Winegrad AI, Porte D, eds. Diabetic Neuropathy. Saunders, Philadelphia, 1987, pp. 162–176.
38. Dyck PJ, O'Brian PC. Meaningful degrees of prevention or improvement of nerve conduction in controlled clinical trials of diabetic neuropathy. Diabetes Care 1989;12:649–652.
39. Consensus Statement. 1996 Standardized measures in diabetic neuropathy. Morphological and biochemical measures. Diabetes Care 1996;19(Suppl 1):S74–S76.
40. Dyck PJ, Karnes JL, Daube J, O'Brien P, Service FJ. Clinical and neuropathological criteria for the diagnosis and staging of diabetic neuropathy. Brain 1985;1985:861–880.
41. Veves A, Malik RA, Lye RH, Masson EA, Sharma AK, Schady W, Boulton AJM. Correlations between sural nerve histology and electrophysiology and quantitative sensory tests in mild diabetic neuropathy. Diabetic Med 1991;8:917–921.
42. Dyck PJ, Bushek W, Spring EM, Karnes JL, Litchy J O'Brien P, Service FJ. Vibratory and cooling detection thresholds compared with other tests in diagnosing and staging diabetic neuropathy. Diabetes Care 1987;10:432–440.
43. Veves A, Young MJ, Manes C, Boulton AJM. Differences in peripheral and autonomic nerve function measurements in painful and painless neuropathy: a clinical study. Diabetes Care 1994;17:1200–1203.
44. Veves A, Manes C, Murray HJ, Young MJ, Boulton AJM. Painful neuropathy in diabetic patients with or without foot ulceration. Diabetes Care 1993;16:1187–1189.
45. Britland ST, Young RJ, Sharma AK, Clarke BF. Association of painful and painless diabetic polyneuropathy with different patterns of nerve fiber degeneration and regeneration. Diabetes 1990;39:898–908.
46. Malik RA, Newrick PG, Sharma AK, Jennings A, Ah-See AK, Mayhew TM, Jakubowski J, Boulton AJM, Ward JD. Microangiopathy in human diabetic neuropathy: relationship between capillary abnormalities and the severity of neuropathy. Diabetologia 1989;32:92–102.

47. Behse F, Buchthal F, Carlsen F. Nerve biopsy and conduction studies in diabetic neuropathy. J Neurol Neurosurg Psychiatry 1977;40:1072–1082.
48. Ward JD, Fisher DJ, Barnes CG, Jessop JD. Improvement in nerve conduction following treatment in newly diagnosed diabetics. Lancet 1971;1:428–430.
49. Dyck PJ. Detection, characterization, and staging of polyneuropathy: assessed in diabetics. Muscle Nerve 1988;11:21–32.

# 5 Histologic Changes
## *Implications for Treatment Strategies*

*Anders AF Sima,* MD, PHD

***Contents***



## INTRODUCTION

Distal symmetric polyneuropathy, often combined with autonomic polyneuropathy, constitutes the most common chronic symptomatic complication of diabetes mellitus and affects approx 17 million people in the United States and Europe *(1)*.

Diabetic peripheral polyneuropathy is a disorder demonstrating progressive nerve fiber loss, atrophy, and nodal changes manifested clinically as deteriorating nerve function with or without accompanying dysesthetic and/or paresthetic symptoms *(2)*. The disease culminates in severe sequelae such as insensitivity to pain, anesthesia, limb deformities, foot ulcerations, infections, and limb amputations. Although sensory loss corresponds to the degree of fiber loss *(3)*, neuropathic symptoms are difficult to assess and unreliable indicators of the degree of nerve fiber injury *(4)*. They tend to be highly variable, transient, and difficult to quantify objectively. Furthermore, symptoms such as pain are of different qualities, each one reflecting processes that may be independent of progressive nerve fiber loss, such as nerve fiber regeneration, neuropeptide imbalances, dispersion of central processing of impulses or to extraneuronal causes such as arthropathy, and mechanical foot deformities. Neuropsychological tests of sensory loss are difficult to standardize and show wide day-to-day variations *(5,6)*. Electrophysiological analyses such as waveform analyses of evoked potentials, neurography or single-fiber electromyography, accurately reflect the functional integrity of peripheral nerve fibers, but suffer from limited sampling and are not well standardized *(7,8)*. On

From: *Contemporary Endocrinology: Clinical Management of Diabetic Neuropathy*
Edited by: A. Veves © Humana Press Inc., Totowa, NJ

the other hand, well-standardized diagnostic nerve conduction studies are readily available and are highly reproducible when correctly performed *(2,9)*.

Measurements such as nerve conduction velocities and amplitudes of evoked potential do indeed correlate relatively well with nerve fiber pathology such as morphometric assessments of nerve-fiber densities and quantitative nodal pathology *(10,11)*. However, nerve function as measured by nerve conduction velocity or amplitudes of evoked responses is sensitive to momentary alterations in glucose control and, therefore may not accurately reflect underlying structural abnormalities of the nerve *(12,13)*.

Sural nerve biopsy is an invasive diagnostic procedure, although safe and well established. This technique has been widely applied over the last decade in clinical trials in an attempt to morphometrically quantify nerve-fiber loss and damage as measures of therapeutic responses *(10,14)*. Although the full potential of quantitative structural assessments has not been utilized in these studies, it is clear that basic morphometric measures such as fiber densities correlate well with electrophysiologic parameters *(15)*. However, in subsets of biopsies in which more detailed morphometric analyses have been performed, specific structural abnormalities show even better correlations with standardized electrophysiologic measures *(16)*. Such detailed analyses in large-scale studies are unfortunately prohibited by the high costs of assessment. In this chapter, the value of morphometric analyses of peripheral nerve biopsies will be discussed, as a potential tool for assessment of drug efficacy and as an opportunity to delineate the natural history of this common and disabling complication of diabetes mellitus.

## PATHOLOGIC CHANGES IN DIABETIC NERVE

The morphological changes seen in human diabetic nerve involve the neural, glial, vascular, and connective tissue elements. In overt diabetic neuropathy, the striking fiber atrophy and loss of myelinated and unmyelinated fibers are associated with segmental demyelination, Wallerian degeneration, and morphologic changes of the node of Ranvier that constitute the hallmarks of human diabetic neuropathy *(9,17–21)*. The proximal-to-distal gradient of these changes together with the topographic and temporal occurrence of neurological deficits and symptoms are in keeping with an axonopathy of dying-back type, affecting preferentially the longest axons. Motor fibers appear to be less severely involved. As to whether this is caused by their shorter axons is not known. Sensory ganglion cells support both a peripheral and central axon, whereas motor neurons only support a peripheral axon. Ultrastructural examination of sural nerve biopsies from individuals with newly detected diabetes demonstrating axonal atrophy is consistent with what appears to be a primary axonopathy *(18,19)*. However, supporting endoneurial tissue components are also involved with proliferation of mesenchymal elements including fibroblast and collagen, endoneurial endothelial cells, and extracellular matrix components such as basement membranes *(22–25)*.

There appears to be a homology between the structural changes and the sequence in which they occur in human and murine diabetic neuropathy *(26,27)*. In diabetic rat models, such as the type I spontaneously diabetic BB/W rat, careful longitudinal studies have delineated a sequence of axonal changes with secondary demyelination and what appear to be relatively independent nodal changes. The earliest demonstrable structural change is evidenced by dispersion of cytoskeletal elements and abnormal axon swelling at the node of Ranvier *(28,29)*. In the diabetic rat, these changes have been associated with intra-axonal sodium accumulation secondary to decreased activity of

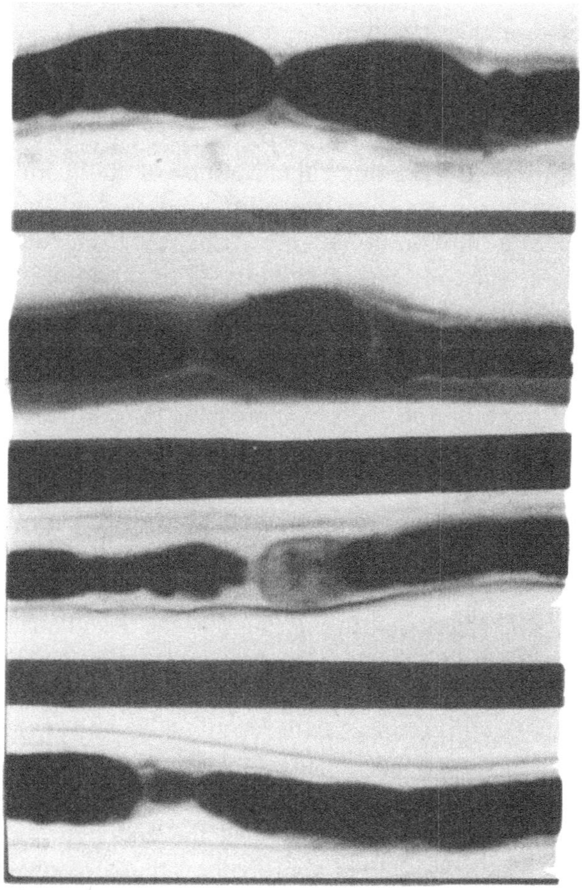

**Fig. 1.** Sequence of nodal changes as seen in single teased-fiber preparation. The top two panels show paranodal swelling, the third panel shows paranodal demyelination, and the bottom panel shows a remyelinated intercalated internode.

$Na^+$-$K^+$-ATPase that is topographically concentrated to the node of Ranvier *(30)*. These changes are followed by axonal dwindling starting at the distal out-reaches of the axon. There is malorientation of cytoskeletal elements that has been associated with impaired polymerization of microfilaments because of nonenzymatic glycation or fructation *(26,28,31)* as well as impaired synthesis of these building blocks by the perikaryon *(32)*. These progressive abnormalities lead eventually to axonal death and Wallerian degeneration. The nodal changes appear to be initiated by a loss of intercellular junctional complexes that adhere the myelin to the axolemma and constitute the functionally important paranodal ion-channel barrier *(29,33)*. The defect in paranodal myelin adhesion to the paranodal axon results in paranodal myelin retraction and demyelination, which may be repaired by the lay down of new myelin resulting in short so-called intercalated internodes (Fig. 1).

This sequence of structural changes demonstrated in experimental diabetes can be reconstructed in human diabetic neuropathy, particularly by the evaluation of single teased fibers *(34)*.

## VASCULAR PATHOLOGY IN DIABETIC POLYNEUROPATHY

Endoneurial vessels in diabetic patients undergo progressive changes with hyalinization and deposition of PAS-positive material in the vessel walls, which in extreme situations may lead to occlusion of the vessel lumina *(22)*. Rarely, microthrombi composed of platelets have been demonstrated in nerve biopsies *(35)*. The most characteristic change is that of basement membrane thickening either because of duplication of basement membranes or homogeneous basement-membrane thickening. Additional changes include proliferation and swelling of endothelial cells *(24,25,36)*. The degree of microangiopathic changes correlate with the severity of nerve-fiber pathology and clinical severity of the neuropathy *(36)*. These findings led to a revitalization of the vascular theory proposed by Fagerberg almost 50 yr ago *(22)*. The basement membrane changes in diabetes have detrimental effects on its normal barrier function, both the charge-selective barrier function as well as its filter function, thereby increasing the permeability of the protective blood–nerve barrier. This defect is probably further enhanced by loss of interendothelial junctional complexes, analogous to axoglial dysjunction of the paranodal apparatus *(24)*. The thickening of the basement membrane may lead to increased diffusion distance for oxygen, potentially leading to endoneurial hypoxemia *(37,38)*.

Dyck and coworkers *(39)* reported multifocal nerve-fiber loss in peripheral nerves from diabetic patients and suggested that ischemia was the main underlying cause for the characteristic nerve-fiber loss. Their ultrastructural studies suggested that endoneurial ischemia was consequent to endothelial-cell hypertrophy causing capillary closure, a measure that correlated with scores of nerve-fiber pathology. Subsequent studies *(24,40,41)* were not able to reproduce these interesting findings by Dyck et al., but suggested that capillary closure, which is seen in venules rather than capillaries, represents a physiological regulation of venous drainage of the endoneurium, seen just as commonly in normal peripheral nerve and in neuropathies that are not considered to have an ischemic basis. In a later study, Giannini and Dyck *(42)* were unable to reproduce their previous results. Nevertheless it appears clear that both structural and functional abnormalities of the endoneurial vasculature contribute to the nerve-fiber pathology seen in diabetic neuropathy. However, these changes may, in part, occur independently from a primary nerve-fiber damage, since focal nerve-fiber loss characteristic of ischemic injury is twice as common in NIDDM patients as in IDDM subjects with the same duration of diabetes *(20)*. These differences may, in part, be caused by age-related changes, pre-existing vascular disease, and accelerated atherosclerosis in the older NIDDM population. It is very likely that early functional changes in vascular tone and perfusion contribute to the nerve-fiber pathology. Mounting evidence from experimental diabetes strongly suggest that imbalances in vasoactive substances such as NO and prostanoids impact on peripheral-nerve blood flow and oxygenation of the endoneurial content *(43)*. Indirect evidence for a functional vascular component in human diabetic nerve was presented by Inone et al. *(44)*, who demonstrated a beneficial effect of a prostaglandin $E_1$ analog on nerve function in diabetic patients.

## DIFFERENCES IN DIABETIC NEUROPATHY IN IDDM AND NIDDM PATIENTS

Since there are marked differences in underlying pathophysiology, metabolic, and hormonal aberrations in IDDM and NIDDM patients who only have hyperglycemia in common, it is not surprising that the pathologic expression of neuropathic changes may be different in the two types of diabetes. Superimposed on these differences, the two groups show differences in age that may impart a varied susceptibility to nerve injury as well as age-related structural changes. Of quantifiable structural changes characterizing diabetic polyneuropathy, axonal atrophy and axoglial dysjunction of the paranode appear to be significantly more severely expressed in IDDM patients than in those with NIDDM with comparable duration of diabetes and hyperglycemic control *(20)*. In experimental diabetes, these changes have been closely related to metabolic abnormalities affecting primarily the neuronal tissue elements. In contrast NIDDM patients with neuropathy show a significantly higher frequency of Wallerian degeneration and increased focality of nerve fiber loss, which may suggest a greater importance of vascular pathophysiological mechanisms with hypoxia and/or ischemia as important contributing factors to nerve-fiber damage and loss *(17,20)*. Elucidation of mechanistic differences in the neuropathies occurring in the two types of diabetes will be of importance, since this may impact upon the design of targeted therapies for this disorder.

## QUANTITATIVE ASSESSMENTS OF PATHOLOGY

Morphometric techniques have been employed in the quantitative assessment of the structural pathology and as a measure of drug efficacy in biopsies obtained from patients participating in clinical diabetic neuropathy trials *(10,14)*.

Mainly two histopathologic techniques have been applied: light-microscopic morphometric assessment of semithin plastic-embedded cross sections of sural nerve; and single-teased-fiber analyses of a minimum of 100 randomly selected myelinated fibers, although this technique has not been used in recent trials. Light-microscopic morphometric analysis provides measures such as mean fiber size, fiber size histograms, fiber density, and coefficient of variation of fiber density between frames, which gives a value for the focality of fiber loss *(14,34)*. Less commonly used measures include the ratio between axonal area and that of the surrounding myelin sheath and index of circularity and frequency of regenerating clusters.

Teased fiber analysis, when accurately performed, is a sensitive and informative technique that provides a different set of information. The sequential nodal pathology characteristic of diabetic polyneuropathy can be assessed by the frequency of fibers exhibiting nodal swelling, paranodal demyelination, and intercalated remyelinated internodes *(34,45)* (Fig. 1). A measure of axonal atrophy is obtained by the frequency of fibers exhibiting excessive myelin wrinkling. Other specific pathologies that are quantitated by teased fiber analysis include segmental and Wallerian degeneration and regenerated fibers.

Each pathologic change is expressed as its frequency among all fibers examined minus those showing regeneration, but including fibers showing the normal structural appearance ("normalcy") *(46)*. The number of normal fibers (frequency of normal teased fibers × fiber density) constitutes the index of normality, which has been shown to be a valuable overall reciprocal measure of pathology that correlates well with electrophysiologic measurements *(3)*. Additional quantitative analyses can be performed using ultrastructural morphometry. However, these techniques are difficult and extremely time consuming, but can be used for research purposes and for detailed analyses of the natural history of the disease. The ultrastructural morphometric techniques include the ratio between axonal cross-sectional area and myelin thickness,

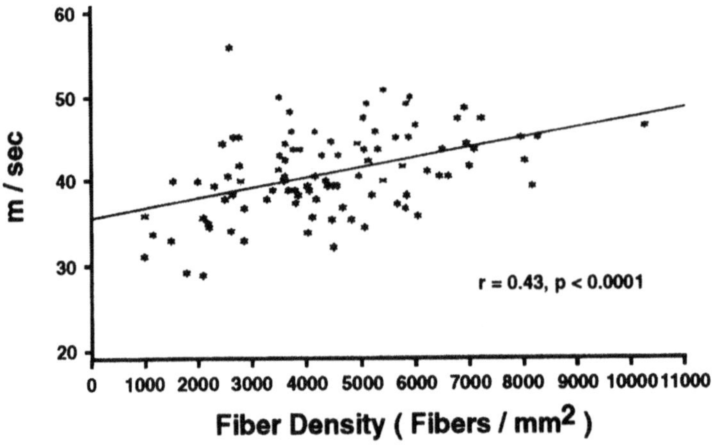


**Fig. 2.** Correlations between sural-nerve conduction velocity and sural-nerve fiber density.

expressed as the number of myelin lamellae. Detailed quantitative analysis can also be applied to axoglial dysjunction, but requires serial sectioning of ultrathin sections of large samples of ultrastructurally identified nodes *(47)*.

## CORRELATIONS BETWEEN MORPHOMETRIC MEASUREMENTS AND ELECTROPHYSIOLOGIC PARAMETERS

Diabetic polyneuropathy is characterized structurally by a progressive loss of myelinated fibers and electrophysiologically by a progressive decrease in nerve conduction velocity and amplitude of evoked responses. It is therefore not surprising that relatively good correlations have repeatedly been established between myelinated fiber density and nerve conduction velocity or amplitude of evoked responses in the sural nerve (Figs. 2 and 3) *(3,10,11,15)*.

Similarly, index of normality obtained from morphometric analysis of sural nerves also correlates with nerve conduction velocity and amplitudes measured in sural nerves *(3)*.

As mentioned earlier, the hallmarks of the pathology in diabetic polyneuropathy appear to be axonal atrophy and nodal changes. Since both these measures would be expected to be determinants for nerve conduction velocity, correlations have been established between the sum of axonal atrophy and magnitude of axoglial dysjunction and nerve conduction velocity *(16)*.

There is evidence to suggest that both the pathologic and electrophysiological deficits characterizing diabetic polyneuropathy do not progress linearly in the same nerve over the duration of diabetes. Furthermore, functional deficits in different nerves start at different time points and may progress at different rates, reflecting the length dependent dying-back nature of the neuropathy. For instance, at a given time point during the disease, the electrophysiologic deficits are worst in sensory nerves of the lower extremity, less so in sensory nerves of the upper extremity, and least affected in upper extremity motor nerves *(48)*. However, despite these differences in the stages of the neuropathy in different nerves, the pathology obtained in the sural nerve correlates well

Table 1
Decreases in Amplitudes of Evoked Responses in Sural, Peroneal, Median Sensory and Median Motor Nerves and Their Correlations with Sural Nerve Fiber Density in 334 Patients

| | *Amplitude (% of normal)* | *Correlation with Sural Nerve Fiber Density* | |
|---|---|---|---|
| | | r⁻ | p-*value* |
| Sural | 38.8 | 0.44 | 0.0001 |
| Peroneal | 68.9 | 0.25 | 0.0001 |
| Median sensory | 57.8 | 0.34 | 0.0001 |
| Median motor | 92.1 (N.S.) | 0.08 | 0.14 |

Note no correlation could be demonstrated between the normal median motor amplitude and the sural nerve fiber density.

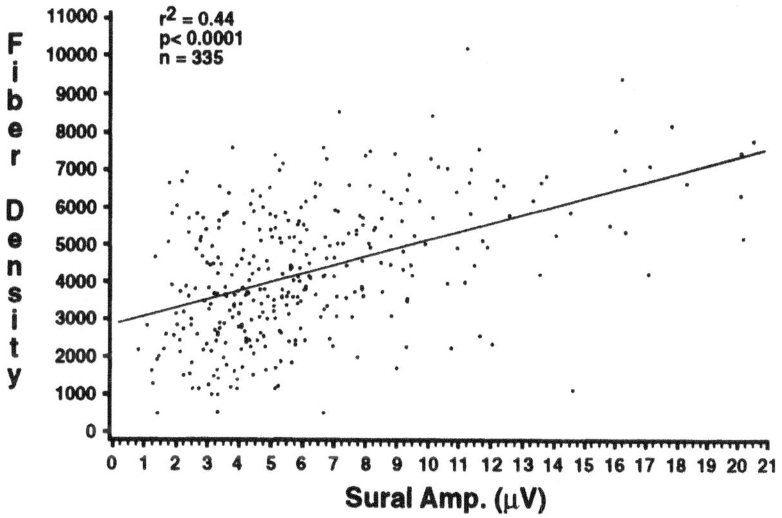


**Fig. 3.** Correlations between sural-nerve fiber density and sural-nerve amplitudes in 334 patients.

with the electrophysiology in any of the affected nerves, suggesting that the neuropathy once established in any given nerve progresses *pari passu* with that of the most severely affected sural nerve, albeit at a less severe stage (Table 1) *(48)*.

## THE UTILITY OF NERVE-FIBER MORPHOLOGY AS A MEASURE OF EFFICACY IN CLINICAL TRIALS

Nerve morphometry, when utilized to its full potential, is an extremely useful technique to assess the nature and the quantity of peripheral-nerve pathology in any neuropathy *(45)*. Early clinical trials of various aldose reductase inhibitors from which nerve biopsies were obtained, clearly established some basic correlations between nerve pathology and functional deficits. Nerve-fiber density, for instance, correlates relatively well with both nerve conduction velocity and amplitudes of evoked potentials, and specific pathologic changes such as axonal atrophy and nodal pathology correlate with nerve conduction velocity. The establishment of these correlations have been important by lending greater confidence to conventional electrophysiologic measures as indicators of the severity of underlying structural pathology, but beyond this has added little to our understanding of the disease process or as to how various interventional therapies may change the course of the disease.

In order to assess and understand this latter phenomenon, different sets of morphometric assessments have to be applied, such as structural changes reflecting reparative phenomena. These can be divided into two groups. First, one in which there is replacement of degenerated fibers by newly regenerated fibers and, second, one in which affected fibers are repaired. For instance, increase in axonal size of previously atrophic fibers or repair of the destructive nodal pathology (axoglial dysjunction and paranodal demyelination) by intercalated remyelinated internodes.

Nerve-fiber regeneration is impaired in diabetic polyneuropathy. Several aldose reductase trials have in fact demonstrated impressive increases in nerve-fiber regeneration following treatment with active drug, which have been interpreted as a positive treatment effect *(10,14)*. However critics *(38)* have raised the question as to whether these regenerated nerves ever reach their target organ and thereby become functional. Evidence in support of reinnervation was demonstrated by Bril and coworkers *(8)*, who showed increased reinnervation of muscle fibers by single-fiber EMG. Unfortunately, however, experimental studies of regenerated fibers in aldose reductase-treated diabetic rats have demonstrated incomplete structural maturation of the nodal apparatus and impaired myelination of regenerated fibers in diabetic rats as compared to nondiabetic control animals. These defects were associated with incomplete functional maturation of regenerated fibers *(49)*. Therefore, it is possible that the burst of regeneration seen following ARI treatment may have some effect as to reinnervation, but may not achieve the full potential of normal regenerated fibers. Hence, the increase in regenerated fibers assessed morphometrically in clinical trials should be interpreted with caution and their significance as a reparative phenomenon at this time is uncertain.

Repair of dwindling axons and structurally impaired nodes has only been investigated in studies with small numbers of patients. However in one such study, repair of both nodal changes and axonal size appeared to correlate with small increases in nerve conduction velocity *(16)*. The functional and clinical significance of these reparative changes of the axon and the node of Ranvier will have to be confirmed in large-scale studies. Therefore, these measures of fiber regeneration and repair should be used as logical indicators of drug efficacy in clinical trials. Unfortunately, except for nerve-fiber regeneration, the significance of which is unsettled, these analyses have not been performed in recent large-scale biopsy trials. For instance, axonal atrophy should be assessed using more sensitive techniques such as ultrastructural assessments and/or teased fiber analysis as mentioned above. Similarly the reparative changes of previous nodal pathology as well as those of segmental demyelination can be accurately assessed and quantitated utilizing single teased fibers.

As mentioned previously, qualitative differences exist in the neuropathology of diabetic neuropathy between IDDM and NIDDM patients. Therefore, it will be paramount in future clinical trials, in which morphometric assessment is contemplated, to separate these two patient groups in the evaluation of morphometric data, since combining data sets from the two groups may mask improvements occurring in one group but not in the other.

In summary, the usefulness of morphometric analyses of peripheral nerve biopsies as indicators of drug efficacy is questionable. This is an invasive procedure associated with extremely high costs of analysis and, as employed today, will not provide any information in addition to what can be obtained from carefully performed electrophysiological measurements. However, the very large biopsy material that has accumulated from several clinical trials and which has been only partially examined, could serve as an extremely valuable source for systematic examinations of the natural history of this diverse and complex disease accompanying the two types of diabetes.

## REFERENCES


1. Sima AAF. Diabetic neuropathy: pathogenesis, natural history and therapeutic potentials. In: Vasselli JR, Maggio CA, Scriabine A, eds. Drugs in Development, vol 1, A-Glucosidase Inhibition: Potential Use in Diabetes. Neva Press, Bradford, CT, 1993, pp. 201–209.
2. Greene DA, Sima AAF, Albers JW, Pfeifer MA. Diabetic Neuropathy. In: Rifkin H, Porte DP Jr, eds. Diabetes Mellitus, Theory and Practice, 4th ed. Elsevier, New York, 1990, pp. 710–755.
3. Sima AAF, Greene DA. Sural nerve fiber density and normality predict clinical sensory deficits and electrophysiology in chronic diabetic neuropathy. Diabetes 1991;40:554A.
4. Britland ST, Young RJ, Sharma AK, Clark BF. Association of painful and painless diabetic polyneuropathy with different patterns of nerve fiber degeneration and regeneration. Diabetes 1990;39:898–908.
5. Dyck PJ, Karnes J, O'Brien PC. Detection of thresholds of cutaneous sensation, in Diabetic Neuropathy, (Dyck PJ, Thomas PK, Asbury AK, Winegrad AL, Porte D Jr, eds), W.B. Saunders, Philadelphia, PA, pp. 107–121.
6. Maser RE, Nielsen VK, Bass EB, Manjoo Q, Dorman JS, Kelsey SF, Becker DJ, Orchard TJ: Measuring diabetic neuropathy: assessment and comparison of clinical examination and quantitative sensory testing. Diabetes Care 1989;12:270–275.
7. Thiele K, Stålberg F. Single fiber EMG findings in polyneuropathies of different etiology. J Neurol Neurosurg Psychiatry 1975;38:881–887.
8. Bril V, Werb MR, Greene DA, Sima AAF. Single fiber electromyography in diabetic peripheral polyneuropathy. Muscle Nerve 1996;19:2–9.
9. Behse F, Buchthal F, Carlsen F. Nerve biopsy and conduction studies in diabetic neuropathy. J Neurol Neurosurg Psychiatry 1977;40:1072–1082.
10. Sima AAF, Greene DA, Brown MB, Hohman TC, Hicks D, Graepel GJ, Bochenek WJ, Beg M, Gonen B: Effect of hyperglycemia and the aldose reductase inhibitor tolrestat on sural nerve biochemistry and morphometry in advanced diabetic peripheral polyneuropathy. J Diab Compl 1993;7:157–169.
11. Sima AAF, Greene DA. Morphologie der peripheren diabetischen Neuropathie und ihre Korrelation mit Funktionstesten. Diabetes und Stoffwechsel 1992;1:45–51.
12. Ward JD, Barnes CG, Fisher DJ, Jessop JD, Baker RW. Improvement in nerve conduction following treatment in newly diagnosed diabetics. Lancet 1971;I:428–430.
13. Pietri A, Ehle A, Raskin P. Changes in nerve conduction velocity after six weeks of gluco-regulation with portable insulin infusion pumps. Diabetes 1980;29:668–671.
14. Sima AAF, Bril V, Nathaniel V, McEwen TA, Brown MB, Lattimer SA, Greene DA: Regeneration and repair of myelinated fibers in sural nerve biopsies from patients with diabetic neuropathy treated with an aldose reductase inhibitor. N Engl J Med 1988;319:548–555.
15. Sima AAF. Structural-functional interactions in the therapeutic response of diabetic neuropathy. J Diab Compl 1992;6:40–44.
16. Sima AAF, Prashar A, Nathaniel V, Bril V, Werb WR, Greene DA: Overt diabetic neuropathy: repair of axoglial dysjunction and axonal atrophy by aldose reductase inhibition and its correlation to improvement in nerve conduction velocity. Diab Med 1993;10:115–121.

17. Dyck PJ, Lais A, Karnes JL, O'Brien P, Rizza R. Fiber loss is primary and multifocal in sural nerves in diabetic polyneuropathy. Ann Neurol 1986;19:425–439.
18. Bischoff A. Diabetic neuropathy. Pathologic anatomy, pathophysiology and pathogenesis on the basis of electron microscopic studies. Dutsch Med Wochenschr 1968;93:237–241.
19. Yagihashi S, Matsunaga M. Ultrastructural pathology of peripheral nerves in patients with diabetic neuropathy. Tohoku J Exp Med 1979;129:357–366.
20. Sima AAF, Nathaniel V, Bril V, McEwen TA, Greene DA: Histopathological heterogeneity of neuropathy in insulin-dependent and non-insulin dependent diabetes, and demonstration of axo-glial dysjunction in human diabetic neuropathy. J Clin Invest 1988;81:349–364.
21. Sima AAF. Diabetic Neuropathy. In: Tze WJ, Sima AAF, eds. Insulin Dependent Diabetes Mellitus Current Concepts and Approaches. Radar Publ Montreal, 1991, pp. 233–244.
22. Fagerberg SE. Diabetic neuropathy, a clinical and histological study on the significance of vascular affection. Acta Med Scand Suppl 1959;345:1–97.
23. Johnson PC, Doll SC, Cromey DW. Pathogenesis of diabetic neuropathy. Ann Neurol 1986;19:450–457.
24. Sima AAF, Nathaniel V, Prashar A, Bril V, Greene DA. Endoneurial microvessels in human diabetic neuropathy: endothelial cell dysjunction and lack of treatment effect by ARI. Diabetes 1991;40:1090–1099.
25. Yasuda H, Dyck PJ. Abnormalities of endoneurial microvessels and sural nerve pathology in diabetic neuropathy. Neurology 1987;37:20–28.
26. Sima AAF, Bouchier M, Christensen H. Axonal atrophy in sensory nerves of the diabetic BB-Wistar rat, a possible early correlate of human diabetic neuropathy. Ann Neurol 1983;13:264–272.
27. Sima AAF. Natural history of structural and functional alterations in diabetic BB-rat peripheral nerve. In Renold AE, Shafrir E, eds. Frontiers in Diabetes Research: Lessons from Animal Diabetes II. John Libbey Comp, London, 1988, pp. 471–476.
28. Sima AAF, Lorusso AC, Thibert P. Distal symmetric polyneuropathy in the spontaneously diabetic BB-Wistar rat. An ultrastructural and teased fiber study. Acta Neuropath (Berl) 1982;58:39–47.
29. Sima AAF, Lattimer SA, Yagihashi S, Greene DA. "Axoglial dysjunction:" a novel structural lesion that accounts for poorly reversible slowing of nerve conduction in the spontaneously diabetic BB-rat. J Clin Invest 1986;77:474–484.
30. Powell HC, Garret RS, Kador PF, Mizisin AP. Fine structural localization of aldose reductase and ouabain-sensitive $K^+$-dependent p-nitro-phenylphosphatase in rat peripheral nerve. Acta Neuropath (Berl) 1991;81:529–539.
31. Williams SK, Howarth NL, Devenny JJ, Britensky NW. Structural and functional consequences of increased tubulin glycosylation in diabetes mellitus. Proc Natl Acad Sci USA 1982;72:6546–6550.
32. Thomas PK, Wright DW, Tzebelikos E. Amino acid uptake by dorsal root ganglia from streptozotocin-diabetic rats. J Neurol Neurosurg Psychiatry 1984;47:912–916.
33. Cherian PV, Kamijo M, Angelides KJ, Sima AAF. Nodal Na+-channel displacement is associated with nerve conduction slowing in the chronically diabetic BB/W-rat. Prevention by an aldose reductase inhibitor. J Diab Compl 1996;10:192–200.
34. Sima AAF, Brown MB, Prashar A, Chakrabarti S, Laudadio C, Greene DA: The reproducibility and sensitivity of sural nerve morphometry in the assessment of diabetic peripheral polyneuropathy. Diabetologia 1992;35:560–569.
35. Williams E, Timperley WR, Ward JD, Duckworth T. Electron microscopic studies of vessels in diabetic peripheral neuropathy. J Clin Path 1980;33:462–470.
36. Malik RA, Newrick PG, Sharma AK, Jennings A, Ah-See AK, Mayhew TM, Jakubowski J, Boulton AJ, Ward JD: Microangiopathy in human diabetic neuropathy: relationship between capillary abnormalities and the severity of neuropathy. Diabetologia 1989;32:92–102.
37. Giannini C, Dyck PJ. Ultrastructural morphometric features of human sural nerve endoneurial microvessels. J Neuropath Exp Neurol 1993;52:361–369.
38. Dyck PJ, Giannini C. Pathologic alterations in the diabetic neuropathies of humans. J Neuropath Exp Neurol 1996;55:1181–1193.
39. Dyck PJ, Hansen S, Karnes J, O'Brien P, Yasuda H, Windebank A, Zimmerman B: Capillary number and percentage closed in human diabetic sural nerve. Proc Natl Acad Sci USA 1985;82:2513–2517.
40. Bradley J, Thomas PK, King RH, et al. Morphometry of endoneurial capillaries in diabetic sensory and autonomic neuropathy. Diabetologia 1990;33:611–618.

41. Llewelyn JG, Thomas PK, Gilbey SG, Watkins PJ, Muddle JR. Pattern of myelinated fibre loss in the sural nerve in neuropathy related to type 1 (insulin-dependent) diabetes. Diabetologia 1988;31:162–167.
42. Giannini C, Dyck PJ. Ultrastructural morphometric abnormalities of sural nerve endoneurial microvessels in diabetes mellitus. Ann Neurol 1994;36:408–415.
43. Cameron NE, Cotter MA. The relationship of vascular changes to metabolic factors in diabetes mellitus and their role in the development of peripheral nerve complications. Diab Metab Rev 1994;10:189–224.
44. Inone S, Yajima Y, Sono T, Greene DA, Bril V, Sima AAF: Effects of prostaglandin $E_1$ on diabetic neuropathy. In: Ward JD, Goto Y, eds. Diabetic Neuropathy. John Wiley, Chichester, 1990; pp. 511–516.
45. Sima AAF, Blaivas M. The pathology of peripheral nerve. In: Garcia J, McKeever P, Sima AAF, eds. Neuropathology: A Diagnostic Approach. Mosby, Philadelphia (in press).
46. Sima AAF, Ristic H, Merry A, Kamijo H, Lattimer SA, Stevens MJ, Greene DA: The primary preventional and secondary interventative effects of acetyl-L-carnitine on diabetic neuropathy in the BB/W-rat. J Clin Invest 1996;97:1900–1907.
47. Yamamoto K, Merry A, Sima AAF. An orderly development of paranodal axoglial junctions and bracelets of Nageotte in the rat sural nerve. Develop Brain Res 1996;96:36–45.
48. Sima AAF, Albers JW, Cherian PV, Greene DA, Hohman TC, Beg M: Structural-functional relationships in diabetic neuropathy. Proc US-Japan Aldose Reductase Workshop, Kona, Hawaii, 1994.
49. Sima AAF, Yamamoto K, Ristic H. Impaired functional maturation of regenerated fibers in diabetic and diabetic ARI-treated rats is due to impaired myelination and incomplete maturation of the paranodal barrier. VIth Annual Neurodiab Meeting, Baden, Austria, 1996.

# 6 Clinical Management of Diabetic Neuropathy

*An Overview*

*Eva L. Feldman,* MD, PHD,
*Martin J. Stevens,* MD,
*and Douglas A. Greene,* MD

**CONTENTS**



## INTRODUCTION

Current estimates suggest there are 14 million people in the United States with diabetes mellitus and the number of afflicted individuals is increasing by 5% per year *(1)*. In 1992, the direct and indirect costs in the United States of diabetes was $92 billion. Neuropathy is a common complication of diabetes and occurs in approximately 50% of diabetic patients during the course of their disease *(2)*. Neuropathic sequelae, including foot infections, nonhealing foot ulcers, and amputations, make diabetic neuropathy the most morbid and costly diabetic complication *(3)*. In this chapter, we will discuss the management strategies we used in our clinics for patients with diabetic neuropathy. As background material, the authors will first briefly review the classification and pathogenesis of diabetic neuropathy (for a more complete discussion of these topics, the reader is referred to Greene and colleagues, ref 2). Then, the therapeutic approach we have used for the care of patients with diabetic neuropathy will be discussed.

## CLASSIFICATION

Diabetic neuropathy comprises a set of distinct clinical syndromes. The signs and symptoms of each syndrome depend on which part of the nervous system is compromised by chronic hyperglycemia. The most common type of diabetic neuropathy is distal, symmetric sensorimotor polyneuropathy (DPN), characterized by progressive distal sensory, and in severe cases, motor dysfunction caused by loss of

From: *Contemporary Endocrinology: Clinical Management of Diabetic Neuropathy*
Edited by: A. Veves © Humana Press Inc., Totowa, NJ

Table 1
Classification of Diabetic Neuropathy

| |
|---|
| Distal symmetric sensorimotor polyneuropathy (DPN) |
| Diabetic autonomic neuropathy (DAN) |
| Diabetic polyradiculopathy |
| L-2, L-3, L-4 roots: diabetic amyotrophy |
| T-4–T-12 roots: diabetic thoracic radiculopathy |
| L-5, S-1 (S-2) roots |
| C-5, C-6 (C-7–T-1) roots |
| Diabetic polyradiculopathy plus DPN |
| Diabetic cranial mononeuropathies |
| Diabetic limb mononeuropathies |
| Upper-extremity mononeuropathies |
| Lower-extremity mononeuropathies |
| Diabetic mononeuropathy multiplex |

Adapted from: Feldman EL, Greene DA, Stevens MJ. Diabetic neuropathy. In: Rose BD, ed. *UpToDate*™ (CD-ROM), vol. 4(3), 1996.

sensory and motor axons. Diabetes also damages: the autonomic nervous system, resulting in diabetic autonomic neuropathy; thoracic and lumbar nerve roots, producing diabetic polyradiculopathy; isolated peripheral nerves, particularly median, ulnar, and femoral nerves, yielding diabetic mononeuropathies; and cranial nerves, especially the third nerve, producing cranial mononeuropathies. Commonly encountered diabetic neuropathies are presented in Table 1. This review will focus on DPN. The reader is referred to reviews by Greene et al. *(2)* and Feldman et al. *(4)* for the author's approach to patients with autonomic neuropathy, polyradiculopathy, and both peripheral and cranial mononeuropathies.

## DISTAL SYMMETRIC SENSORIMOTOR POLYNEUROPATHY (DPN)

Estimates of the prevalence of DPN vary, depending on which criteria are used for diagnosis and which patient population is examined *(5–7)*. Review of multiple studies suggests that 50% is a reasonable estimate. Pirart examined 4400 outpatients with diabetes over a period of 25 yr. Twelve percent of patients had neuropathy at the onset of their diagnosis. Prevalence of neuropathy correlated with diabetes duration, and, by the end of the study, 50% of patients had DPN *(8)*. In the United Kingdom, a multicenter study of 6487 patients reported the prevalence of DPN reached 44% in patients 70 yr of age or older *(9)*. In the Rochester Diabetic Neuropathy Study, 45% of type I and 54% of type II diabetic patients had DPN *(10)*. In the Pittsburgh Epidemiology of Diabetes Study, 58% of type I patients 30 yr of age or older had DPN *(11)*. Fedele and colleagues examined 8757 diabetic patients from 109 clinics in Italy and diagnosed DPN in 32.3% of patients; severity of DPN correlated with duration of diabetes *(12)*.

DPN is initially manifested as a sensory disorder of the feet, reflecting distal axon loss. With disease progression, sensation loss ascends up the legs. When DPN reaches midcalf, patients commonly notice sensory loss in the hands. This slow progression over time results in the classical "stocking-glove" sensory loss. Early altered sensation in DPN commonly reflects the loss of large and small myelinated as well as unmyelinated nerve fibers. Large myelinated fibers carry vibration and proprioception, whereas small myelinated and unmyelinated nerve fibers transmit pain, light touch, and temperature sensation. Patients with DPN usually have signs corresponding to loss of all three fiber types. These signs include decreased vibration and light touch, altered temperature sensation, and poor pain perception. Symptoms are highly variable in patients with DPN *(10,13)*. Patients with "positive" symptoms complain of pain, paresthesias, and/or dysesthesias. More frequently, patients have "negative" symptoms with few or no sensory complaints, but identifiable sensory loss on examination *(10,13)*.

Weakness, especially of the toes and ankles, is a late sequelae of DPN seen in severe cases. Progression of sensory loss with onset of weakness predisposes to ulceration formation. Ulceration is commonly divided into two categories: acute and chronic. Acute foot ulcers occur when improper footwear results in dermal abrasion in a patient with poor or absent sensation. Chronic ulceration is more likely multifactorial, occurring in patients with not only DPN, but also autonomic neuropathy and compromised vascular supply. Motor axonal loss produces atrophy of intrinsic foot muscles and a disparity in the strength between toe extensors and flexors. Over time, afflicted patients develop chronic metatarsal-phalangeal flexion, commonly referred to as a claw-toe deformity. This change in foot structure shifts much of the patient's weight-bearing to his or her metatarsal heads. This shift can result in callus formation that can fissure, become infected, and ulcerate. Callus formation and its sequelae are further promoted by sensory loss and vascular insufficiency. Resulting ulcers can, in turn, lead to amputation. The lifetime risk of amputation in a diabetic patient is estimated at 15% *(14)* and, in the United States, approximately 60,000 lower-extremity amputations per year are caused by the sequelae of DPN *(15)*. Indeed, the most frequent reason for hospitalization of a diabetic patient is one or more of these complications of neuropathy *(16)*.

## *Pathogenesis of DPN*

Despite intensive investigations, the pathogenesis of DPN remains unknown *(2,16,17)*. The Diabetes Control and Complications Trial (DCCT) has proven that hyperglycemia, and not the diabetic state *per se*, is essential for the development of DPN *(18)*. Commonly proposed theories for DPN include alterations in the polyol pathway, vascular insufficiency, abnormal glycation of proteins and lipids, enhanced oxidative stress, altered nitric oxide synthesis, impaired axonal transport, and faulty neurotrophism *(2,16,17)*. Classically, these theories regarding the pathogenesis of DPN are placed into one of two categories: *metabolic* or *vascular*. It is increasingly accepted that these defects are interrelated and their cumulative interactions result in the development of DPN *(2,16,17)*.

The most popular metabolic theory proposes that aldose reductase converts glucose to sorbitol as part of the polyol pathway. In the diabetic microenvironment, elevated sorbitol results in reciprocal decreases of myo-inositol and taurine, which become rate-limiting for essential intracellular metabolism *(2,19–21)*. The vascular theory, once considered separate from the metabolic theory, contends that reduced nerve blood flow and resulting hypoxia/ischemia account for the development of DPN *(22–25)*. It is now clear that the metabolic and vascular theories are linked on many levels (Fig. 1). Glucose flux through the polyol pathway results in depletion of NADPH and $NAD^+$ *(26)*.

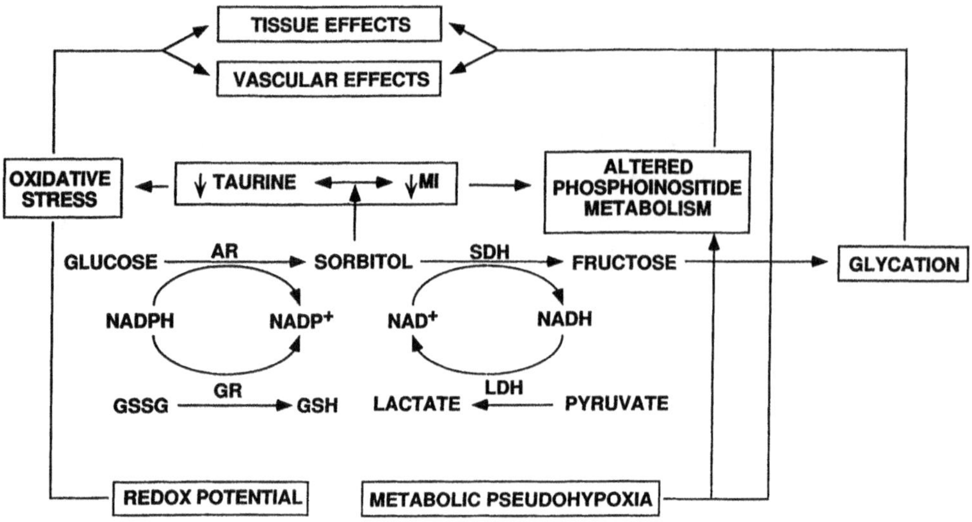


**Fig. 1.** Pathogenesis of diabetic neuropathy: Unification of metabolic and vascular theories. AR, aldose reductase; MI, myo-inositol; LDH, lactate dehydrogenase; GSSG, oxidized glutathione; GR, glutathionine reductase; GSH, reduced glutathionine. (Used with permission from Feldman EL, Stevens MJ, Greene DA. Pathogenesis of diabetic neuropathy. Clinical Neuroscience, 4:365–370, 1997).

Without sufficient NADPH, neuroglial cells can not regenerate the glutathionine needed to detoxify reactive oxygen species. As a result, nervous tissue sustains oxidative damage that decreases nerve endoneurial blood flow and promotes nerve ischemia *(27,28)*. Activity of the potent vasodilator, nitric oxide (NO), is also tightly linked to NADPH. NO is synthesized by NO synthase, an NADPH-dependent reaction. Thus, depletion of NADPH limits NO synthesis, which results in vasoconstriction, ischemia, and slowing of nerve conduction *(29,30)*.

Currently, treatment strategies based on these theories are testable in the diabetic rodent. A wide range of interventions in the diabetic rodent are linked with improved nerve conduction velocity, restoration of blood flow, or return of normal axonal transport rates. Currently, both aldose reductase inhibitors as well as nerve growth factor are in phase 3 human clinical trials for the treatment of DPN. Recent studies on antioxidant therapies in rodents are promising and have led to a proposed clinical trial in humans with the antioxidant α-lipoic acid.

This review will focus on the therapeutic strategies currently available for the treatment of DPN. Further discussion on the use of aldose reductase inhibitors, growth factors, and antioxidants awaits successful completed clinical trials of these compounds.

## TREATMENT

The authors have three treatment strategies in their clinic. They aim first for early diagnosis of DPN. Early diagnosis allows the authors to implement their second strategy: good glycemic control and foot care. The third approach is focused on the treatment of painful DPN. This strategy is superimposed upon good glycemic control and foot care.

Table 2
The Differential Diagnosis of Diabetic Neuropathy

- I. Distal symmetrical polyneuropathy
  - A. Metabolic
    1. Diabetes mellitus
    2. Uremia
    3. Folic acid/cyanocobalamin deficiency
    4. Hypothyroidism
    5. Acute intermittent porphyria
  - B. Toxic
    1. Alcohol
    2. Heavy metals (lead, mercury, arsenic)
    3. Industrial hydrocarbons
    4. Various drugs
  - C. Infectious or inflammatory
    1. Sarcoidosis
    2. Leprosy
    3. Periarteritis nodosa
    4. Other connective-tissue diseases (e.g., systemic lupus erythematosus)
  - D. Other
    1. Dysproteinemias and paraproteinemias
    2. Paraneoplastic syndrome
    3. Leukemias and lymphomas
    4. Amyloidosis
    5. Hereditary neuropathies
- II. Pains and paresthesias without neurologic deficit
  - A. Early small-fiber sensory neuropathy
  - B. Psychophysiologic disorder (e.g., severe depression, hysteria)
- III. Autonomic neuropathy without somatic component
  - A. Shy-Drager syndrome (progressive autonomic failure)
  - B. Diabetic neuropathy with mild somatic involvement
  - C. Riley-Day syndrome
  - D. Idiopathic orthostatic hypotension
- IV. Diffuse motor neuropathy without sensory deficit
  - A. Guillain-Barre syndrome
  - B. Primary myopathies
  - C. Myasthenia gravis
  - D. Heavy-metal toxicity
- V. Femoral neuropathy (sacral plexopathy)
  - A. Degenerative spinal-disc disease (e.g., Paget's disease of the spine)
  - B. Intrinsic spinal-cord-mass lesion
  - C. Equina cauda lesions
  - D. Coagulopathies
- VI. Cranial neuropathy
  - A. Carotid aneurysm
  - B. Intracranial mass
  - C. Elevated intracranial pressure
- VII. Mononeuropathy multiplex
  - A. Vasculidites
  - B. Amyloidosis
  - C. Hypothyroidism
  - D. Acromegaly
  - E. Coagulopathies

Adapted from: Greene DA, Feldman EL, Stevens MJ, Sima AAF, Albers JW, Pfeifer MA. Diabetic neuropathy. In: Porte Jr D, Sherwin RS, Rifkin H ed. Ellenberg and Rifkin's Diabetes Mellitus, 5th ed. Appleton and Lange, Stamford, CT 1997, pp. 1009–1076.

### *Early Diagnosis of DPN*

The early diagnosis of DPN is imperative; it allows for early intervention that significantly decreases patient morbidity. Unfortunately, there is no one test to diagnose DPN. It is essential that other causes of neuropathy are excluded before DPN is ascribed to the diabetic state (Table 2) *(2)*. This is particularly important if there are any atypical features of the neuropathy, such as rapid progression, marked asymmetry, or motor greater than sensory weakness.

Historically, DPN was diagnosed based on a pattern of symptoms and signs, including loss of light touch or vibratory sensation in the feet and depressed or absent ankle reflexes *(31)*. In the last 10 yr, several groups have proposed more strict, quantifiable criteria for the diagnosis of DPN. In 1988, the San Antonio Consensus panel, consisting of endocrinologists and neurologists, recommended that a patient undergo a panel of five quantifiable measures for the accurate diagnosis of DPN. These included: a symptom questionnaire, a standardized clinical examination, quantitative sensory testing, nerve conduction studies, and autonomic function testing. Patients are then classified as either stage I (no symptoms) or stage II (symptoms) neuropathy and within each stage are further grades from a to c depending on the number of positive test results and the severity of their clinical impairment (Table 3) *(32)*. These criteria are currently utilized in studying the Rochester Diabetic cohort *(6,33)*, and modified criteria have been employed in several clinical trials, including the DCCT *(18,34)*.

Simpler screening instruments for DPN are also available. These instruments were developed because patient and physician resources are frequently limited, making completion of the San Antonio criteria difficult. In the United Kingdom, a two-part symptom and sign score is utilized, yielding a neuropathy disability score. DPN is diagnosed if patients present with mild signs and moderate symptoms or moderate signs alone, in the absence of symptoms *(9)*. The authors utilize a similar screening instrument, developed in their institution *(13)*. The Michigan Neuropathy Screening Instrument, presented in Fig. 2, is used by to screen large numbers of patients. In this simple examination, the feet are inspected for dry skin, callus, fissure, or ulceration. Then vibratory sensation is assessed in the great toes and ankle reflexes are tested. A score of $> 2$ indicates neuropathy with both a high sensitivity (80%) and specificity (95%) *(13)*. Because of its simplicity, the Michigan Neuropathy Screening Instrument is also highly reproducible *(35)*. If appropriate resources exist, the authors grade the severity of a patient's neuropathy with a standardized neurological examination (Fig. 3A) and nerve conduction studies (Fig. 3B). Results of these two examinations give a summated Michigan Diabetic Neuropathy Score, which can be plotted over time (Fig. 4). Fedele and colleagues administered the Michigan Neuropathy Screening Instrument to 8757 patients and found that 32% were positive for DPN. Quantification of the severity of DPN in these patients found that 16% had no neuropathy, 41% mild, 29% moderate, and 13% severe DPN. Severity of disease correlated with duration of diabetes *(12)*.

Another simple method to screen patients for the presence of DPN is the use of a 10-g nylon monofilament. The filament is pressed against the skin of the sole of the foot until the filament buckles, indicating a known force has been applied to the sole. If a patient is unable to perceive the filament, he or she is at increased risk for the complications of DPN *(36,37)*.

**Table 3**
**Classification and Staging of Diabetic Neuropathy**

CLASS I: Subclinical neuropathy[a]
- A. Abnormal electrodiagnostic tests (EDX)
  - 1. Decreased nerve conduction velocity
  - 2. Decreased amplitude of evoked muscle or nerve action potential
- B. Abnormal quantitative sensory testing (QST)
  - 1. Vibratory/tactile
  - 2. Thermal warming/cooling
  - 3. Other
- C. Abnormal autonomic function tests (AFT)
  - 1. Diminished sinus arrhythmia (beat-to-beat heart-rate variation)
  - 2. Diminished sudomotor function
  - 3. Increased pupillary latency

CLASS II: Clinical neuropathy
- A. Diffuse neuropathy
  - 1. Distal symmetric sensorimotor polyneuropathy
    - a. Primarily small-fiber neuropathy
    - b. Primarily large-fiber neuropathy
    - c. Mixed
  - 2. Autonomic neuropathy
    - a. Abnormal pupillary function
    - b. Sudomotor dysfunction
    - c. Genitourinary autonomic neuropathy
      - 1. bladder dysfunction
      - 2. sexual dysfunction
    - d. Gastrointestinal autonomic neuropathy
      - 1. gastric atony
      - 2. gall bladder atony
      - 3. diabetic diarrhea
      - 4. hypoglycemic unawareness (adrenal medullary neuropathy)
    - e. Cardiovascular autonomic neuropathy
    - f. Hypoglycemic unawareness
- B. Focal neuropathy
  - 1. Mononeuropathy
  - 2. Mononeuropathy multiplex
  - 3. Plexopathy
  - 4. Radiculopathy
  - 5. Cranial neuropathy

[a] Neurological function tests are abnormal but no neurological symptoms or clinically detectable neurological deficits indicative of a diffuse or focal neuropathy are present. Class I subclinical neuropathy is further subdivided into Class Ia if an AFT or QST abnormality is present, Class Ib if EDX or AFT and QST abnormalities are present, and Class Ic if an EDX and either AFT or QST abnormalities or both are present.

Adapted from: Consensus panel: report and recommendations of the San Antonio Conference on Diabetic Neuropathy. Diabetes 1988; 37:1000–1004.

Pt. Name: ______________________

Pt. Identification #: ______________________

Date: ______________________

## MICHIGAN NEUROPATHY SCREENING INSTRUMENT

**B. Physical Assessment** (To be completed by health professional)

1. Appearance of Feet

| | Right | | Left | |
|---|---|---|---|---|
| a. Normal | ☐ 0 Yes | ☐ 1 No | ☐ 0 Yes | ☐ 1 No |
| b. If no, check all that apply: | | | | |
| Deformities | ☐ | | ☐ | |
| Dry skin, callus | ☐ | | ☐ | |
| Infection | ☐ | | ☐ | |
| Fissure | ☐ | | ☐ | |
| Other | ☐ | | ☐ | |
| specify: ______ | | | specify: ______ | |

| | Right | | | Left | | |
|---|---|---|---|---|---|---|
| 2. Ulceration | Absent ☐ 0 | | Present ☐ 1 | Absent ☐ 0 | | Present ☐ 1 |
| 3. Ankle Reflexes | Present ☐ 0 | Present/ Reinforcement ☐ 0.5 | Absent ☐ 1 | Present ☐ 0 | Present/ Reinforcement ☐ 0.5 | Absent ☐ 1 |
| 4. Vibration perception at great toe | Present ☐ 0 | Decreased ☐ 0.5 | Absent ☐ 1 | Present ☐ 0 | Decreased ☐ 0.5 | Absent ☐ 1 |

Signature: ______________________ Total Score __________ /8 Points

**Fig. 2.** Michigan Neuropathy Screening Instrument. A score of > 2 indicates DPN. (Used with permission from Feldman EL, Stevens MJ, Thomas PK, Brown MB, Canal N, Greene DA. A practical two-step quantitative clinical and electrophysiological assessment for the diagnosis and staging of diabetic neuropathy. Diabetes Care 1994;17:1281–1289).

## A

| Sensory Impairment | | | |
|---|---|---|---|
| Right | Normal | Decreased | Absent |
| Vibration at big toe | 0 | 1 | 2 |
| 10 gr filament | 0 | 1 | 2 |
| Pin prick on dorsum of great toe | Painful 0 | Not Painful 2 | |
| Left | Normal | Decreased | Absent |
| Vibration at big toe | 0 | 1 | 2 |
| 10 gr filament | 0 | 1 | 2 |
| Pin prick on dorsum of great toe | Painful 0 | Not Painful 2 | |

| Muscle Strength Testing | | | | |
|---|---|---|---|---|
| Right | Normal | Mild to Moderate | Severe | Absent |
| Finger spread | 0 | 1 | 2 | 3 |
| Great toe extension | 0 | 1 | 2 | 3 |
| Ankle dorsiflexion | 0 | 1 | 2 | 3 |
| Left | Normal | Mild to Moderate | Severe | Absent |
| Finger spread | 0 | 1 | 2 | 3 |
| Great toe extension | 0 | 1 | 2 | 3 |
| Ankle dorsiflexion | 0 | 1 | 2 | 3 |

| Reflexes | | | |
|---|---|---|---|
| Right | Present | Present with Reinforcement | Absent |
| Biceps brachii | 0 | 1 | 2 |
| Triceps brachii | 0 | 1 | 2 |
| Quadriceps femoris | 0 | 1 | 2 |
| Achilles | 0 | 1 | 2 |
| Left | Present | Present with Reinforcement | Absent |
| Biceps brachii | 0 | 1 | 2 |
| Triceps brachii | 0 | 1 | 2 |
| Quadriceps femoris | 0 | 1 | 2 |
| Achilles | 0 | 1 | 2 |

TOTAL: ______/46 Pts.

## B

Sensory

Sural
Median
Ulnar

Motor

Peroneal
Median

**Fig. 3.** Diabetic neuropathy score. **(A)** A 46-point quantitative neurological examination is combined with **(B)** nerve conduction studies. (Used with permission from Feldman EL, Stevens MJ, Thomas PK, Brown MB, Canal N, Greene DA. A practical two-step quantitative clinical and electrophysiological assessment for the diagnosis and staging of diabetic neuropathy. Diabetes Care 1994; 17:1281–1289).

| CRTN | PATIENT INTITALS | PATIENT STUDY NUMBER | VISIT DATE |
|---|---|---|---|
| _ _ _ _ _ | ___ ___ ___ | ___ ___ ___ ___ | DAY MONTH YEAR |

| VISIT | | Date | Date | Date | Date | Date | |
|---|---|---|---|---|---|---|---|
| Abnormal Nerves | Clinical rate | Score | Score | Score | Score | Score | CLASS |
| 0-1 | 0 - 6: 0 | | | | | | 0 no neuropathy |
| | 1 | | | | | | |
| | 2 | | | | | | |
| | 3 | | | | | | |
| | 4 | | | | | | |
| | 5 | | | | | | |
| | 6 | | | | | | |
| | >6 | | | | | | |
| 2 | <7 | | | | | | 1 mild neuropathy |
| | 7 - 12: 7 | | | | | | |
| | 8 | | | | | | |
| | 9 | | | | | | |
| | 10 | | | | | | |
| | 11 | | | | | | |
| | 12 | | | | | | |
| | >12 | | | | | | |
| 3-4 | <13 | | | | | | 2 moderate neuropathy |
| | 13-29: 13 | | | | | | |
| | 14 | | | | | | |
| | 15 | | | | | | |
| | 16 | | | | | | |
| | 17 | | | | | | |
| | 18 | | | | | | |
| | 19 | | | | | | |
| | 20 | | | | | | |
| | 21 | | | | | | |
| | 22 | | | | | | |
| | 23 | | | | | | |
| | 24 | | | | | | |
| | 25 | | | | | | |
| | 26 | | | | | | |
| | 27 | | | | | | |
| | 28 | | | | | | |
| | 29 | | | | | | |
| | >29 | | | | | | |
| 5 | <30 | | | | | | 3 severe neuropathy |
| | 30-46: 30 | | | | | | |
| | 31 | | | | | | |
| | 32 | | | | | | |
| | 33 | | | | | | |
| | 34 | | | | | | |
| | 35 | | | | | | |
| | 36 | | | | | | |
| | 37 | | | | | | |
| | 38 | | | | | | |
| | 39 | | | | | | |
| | 40 | | | | | | |
| | 41 | | | | | | |
| | 42 | | | | | | |
| | 43 | | | | | | |
| | 44 | | | | | | |
| | 45 | | | | | | |
| | 46 | | | | | | |

**Fig. 4.** The Michigan Diabetes Neuropathy Score (MDNS). Each patient is given a composite score based on the number of abnormal nerve conductions and the number of points scored on the clinical examination. For example, if a patient had abnormal conduction in two nerves and 12 points on the clinical examination, he would have received a score of 2.12. (Used with permission from Feldman EL, Stevens MJ, Thomas PK, Brown MB, Canal N, Greene DA. A practical two-step quantitative clinical and electrophysiological assessment for the diagnosis and staging of diabetic neuropathy. Diabetes Care 1994;17:1281–1289).

### *Glycemic Control and Foot Care*

Once DPN is diagnosed, glycemic control and foot care is emphasized. The DCCT clearly demonstrates that improved glycemic control decreases the frequency of DPN in patients with type I diabetes mellitus. A 60% decrease of the incidence of clinical DPN was reported in the combined primary- and secondary-prevention cohorts *(18)*. Good glycemic control requires patient education. The authors instruct their patients on the importance of diet and regular glucose monitoring. This is done using a team approach consisting of a diabetes nurse educator, a dietitian, and a physician.

The authors also teach good foot care *(38–40)*. Patients are instructed to inspect their feet each night. The importance of examining the feet for evidence of dry skin, cracking or fissuring of the skin is explained. They also educate the patients to look for plantar callus formation. Patients are taught to inspect the area between the toe nails and toes for evidence of redness or early infection. All patients are sent to a podiatrist who regularly cuts their toe nails and trims any calluses. Patients use a mirror to examine the bottom of their feet if it is difficult for them to visualize their feet otherwise.

The authors emphasize proper footwear. The importance of footwear is well-documented *(2,41–43)*. Shoes must offer cushioning at the points of contact between the foot and the shoe and must also accommodate any inherent or acquired foot deformities *(41–43)*. For patients with mild neuropathy, cushioned socks *(44)* and high-quality athletic shoes with adequate room for the forefoot and toes are suggested *(45)*. In more severe cases, patients require customized inserts or molded shoes *(41–43)*.

If, despite the current program, the patient develops an ulcer, the authors utilize a regimen developed at Milton S. Hershey Medical Center, Hershey, Pennsylvania by Caputo, Cavanagh, and Ulbrecht *(46)*. This regimen was adapted to meet their own preferences for routine screening for DPN. We first determine if the ulcer appears infected. If there are no signs of infection or inflammation, we begin a program of strict nonweight bearing and meticulous wound care. A total-contact cast is used in some cases. Signs and symptoms of a mildly infected ulcer include a superficial appearance with limited cellulitis and no evidence of bone or joint involvement. Aerobic gram-positive cocci or streptococci are the most common pathogens of mild foot infections *(47,48)*. In these patients, we couple a program of strict nonweight bearing and meticulous wound care with antibiotic therapy. We define a limb-threatening infection as a full-thickness ulcer with $> 2$ cm of cellulitis. Many of these patients do not appear systematically ill and are not febrile, but do experience more difficulty with hyperglycemia. In parallel, affected patients may or may not have signs of bone or joint involvement or serious ischemia *(36,48)*. Aerobic gram-positive cocci are also pathogenic in these deeper, limb-threatening infections, along with gram-negative bacilli and anerobes *(47–49)*. We aggressively treat these patients. Our plan includes admission to the hospital, when needed, coupled with meticulous wound care, strict nonweight bearing, antibiotic therapy, early surgical debridement, drainage and, if required, amputation. In cases of both mild and limb-threatening infections, we obtain cultures prior to beginning empirical treatment, and modify our antibiotic regimen as needed. Our approach is outlined in a flow diagram, adapted from Caputo and colleagues *(36)* (Fig. 5).

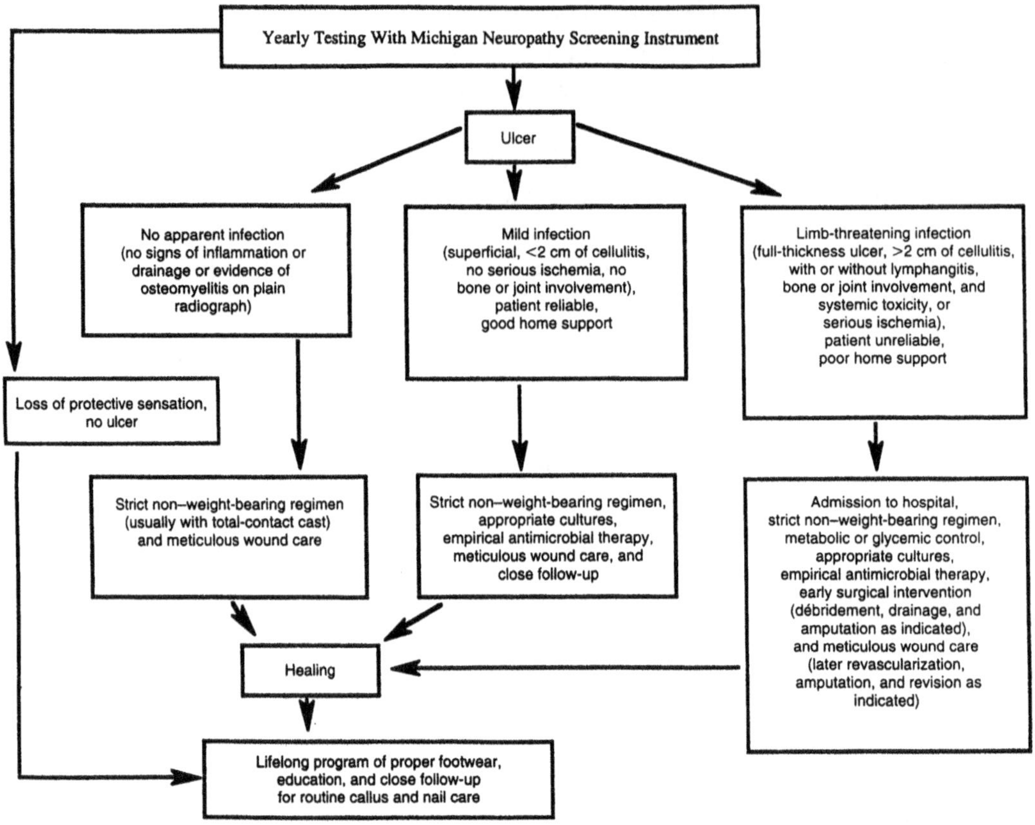


**Fig. 5.** Management of prevention of neuropathic foot ulcers in patients with diabetes mellitus. (Used with permission from Caputo GM, Cavanagh PR, Ulbrecht JS, Gibbons GW, Karchmer AW. Assessment and management of foot disease in patients with diabetes. New Engl J Med 1994;331:854–860).

## *Acute and Chronic Painful DPN*

We utilize a stepwise treatment protocol for our patients with painful DPN *(2,50)*. We *(2,50)* and others *(51,52)* find that patients with acute painful DPN (defined as pain of less than 6-mo duration) have a better long-term prognosis than chronic painful DPN (symptoms of greater than 6-mo duration). We use the same management guidelines for glycemic control and foot care in all patients, regardless of their degree of pain.

Table 4 lists the drugs that we use in our clinics for the treatment of painful DPN. Generally, we restrict our use to those therapies that have been shown to be effective in double-blind, placebo-controlled trials. We find that nonsteroidal anti-inflammatory drugs provide relief, particularly in patients with chronic painful DPN. In these patients, we believe that joint pain is a major contributor to their discomfort *(2)*. In a double-blind, placebo-controlled trial, both ibuprofen (600 mg four times per day) and sulindac (200 mg two times per day) effectively decreased pain associated with DPN *(53)*. This study parallels our own clinical experience. A note of caution, however, is that this class of drugs cannot be used in patients with renal impairment.

Table 4
Drugs Used in the Treatment of Painful Diabetic Neuropathy

| | |
|---|---|
| 1. Nonsteroidal drugs | 3. Nonaddicting analgesics |
| Ibuprofen 600 mg qid | Carbamazipine 200 mg qid |
| Sulindac 200 mg bid | Garbapentin 900 mg tid |
| 2. Tricyclic antidepressant drugs | Mexiletine 150–450 mg/qd |
| Amitryptiline 50–150 mg at night | 4. Others |
| Nortriptiline 50–150 mg at night | Capsacin 0.075% qid |
| Imipramine 100 mg qd | Fluphenazine 1 mg tid |
| Paroxetine 40 mg qd | Transcutaneous nerve stimulation |

Adapted from: Feldman EL, Stevens MJ, Greene DA. Treatment of Diabetic Neuropathy. In: *Advances in Endocrinology and Metabolism,* Mazzaferri EL, Bar RS, and Kreisberg RA, eds, vol. 5, pp. 393–428, 1994.

The tricyclic antidepressants are the best-studied class of drugs for the treatment of painful DPN. These drugs prolong norepinephrine inhibition of pain pathways by blocking norepinephrine uptake in the brain stem and spinal cord *(54)*. In double-blind, placebo-controlled trials, amyitriptyline, nortriptyline, and imipramine are each effective in the treatment of painful DPN *(50,55,56)*. If a patient has no history of cardiac disease or prostatism, we prescribe amyitriptyline, beginning at 10 mg per night. We increase the dose by 10 mg every 3 days, until the patient is free of symptoms, becomes intolerant of side effects (sedation and dry mouth) or reaches 100 mg. We keep patients at 100 mg per night for 1 month. If they continue to experience pain, we use the same regimen to reach a dose of 150 mg. We rarely use higher doses (up to 300 mg). We have not observed any increased efficacy at doses greater than 300 mg and we inform patients that there are reports of worsening neuropathy with amyitriptyline abuse *(57)*. If a patient is intolerant of amyitriptyline, we substitute nortriptyline. Compared to amyitriptyline, nortriptyline is less sedating and its use causes fewer episodes of urinary retention and orthostasis *(50)*. In patients with cardiac disease, the tricyclic antidepressant of choice is doxepin; we use the same paradigm for doxepin as for amyitriptyline. There are isolated examples of the efficacy of other antidepressant medications in the treatment of DPN. Of these, two serotonin-uptake inhibitors, trazadone *(58)* and paroxetine *(59)*, are effective. We use paroxetine, up to doses of 40 mg and have observed good relief of symptoms *(59,60)*. We do not combine a tricyclic antidepressant with a serotonin-uptake inhibitor.

If a patient continues to experience disabling pain, a second drug is added to their therapeutic regimen. We have recently begun adding gabapentin. We begin at 300 mg three times per day, and double the dose at weekly intervals until we reach 900 mg three times per day or the patient becomes intolerant of side effects (unsteadiness, sleepiness). In many patients, this therapy has proven so effective that we discontinue the antidepressant medication. Carbamazepine also is a good drug to add to either a tricyclic antidepressant or a serotonin-uptake inhibitor. Double-blind, placebo-controlled trials reveal it provides symptomatic relief to a large percentage of afflicted patients *(61,62)*. We initiate therapy at 100 mg two times per day and increase by 100 mg each week until the patient reaches a dose of 200 mg three times per day or becomes intolerant of the common side effects: nausea, dizziness, and a truncal rash *(63)*. Patients must have total blood counts after the first month of therapy and monthly thereafter for 3 months because of reported cases of leukopenia and even pancytopenia *(63)*. Blood levels of carbamazepine can be measured and we aim for levels between 8–12 mg/mL. We have not found phenytoin to be useful as a substitute for carbamazepine in the treatment of painful DPN *(64)*.

In patients who are on two medications and are still experiencing significant discomfort, we frequently add capsaicin cream, a topical therapy that inhibits the uptake of substance P at sensory endings *(65,66)*. Patients are instructed to apply capsaicin cream (0.075%) four times per day, the same regimen that was successful in a double-blind, placebo-controlled trial *(65,66)*. We warn our patients that for the first 1 to 3 days of therapy, they might experience an increase in pain, prior to experiencing any pain relief.

If these therapeutic strategies fail, we discontinue the second drug (gabapentin or tegretol) and institute a new, third drug. Our first choice is the cardiac antiarrhythmic drug mexiletine *(67,68)*. After the patient is seen by a cardiologist who agrees to administration of the drug, mexiletine is begun at 150 mg per day and increased in 150 mg increments until the patient reaches 450 mg per day or becomes intolerant of side effects (nausea, rash). We find mexiletine is effective in a percentage of our patients who otherwise were refractory to treatment *(69)*. We rarely use iv lidocaine, although this cardiac antiarrhythmic drug is also effective in the treatment of painful DPN *(70,71)*. Our patients dislike the hospitalization and cardiac monitoring required to administer the drug. In parallel, although there are reports that phenothiazines are also effective in the treatment of painful DPN *(72)*, we do not use this class of drugs. The long-term side effects, particularly the facial and oral dyskinesias, are not acceptable to our patients.

If a patient remains refractory to these treatment strategies, we refer them to our Comprehensive Pain Clinic. There our patients frequently receive local nerve blocks, a TENS unit, or, in certain patients, acupuncture. Unfortunately, the prognosis for good pain relief in our patients who require a pain clinic referral is low.

## SUMMARY

In summary, we take a systematic, stepwise approach to patients with DPN *(2,13,50,73,74)*. This approach ensures optimal patient care and decreases the risks for both short- and long-term disability. We are optimistic that future therapies hold promise, particularly those therapies targeted towards ameliorating the metabolic and vascular compromise imposed upon the peripheral nervous system by continued hyperglycemia.

## ACKNOWLEDGMENTS

This work was supported by NIH grant R29 NS32843 (EF), United States Public Health Service grant RO1 DK38304 DG, the Michigan Diabetes and Research Training Center grant P60 DK20572 (EF, MS, DG), and grants from the American Diabetes Association (EF, MS), Juvenile Diabetes Foundation International (EF) and the Muscular Dystrophy Association (EF). The authors would like to thank Judy Boldt for expert secretarial assistance.

## REFERENCES


1. Herman WH, Sinnock P, Brenner E, Brimberry JL, Langford D, Nakashima A, Sepe SJ, Teutsch SM, Mazze RS. An epidemiologic model for diabetes mellitus: incidence, prevalence, and mortality. Diabetes Care 1984;7:367–371.
2. Greene DA, Feldman EL, Stevens MJ, Sima AAF, Albers JW, Pfeifer MA. Diabetic Neuropathy. In: Porte Jr D, Sherwin R, Rifkin H, eds. Diabetes Mellitus Appleton & Lange, East Norwalk, CT, 1997, pp. 1009–1076.
3. Ward JD. The cost of diabetic neuropathy. Pharmacoeconomics 1995;8(Suppl. 1):52–54.
4. Feldman EL, Greene DA, Stevens MJ. Diabetic neuropathy. In: Rose BD, ed. UpToDate™ (CD-ROM), 1996.
5. Dyck PJ, Litchy WJ, Lehman KA, Hokanson JL, Low PA, O'Brien PC. Variables influencing neuropathic endpoints. the Rochester Diabetic Neuropathy Study of Healthy Subjects. Neurol 1995;45:1115–1121.
6. Dyck PJ, Kratz KM, Lehman KA. The Rochester Diabetic Neuropathy Study: design, criteria for types of neuropathy, selection bias, and reproducibility of neuropathic tests. Neurol 1991;41:799–807.
7. Dyck PJ, Karnes JL, O'Brien PC. The Rochester Diabetic Neuropathy Study: reassessment of tests and criteria for diagnosis and staged severity. Neurol 1992;42:1164–1170.
8. Pirart J. Diabetes mellitus and its degenerative complications; a prospective study of 4400 patients observed between 1947 and 1973. Diabetes Care 1978;1:168–188.
9. Young MJ, Boulton AJM, Macleod AF, Williams DRR, Sonksen PH. A multicentre study of the prevalence of diabetic peripheral neuropathy in the United Kingdom hospital clinic population. Diabetologia 1993;36:150–154.
10. Bondy C, Zhou J. Insulin-like growth factor system gene expression in the postpubertal human ovary. Ann NY Acad Sci 1993;687:65–76.
11. Maser RE, Steenkiste AR, Dorman JS, Nielsen VK, Bass EB, Manjoo Q, Drash AL, Becker DJ, Kuller LH, Greene DA, Orchard TJ. Epidemiological correlates of diabetic neuropathy. Report from Pittsburgh Epidemiology of Diabetes Complications Study. Diabetes 1989;38:1456–1461.
12. Fedele D, Comi G, Coscelli C, Cucinotta D, Feldman EL, Ghirlanda G, Greene DA, Negrin P, Santeusanio F, Italian Diabetic Neuropathy Committee. A multicenter study on the prevalence of diabetic neuropathy in Italy. Diabetes Care 1997; 620:836–843.
13. Feldman EL, Stevens MJ, Thomas PK, Brown MB, Canal N, Greene DA. A practical two-step quantitative clinical and electrophysiological assessment for the diagnosis and staging of diabetic neuropathy. Diabetes Care 1994;17:1281–1289.
14. Moss SE, Klein R, Klein BEK. The prevalence and incidence of lower extremity amputation in a diabetic population. Arch Intern Med 1992;152:610–616.
15. Brand PW. The diabetic foot. In: Ellenberg M, Rifkin H, eds. Diabetes Mellitus. Medical Examination Publishing, New York, 1983, pp. 829–849.
16. Greene DA, Sima AAF, Stevens MJ, Feldman EL, Lattimer SA. Complications: neuropathy, pathogenetic considerations. Diabetes Care 1992;15:1902–1925.
17. Feldman EL, Stevens MJ, Greene DA. The pathogenesis of diabetic neuropathy. J Clin Neurosci 1997; 4:365–370.
18. The Diabetes Control and Complications Trial Research Group. The effect of intensive treatment of diabetes on the development and progression of long-term complications in insulin-dependent diabetes mellitus. N Engl J Med 1993;329:977–986.
19. Greene DA, Lattimer SA. Sodium- and energy-dependent uptake of myo-inositol by rabbit peripheral nerve. J Clin Invest 1982;70:1009–1018.
20. Greene DA, Lattimer SA. Impaired rat sciatic nerve sodium-potassium adenosine triphosphatase in acute streptozocin diabetes and its correction by dietary myo-inositol supplementation. J Clin Invest 1983;72:1058–1063.
21. DelMonte MA, Rabbani R, Diaz TC, Lattimer SA, Nakamura J, Brennan MC, Greene DA. Sorbitol, myo-inositol, and rod outer segment phagocytosis in culture hRPE cells exposed to glucose. Diabetes 1991;40:1335–1345.
22. Tuck RR, Schmelzer JD, Low PA. Endoneurial blood flow and oxygen tension in the sciatic nerves of rats with experimental diabetic neuropathy. Brain 1984;107:935–950.
23. Low PA, Tuck RR, Takeuchi M. Nerve microenvironment in diabetic neuropathy. Dyck PJ, Thomas PK, Asbury AK, Winegrad AI, Porte D, eds. In: Diabetic Neuropathy. Saunders, Philadelphia, 1987, pp. 266–278.

24. Dyck PJ, Lais A, Karnes JL, O'Brien P, Rizza R. Fiber loss is primary and multifocal in sural nerves in diabetic polyneuropathy. Ann Neurol 1986;19:425–439.
25. Johnson PC, Doll SC, Cromey DW. Pathogenesis of diabetic neuropathy. Ann Neurol 1986;19:450–457.
26. van Dam PS, Van Asbeck BS, Erkelens DW, Marx JJ, Gispen WH, Bravenboer B. The role of oxidative stress in neuropathy and other diabetic complications. Diabetes/Metab Rev 1995;11:181–192.
27. Gallo G, Pollack ED. Cyclic remodelling of growth cone lamellae and the effect of target tissue. Dev Brain Res 1995;85:140–145.
28. Cameron NE, Cotter MA. Potential therapeutic approaches to the treatment or prevention of diabetic neuropathy: evidence from experimental studies. Diab Med 1993;10:593–605.
29. Stevens MJ, Dananberg J, Feldman EL, Lattimer SA, Kamijo M, Thomas TP, Shindo H, Sima AAF, Greene DA. The linked roles of nitric oxide, aldose reductase and ($Na^+$, $K^+$)-ATPase in the slowing of nerve conduction in the streptozotocin diabetic rat. J Clin Invest 1994;94:853–859.
30. Stevens MJ. Nitric oxide as a potential bridge between the metabolic and vascular hypotheses of diabetic neuropathy. Diab Med 1995;12:292–295.
31. Mulder DW, Lambert EH, Bastian JA. The neuropathies associated with diabetes mellitus: a clinical and electromyographic study of 103 unselected diabetic patients. Neurol 1961;11:275–284.
32. American Diabetes Association and American Academy of Neurology. Report and recommendations of the San Antonio Conference on Diabetic Neuropathy. Diabetes Care 1988;11:592–597.
33. Dyck PJ, Kratz KM, Karnes JL, Litchy WJ, Klein R, Pach JM, Wilson DM, O'Brien PC, Melton III LJ. The prevalence by staged severity of various types of diabetic neuropathy, retinopathy, and nephropathy in a population-based cohort: The Rochester Diabetic Neuropathy Study. Neurology 1993;43:817–824.
34. Maser RE, Becker DJ, Drash AL, Ellis D, Kuller LH, Greene DA, Orchard TJ. Pittsburgh Epidemiology of Diabetes Complications Study. Measuring diabetic neuropathy follow-up study results. Diabetes Care 1992;15:525–527.
35. Bax G, Fagherazzi C, Piarulli F, Nicolucci A, Fedele D. Reproducibility of Michigan Neuropathy Screening Instrument (MNSI). Diabetes 1996;45:1309–1310.
36. Caputo GM, Cavanagh PR, Ulbrecht JS, Gibbons GW, Karchmer AW. Assessment and management of foot disease in patients with diabetes. N Engl J Med 1994;33:854–860.
37. Duffy JC, Patout CA. Management of the insensitive foot in diabetes: lessons learned from Hansen's Disease. Milit Med 1990;155:575–579.
38. Hollingshead TS. Pathophysiology and treatment of diabetic foot ulcer. Clin Podiatr Med Surg 1991;8:843–855.
39. Joseph R, Cavuoto JW. The latest theories and treatment for diabetic foot complications. Clin Podiatr Med Surg 1991;8:249–272.
40. Apelqvist J, Larsson J, Agardh CD. The influence of external precipitating factors and peripheral neuropathy on the development and outcome of diabetic foot ulcers. J Diabet Complications 1990;4:21–25.
41. Cavanagh PR, Ulbrecht JS. Biomechanics of the foot in diabetes mellitus. In: Levin ME, O'Neal LW, Bowker JH, eds. The Diabetic Foot. Mosby Year Book, St. Louis, 1993, pp. 199–232.
42. Ulbrecht JS, Perry JE, Hewitt FG, Cavanagh PR. Controversies in footwear for the diabetic foot at risk. In: Kominsky SJ, ed. The Diabetic Foot. Mosby Year Book, Chicago, 1994, pp. 441–453.
43. Coleman WC. Footwear in a management program for injury prevention. In: Levin ME, O'Neal LW, Bowker JH, eds. The Diabetic Foot Mosby Year Book, St. Louis, 1993, pp. 531–547.
44. Veves A, Masson EA, Fernando DJS, Boulton AJM. Use of experimental padded hosiery to reduce abnormal foot pressures in diabetic neuropathy. Diabetes Care 1989;12:653–655.
45. Soulier SM. The use of running shoes in the prevention of plantar diabetic ulcers. J Am Podiatr Med Assoc 1986;76:395–400.
46. Sarma V, Lin Z, Clark L, Rust BM, Tewari M, Noelle RJ, Dixit VM. Activation of the B-cell surface receptor CD40 induces A20, a novel zinc finger protein that inhibits apoptosis. J Biol Chem 1995;270:12,343–12,346.
47. Jones EW, Edwards R, Finch R. A microbiologic study of diabetic foot lesions. Diab Med 1984;2:213–215.
48. Lipsky BA, Pecoraro RE, Wheat LJ. The diabetic foot: soft tissue and bone infection. Infect Dis Clin North Am 1990;4:409–432.
49. Wheat LJ, Allen SD, Henry M, Kernek CB, Siders JA, Kuebler T, Fineberg N, Norton J. Diabetic foot infections: bacteriologic analysis. Arch Int Med 1986;146:1935–1940.

50. Feldman EL, Stevens MJ, Greene DA. Treatment of diabetic neuropathy. In: Mazzaferri EL, Bar RS, Kreisberg RA, eds. Advances in Endocrinology and Metabolism. Mosby Year Book, Chicago, 1994, pp. 393–428.
51. Said G, Goulon-Goeau C, Slama G, Tchobroutsky G. Severe early-onset polyneuropathy in insulin-dependent diabetes mellitus. A clinical and pathological study. N Engl J Med 1992;326:1257–1263.
52. Boulton AJM, Scarpello JHB, Armstrong WD, Ward JD. The natural history of painful diabetic neuropathy—a 4-year study. Postgrad Med J 1983;59:556–559.
53. Cohen KL, Harris S. Efficacy and safety of nonsteroidal anti-inflammatory drugs in the therapy of diabetic neuropathy. Arch Intern Med 1987;147:1442–1444.
54. Gregory I, Smeltzer DJ. Psychotherapeutic drugs and electrotherapy. In: Psychiatry. Essentials of Clinical Practice With Examination Questions, Answers, and Comments. Little, Brown and Company, Boston, 1983, pp. 93–138.
55. Max MB, Culnane M, Schafer SC, Gracely RH, Walther DJ, Smoller B, Dubner R. Amitriptyline relieves diabetic neuropathy pain in patients with normal or depressed mood. Neurology 1987;37:589–596.
56. Hoogwerf BJ. Amitriptyline treatment of painful diabetic neuropathy: an inadvertent single-patient clinical trial [letter]. Diabetes Care 1985;8:526, 527.
57. LeWitt PA. Forno LS. Peripheral neuropathy following amitriptyline overdose. Muscle Nerve 1985;8:723, 724.
58. Davis. JAMA 1977;238:2291.
59. Sindrup SH, Gram LF, Brosen K, Eshoj O, Mogensen EF. The selective serotonin reuptake inhibitor paroxetine is effective in the treatment of diabetic neuropathy symptoms. Pain 1990;42:135–144.
60. Sindrup SH, Grodum E, Gram LF, Beck-Nielsen H. Concentration-response relationship in paroxetine treatment of diabetic neuropathy symptoms: a patient-blinded dose-escalation study. Ther Drug Monit 1991;13:408–414.
61. Rull JA, Quibrera R, Gonzalez-Millan H, Lozano CO. Symptomatic treatment of peripheral diabetic neuropathy with carbamazepine (Tegretol): double blind crossover trial. Diabetologia 1969;5:215–218.
62. Chakrabarti AK, Samantaray SK. Diabetic peripheral neuropathy: nerve conduction studies before, during and after carbamazepine therapy. Aust NZ J Med 1976;6:565–568.
63. Rodin EA. Carbamazepine (tegretol). In: Browne TR, Feldman RG, eds. Epilepsy. Diagnosis and Management Little, Brown, Boston, 1983, pp. 203–213.
64. Saudek CD, Werns S, Reidenberg MM. Phenytoin in the treatment of diabetic symmetrical polyneuropathy. Clin Pharmacol Ther 1977;22:196–199.
65. Capsaicin Study Group. Effect of treatment with capsaicin on daily activities of patients with painful diabetic neuropathy. Diabetes Care 1992;15:159–165.
66. Capsaicin Study Group. Treatment of painful diabetic neuropathy with topical capsaicin. Arch Int Med 1991;151:2225–2229.
67. Ackerman III WE, Colclough GW, Juneja MM, Bellinger K. The management of oral mexiletine and intravenous lidocaine to treat chronic painful symmetrical distal diabetic neuropathy. KMA 1991;89:500,501.
68. Stracke H, Meyer UE, Schumacher HE, Federlin K. Mexiletine in the treatment of diabetic neuropathy. Diabetes Care 1992;15:1550–1555.
69. Ameisen JC. Programmed cell death (apoptosis) and cell survival regulation: relevance to AIDS and cancer. AIDS 1994;8:1197–1213.
70. Kastrup J, Angelo H, Petersen P, Dejard A, Hilsted J. Treatment of chronic painful diabetic neuropathy with intravenous lidocaine infusion. Br Med J 1986;292:173.
71. Kastrup J, Petersen P, Dejgard A, Angelo HR, Hilsted J. Intravenous lidocaine infusion—a new treatment of chronic painful diabetic neuropathy? Pain 1987;28:69–75.
72. Gomez-Perez FJ, Rull JA, Dies H, Rodriquez-Rivera JG, Gonzalez-Barranco, J, Lozano-Castaneda O. Nortriptyline and fluphenazine in the symptomatic treatment of diabetic neuropathy. A double-blind cross-over study. Pain 1985;23:395–400.
73. Stevens MJ, Feldman EL, Funnell MM, Sima AAF, Greene DA. Optimal methods for detecting early neuropathy and its progression. In: Mogensen, Standl, eds. Diabetes Forum IV. Concepts for the Ideal Diabetes Clinic. 1993, pp. 315–332.
74. Greene DA, Feldman EL, Stevens MJ. Neuropathy in the diabetic foot: new concepts in etiology and treatment. In: Levin M, O'Neal L, eds. The Diabetic Foot Mosby, New York, 1993, pp. 135–148.

# 7 Implications of the DCCT in the Management of Diabetic Neuropathy

*David A. Gelber,* MD, *and Michael Pfeifer,* MD

***Contents***



## INTRODUCTION

Neuropathy is a common complication of diabetes mellitus; up to 50% of diabetic patients show clinical evidence of neuropathy after 25 yr of the disease *(1)*. In the past, the etiology of diabetic neuropathy had been widely debated, although a correlation with hyperglycemia had been suggested *(2)*. Whether tight blood glucose control could prevent the development of neuropathy and other complications of diabetes had not been convincingly proven. The recently completed prospective multicenter Diabetes Control and Complications Trial (DCCT) was designed to specifically evaluate whether intensive insulin treatment would delay the appearance of or slow the progression of diabetic retinopathy, nephropathy, and neuropathy *(3)*. This chapter reviews the design and results of the DCCT and discusses the clinical implications of the findings.

## CLASSIFICATION OF DIABETIC NEUROPATHY

For classification purposes, diabetic neuropathy can be divided into focal and diffuse neuropathies. The focal neuropathies, including mononeuropathies, mononeuropathy multiplex, brachial and lumbosacral plexopathies, radiculopathies, and cranial neuropathies are caused by occlusion of the vasa nervora causing microinfarcts in the nerve fascicles *(4)*. Patients with diabetes are also more prone to developing focal compressive neuropathies, such as carpal- and cubital-tunnel syndrome, caused by swelling of the endoneurial tissues.

From: *Contemporary Endocrinology: Clinical Management of Diabetic Neuropathy*
Edited by: A. Veves © Humana Press Inc., Totowa, NJ

The diffuse neuropathies include distal symmetrical polyneuropathy (DSP) and autonomic neuropathy. In DSP the long myelinated axons are primarily affected *(5)*, resulting in involvement of the feet initially, and later the hands (stocking and glove distribution). Sensory nerves demonstrate more clinically obvious abnormalities than motor nerves *(6)*. Involvement of large-nerve fibers results in pain, impairment of light touch, vibration, and proprioception, with loss of ankle reflexes and impairment in balance. Weakness and atrophy of the intrinsic muscles of the hands and feet may result in impaired dexterity and ambulation. If small-nerve fibers are affected, pain and temperature sensation may be impaired leading to paresthesias, dysesthesias, and autonomic abnormalities. Late complications include development of foot deformities, foot ulcers, and neuroarthropathy with Charcot joints *(7)*.

Diabetic patients may develop autonomic neuropathy (parasympathetic and/or sympathetic involvement) with sudomotor dysfunction, cardiac arrhythmias, impaired night vision, urinary retention, orthostatic hypotension, sexual dysfunction, and gastrointestinal disturbances *(7)*. Pathological abnormalities have been noted in the paravertebral sympathetic chain, intrinsic nerves of the bladder, vagus nerve, and esophageal and splanchnic nerves *(8–11)*.

## PATHOLOGY AND PATHOGENESIS OF DIABETIC NEUROPATHY

The pathologic abnormalities seen in the peripheral nerves include atrophy and loss of both large and small myelinated nerve fibers, with evidence of Wallerian degeneration, paranodal demyelination, and swelling of endoneurial connective tissue *(12)*. There may be several pathogenetic events. The preferential involvement of large myelinated fibers suggests a primary axonopathy *(5,13)*. The finding of segmental demyelination and remyelination in the nerves of some diabetic individuals also suggests an abnormality of Schwann cells *(14,15)*. In addition, neural ischemic changes may result from endoneurial vascular abnormalities and vessel occlusion *(16)*.

Although there are thought to be several pathogenetic mechanisms involved in the development of DSP and autonomic neuropathy, hyperglycemia appears to be the primary initiating factor causing a number of biochemical abnormalities that result in nerve injury *(7)*. For example, chronic hyperglycemia can lead to glycation of neural proteins, resulting in decreased axonal transport and impaired nerve conduction *(17)*. Hyperglycemia can also competitively inhibit the neural uptake of myo-inositol, a neural membrane component, leading to an impairment in nerve function *(18)*. In addition, elevated blood-glucose levels causes a shunting of glucose to the polyol metabolic pathway, resulting in an accumulation of sorbitol and a decrease in neural myo-inositol *(19)*. Furthermore, an increase in glucose metabolism through the polyol pathway leads to decreased formation of nitric oxide, causing reduced neural blood flow and nerve ischemia *(20)*.

## STUDIES SUPPORTING THE CORRELATION BETWEEN HYPERGLYCEMIA AND DIABETIC NEUROPATHY

Several early animal studies suggested a correlation between hyperglycemia and impaired nerve function. Nerves of diabetic animals were shown to contain elevated levels of glucose, sorbitol, and fructose, and decreased levels of myo-inositol, that correlated with slowed nerve conduction velocities *(21–24)*. In at least one study, nerve conduction slowing could be prevented with insulin administration and improved glucose control *(24)*.

In humans, the frequency of diabetic microvascular complications, including neuropathy has been shown to correlate with the duration and severity of hyperglycemia *(1,25,26)*. Several series of diabetic patients have noted a correlation between hyperglycemia and nerve conduction velocities *(27–29)* and demonstrated an improvement in velocities following insulin treatment *(30–36)*.

Overall, many early series supported the notion that the development and severity of peripheral neuropathy was directly related to glycemic control, and that treatment could prevent or slow the progression of clinical neuropathy. Unfortunately, these series were generally limited by factors including retrospective and uncontrolled study design, and small patient numbers *(2)*.

## DCCT METHODOLOGY

The DCCT, initiated in 1982, was a multicenter National Institutes of Health-sponsored randomized clinical trial designed to compare the effects of intensive insulin therapy with conventional diabetes treatment on the development and progression of vascular and neurologic complications in patients with insulin-dependent diabetes mellitus (IDDM) *(37)*. Retinopathy was chosen as the principal outcome measure; nephropathy, cardiovascular disease, and neuropathy were assessed conjointly *(38)*. Patients were divided into two study cohorts based on whether they had evidence of retinopathy at study onset. A primary-prevention cohort was evaluated to determine whether intensive insulin therapy could prevent the development of long-term complications in patients with no evidence of retinopathy at baseline. A secondary-intervention cohort was studied to determine whether intensive insulin treatment could affect the progression of complications in patients who already had mild-to-moderately severe nonproliferative retinopathy at study onset *(39)*.

Prior to initiation of the full-scale DCCT, a 1 yr feasibility study was undertaken *(38,40,41)*. Two hundred seventy-eight patients (191 adults and 87 adolescents with IDDM) were enrolled. The DCCT methodology was shown to be reliable, reproducible, and precise, and adherence to study protocol was > 95% *(38)*.

Based on these findings the full-scale, multicenter DCCT was initiated. Patients from 29 centers were enrolled from 1983–1989; the trial was terminated in 1993. To be eligible for study inclusion, subjects were to be 13–39 yr old with IDDM diagnosed by deficient C peptide secretion. Subjects had to have glycosylated hemoglobin levels greater than 6.6% and either serum creatinine ≤ 1.2 mg/dL or creatinine clearance > 100 mL/min/1.73 $m^2$ body surface area. In addition, subjects had to be free of advanced microvascular complications of diabetes, including diabetic somatic or autonomic neuropathy severe enough to warrant treatment *(41)*. Criteria for the primary-prevention cohort included IDDM duration 1–5 yr, no evidence of retinopathy based on seven-field steroscopic fundus photography, and urinary albumin excretion < 40 mg/24 h. Eligibility criteria for the secondary-intervention cohort included duration of IDDM 1–15 yr, very mild-to-moderate nonproliferative retinopathy *(42)*, and urinary albumin excretion < 200 mg/24 h *(37,40)*. Subjects in both the primary-prevention and secondary-intervention cohorts were randomly assigned to one of two treatment regimens, conventional treatment, or intensive insulin therapy.

The goal of conventional (standard) therapy was to keep the patient free from symptoms of hypo- or hyperglycemia, avoid development of ketonuria, maintain normal growth, and development in adolescents, and maintain ideal body weight in all subjects *(37)*. The conventional treatment regimen consisted of 1–2 daily injections of any mixture of short-acting, intermediate, or long-acting pork, beef/pork, or human insulin *(43)*. Clinic visits were every 3 mo; routine education regarding diet, exercise, and insulin administration was provided. Patients were to monitor their urine or blood glucose on a daily basis, although no predetermined metabolic targets were set, and insulin dosage was not routinely adjusted based on this monitoring. Glycosylated hemoglobin levels were drawn every 3 mo. Although the investigators and patients were masked to the results, the investigators were notified if the $HbA_{1c}$ rose above 13.1%. The insulin dosage was subsequently adjusted and $HbA_{1c}$ was then measured monthly until it was again $< 13.1\%$ *(43)*. If female patients became pregnant or planned to become pregnant, the protocol mandated that they switch to intensive therapy; they were switched back to conventional therapy after delivery *(43)*.

The goal of intensive therapy was to maintain glycemic control as nearly normal as possible, avoiding significant hypoglycemic episodes. Specific metabolic targets included maintenance of preprandial blood glucose 70–120 mg/dL, postprandial blood glucose $< 180$ mg/dL, a weekly 3:00 AM measurement $> 65$ mg/dL, and $HbA_{1c}$ within normal range ($< 6.05\%$). Subjects were seen in the clinic on a weekly basis, until metabolic targets were reached, and monthly thereafter. They were contacted by phone at least on a weekly basis. More intensive dietary instruction was provided in contrast to the conventional treatment group.

Subjects were administered insulin subcutaneously, by three or more injections per day, or by continuous subcutaneous infusion via an external pump. The latter was maintained at a basal rate and supplemented by bolus doses before meals, and if necessary, before large snacks *(40)*. Patients could switch from one route of administration to the other if their glycemic control was inadequate or if they preferred. Subjects monitored their blood glucose at least four times per day. Insulin dosage was adjusted based on the metabolic targets detailed above *(43)*.

A standardized neurologic history and examination was performed on all subjects by blinded DCCT neurologists at baseline, 5 yr, and study end *(44)*. Uniform criteria were established for the diagnosis of diabetic somatic neuropathy, and consisted of symptoms (paresthesias, dysesthesias, burning pain, or hypersensitivity to touch), signs (abnormal light touch, joint position sense, temperature, and pinprick), and absent or decreased muscle stretch reflexes. Abnormal findings in any two of these three categories was considered to indicate definite clinical neuropathy *(44)*.

Following the clinical examination, nerve conduction studies were performed. These included evaluation of median motor, median sensory, peroneal motor, and sural sensory distal latencies, amplitudes, and conduction velocities, and median and peroneal F-wave latencies according to a standard protocol *(41)*. Results were reviewed at a coordinating center. Nerve conduction was considered abnormal if there were abnormalities in at least two distinct nerves in two different limbs *(44)*.

Three autonomic nervous system (ANS) tests were performed at baseline and every 2 years thereafter. Studies included heart-rate variation during deep breathing (RR variation) and during a Valsalva maneuver (Valsalva ratio), and postural blood pressure testing *(44)*. ANS testing was considered abnormal if RR variation was $< 15$, Valsalva

Table 1
Baseline Demographics of the Study Cohorts *(44)*

| | *Primary Prevention Cohort* | | *Secondary Intervention Cohort* | |
|---|---|---|---|---|
| | *Conventional Therapy* | *Intensive Therapy* | *Conventional Therapy* | *Intensive Therapy* |
| Patients (*n*) | 378 | 348 | 352 | 363 |
| Age (yr) | 26 ± 8 | 27 ± 7 | 27 ± 7 | 27 ± 7 |
| Gender | | | | |
| Males | 54% | 49% | 54% | 53% |
| Females | 46% | 51% | 46% | 47% |
| Duration of IDDM (yr) | 2.6 ± 1.4 | 2.6 ± 1.4 | 8.6 ± 3.7 | 8.9 ± 3.8 |
| $HbA_{1c}$ | 8.8 ± 1.7% | 8.8 ± 1.6% | 8.9 ± 1.5% | 9.0 ± 1.5% |

Values are expressed as mean ± SD.

ratio < 1.5 with an RR variation < 20, or postural hypotension (10 mmHg drop in diastolic blood pressure) with a blunted catecholamine response *(44)*.

The development and progression of diabetic retinopathy and nephropathy were also evaluated. The related protocols are detailed elsewhere *(37)*.

In the DCCT, the main neurologic endpoint was the development of confirmed clinical neuropathy, defined as clinical neuropathy plus abnormal nerve conduction studies or ANS testing.

## DCCT RESULTS

### *Patient Demographics and Adherence to Study Protocol*

A total of 1441 patients with IDDM were enrolled in the DCCT; 726 had no retinopathy at baseline (primary-prevention cohort) and 715 had mild retinopathy (secondary-intervention cohort). Pertinent baseline demographics are detailed in Table 1.

The mean duration of follow-up for the entire study population was 6.5 yr (range 3–9 yr) *(37)*. Ninety-nine percent of the patients completed the study, yielding a total of 9300 patient-years of observation *(44)*. Two hundred seventy-eight patients (19%) were studied for a total of 9 yr, 1088 patients (76%) for 5 yr. Eleven patients died and 8 dropped out of the study *(37)*.

Forty-nine patients switched from intensive to conventional therapy during the study, whereas 106 patients switched from conventional to intensive therapy. Most in the latter group were pregnant women required to do so by the study protocol *(44)*.

### *Metabolic Control*

At baseline, there was no difference between glycosylated hemoglobin levels for patients treated with conventional vs intensive therapy (mean 8.9 ± 1.6% for both groups). However, by 3 mo, patients treated with intensive therapy had significantly lower $HBA_{1c}$ levels (7.2 vs 9.1%, $p < 0.001$); this persisted for the 5 yr of follow-up *(44)*. A significant difference was evident for both the primary-prevention and secondary-intervention cohorts. The blood glucose concentrations also differed signifi-

Table 2
Incidence of Somatic Neuropathy at Study Baseline *(44)*

| | *Primary Prevention Cohort* | | *Secondary Intervention Cohort* | |
|---|---|---|---|---|
| | *Conventional Therapy* n *(%)* | *Intensive Therapy* n *(%)* | *Conventional Therapy* n *(%)* | *Intensive Therapy* n *(%)* |
| No neuropathy | 281 (74.5) | 264 (76.3) | 219 (62.2) | 216 (59.5) |
| Definite clinical neuropathy[a] | 17 (4.5) | 22 (6.4) | 46 (13.1) | 49 (13.5) |
| Confirmed clinical neuropathy[b] | 8 (2.1) | 17 (4.9) | 33 (9.4) | 34 (9.4) |

[a] Defined as abnormalities in at least two of the following: symptoms, sensory examination, or decreased or absent muscle stretch reflexes.

[b] Defined as clinical neuropathy plus either abnormal nerve conduction studies or autonomic nervous system tests

cantly between treatment groups; the mean blood glucose level for the intensive therapy group was 155 ± 30 mg/dL compared to 231 ± 55 mg/dL for the conventional treatment group ($p < 0.001$) *(37)*.

### *Retinopathy and Nephropathy*

For the primary-prevention cohort, intensive therapy reduced the risk for the development of retinopathy by 76% (95% CI, 62–85%) compared to conventional therapy. In the secondary-intervention cohort, intensive therapy slowed the progression of retinopathy by 54% (95% CI, 39–66%). Progression to laser photocoagulation was reduced by 56%. For the entire study population, intensive therapy reduced the development of microalbuminuria by 39% (95% CI, 21–52%) and of albuminuria by 54% (95% CI, 19–74%) *(37)*.

### *Macrovascular Complications*

For the combined study cohort, intensive therapy significantly reduced the development of mean total cholesterol, low-density lipoprotein cholesterol, and triglycerides. Although not statistically significant, in part because of the small number of outcome events, intensive therapy reduced the risk of cardiovascular and peripheral vascular events by 41% *(39)*.

### *Neurologic Outcomes*

The presence of somatic neuropathy at baseline is detailed in Table 2. Ninety-two patients (6%) had confirmed clinical neuropathy at study onset. For the patients without neuropathy at baseline, there was a significant reduction in the risk for the development of neuropathy over a 5-yr period for patients treated with intensive therapy (Table 3). In the primary-prevention cohort, only 2.8% of patients treated with intensive therapy developed confirmed clinical neuropathy compared to 9.6% of the conventional treatment group (risk reduction of 71%, $p < 0.01$). For the secondary-intervention cohort, 6.7% of patients in the intensive therapy group developed neuropathy compared to

Table 3
Risk of Developing Somatic Neuropathy at 5 Years *(44)*

| | *Primary Prevention Cohort* | | | *Secondary Intervention Cohort* | | *Combined Cohort* | |
|---|---|---|---|---|---|---|---|
| | *Conventional Therapy* n *(%)* | *Intensive Therapy* n *(%)* | *Risk Reduction (95%* CI*)* | *Conventional Therapy* n *(%)* | *Intensive Therapy* n *(%)* | *Risk Reduction (95%* CI*)* | *Risk Reduction (95%* CI*)* |
| Patients (n)[a] | 291 | 248 | | 307 | 315 | | |
| Definite clinical neuropathy | 44 (15.2) | 17 (6.9) | 54 (22–73) | 85 (21.2) | 37 (11.8) | 45 (20–62) | 48 (29–62) |
| Confirmed clinical neuropathy | 28 (9.6) | 7 (2.8) | 71 (34–87) | 52 (16.9) | 21 (6.7) | 61 (36–76) | 64 (45–76) |

[a] Patients without neuropathy at study onset.

16.9% in the conventional treatment group (risk reduction of 64%, $p < 0.01$) *(37,44)*. The risk reduction was evident even when subjects were stratified for age, gender, renal status, alcohol, and tobacco use *(37,44)*.

Of the ninety-two patients with confirmed clinical neuropathy at study baseline 5-yr data was available for eighty-four. Forty-one patients (48.8%) again met the criteria for clinical neuropathy at 5 yr; in the primary-prevention cohort this included 6 of 12 (50%) of patients in the intensive-treatment group and 2 of 6 (33%) in the conventional-treatment group, whereas in the secondary-intervention cohort this included 13 of 33 (39%) of patients in the intensive-treatment group and 20 of 33 (61%) in the conventional-treatment group *(44)*. Forty-three patients initially diagnosed with neuropathy were found to have no evidence of clinical neuropathy at 5 yr. Despite what was felt to represent clinical improvement in these patients, approximately two thirds had no improvement in nerve conduction studies or autonomic nervous system tests *(44)*.

### *Effect of Therapy on Nerve Function*

At baseline, there was no significant difference between the intensive and conventional treatment groups for any nerve conduction measures *(45)*. Patients in the conventional-therapy group showed significant decreases in sensory and motor-nerve conduction velocities over the 5 yr of treatment, whereas nerve conduction velocities either improved or decreased only slightly in the intensive-therapy cohort *(44)*. Treatment had little effect on sensory or motor amplitudes *(45)*. The intensive-therapy group showed less prolongation of F wave latencies in comparison to the conventional-treatment group ($p < 0.001$) *(44)*.

Overall, patients in the intensive-therapy group had significantly higher sensory and motor conduction velocities compared to the conventional-treatment group at 5 yr *(45)*. Differences between the two treatment groups became apparent after 1 yr of treatment in the primary-prevention cohort ($p = 0.0038$) and after 2 yr of treatment in the secondary-intervention cohort ($p = 0.0040$) *(44)*.

Intensive therapy was also shown to slow the progressive decrease in RR variation. This was evident in the primary-prevention ($p = 0.035$) and combined study cohorts ($p < 0.005$), where the rate of decrease in RR variation was twice as great in patients treated with conventional therapy *(44,46)*. Although there was no significant therapy effect on the Valsalva ratio for the individual cohorts, the rate of decrease was three times greater for the combined cohorts treated with conventional therapy ($p = 0.0075$) *(46)*.

### *Glycemic Threshold*

The risk of all of the complications studied in DCCT, including retinopathy, microalbuminuria, and confirmed clinical neuropathy, were found to be continuous over the entire range of $HBA_{1c}$ values, and was evident for both of the study cohorts and the combined-study group. The relationship between a decrease in glycosylated hemoglobin levels and reduced risk of these complications was nonlinear and suggested a constant relative-risk gradient in which proportional reductions in $HbA_{1c}$ levels were associated with a proportional reduction in the risk of complications. For every reduction of 10% in $HbA_{1c}$, the risk reductions for the various complications ranged from 21–49% (approx 30% for neuropathy) *(47)*. No glycemic threshold could be determined; i.e., there was a definable risk for the development of microvascular complications at all $HbA_{1c}$ levels above the normal range *(47)*.

### *Complications of Treatment*

The major complication in the DCCT trial was severe hypoglycemia. Hypoglycemic episodes occurred three time more frequently in the intensive-treatment group ($p < 0.001$). As well, intensive therapy was associated with a greater frequency of hypoglycemia-related seizures and coma with 16 episodes per 100 patient-years in the intensive-therapy group vs 5 in the conventional-therapy group. Hypoglycemic episodes severe enough to require hospitalization occurred 54 times in the intensive-treatment group and 36 times in the conventional-therapy group. Mortality did not differ significantly between treatment groups.

Weight gain was more commonly associated with intensive therapy. The mean adjusted risk of becoming overweight was increased by 33% in this cohort. After 5 yr of treatment, patients in the intensive-therapy group had gained a mean of 4.6 kg more than patients receiving conventional therapy *(37)*.

### *Cost-Effectiveness of Intensive Insulin Therapy*

A recent analysis of DCCT data evaluated the lifetime costs and benefits of intensive therapy in comparison to conventional treatment *(48,49)*. The annual cost of intensive therapy was $4000 for multiple daily injections and $5800 for continuous subcutaneous insulin infusion; conventional therapy cost only $1700 *(48)*. Much of the increased cost associated with intensive therapy was related to the high frequency of outpatient clinic visits and self-monitoring of blood glucose.

On the benefit side, assuming that there are 120,000 patients with IDDM in the United States, implementation of intensive insulin therapy was estimated to result in a gain of 920,000 years of sight, 691,000 years free from end-stage renal disease, 678,000 years free from lower-extremity amputation, and 611,000 years of life *(49)*. Based on this data, the DCCT Research Group concluded that an intensive therapy approach was cost-effective in the management of type I diabetes *(48)*.

## SUMMARY AND IMPLICATIONS

The DCCT was the first well-designed, large, multicentered, prospective trial to demonstrate convincingly that intensive diabetes treatment could delay the onset and slow the progression of retinopathy, nephropathy, and neuropathy in patients with IDDM. For the combined study cohort, intensive therapy reduced the risk of developing definite clinical neuropathy by 48% and slowed the decline in sensory and motor nerve conduction velocities, RR variation, and the Valsalva ratio in comparison to patients treated with conventional insulin therapy.

Several parallel studies have also evaluated the effect of intensive insulin therapy on the long-term risk of the development and progression of diabetic complications in patients with IDDM. A recently reported meta-analysis study of 16 smaller randomized trials showed a significant reduction in the risk of progression of retinopathy (49%) and nephropathy (34%) in patients treated with over 2 yr of intensive insulin therapy *(50)*. Similar findings were reported by the Stockholm Diabetes Intervention Study, which was initiated in 1982 *(51)*. One hundred two patients with IDDM and nonproliferative retinopathy were randomized to receive either intensive insulin therapy or conventional insulin treatment and were followed for the development of microvascular complications over a 7.5-yr period. Mean glycosylated hemoglobin levels fell from 9.5 ± 1.3% to 7.1 ± 0.7% in the intensive-therapy group and from 9.4 ± 1.4% to 8.5 ± 0.7% in the standard-treatment group. Although the evaluation for neuropathy was less rigorous than the DCCT, the Stockholm study did demonstrate a trend toward less development of neuropathic symptoms in the intensive-therapy group. In addition, patients in the intensive-therapy cohort showed less of a decline in nerve conduction velocities in comparison to the conventional-treatment group ($p < 0.05$) *(51)*.

In diabetic neuropathy, although there is often an irreversible structural component, caused by permanent axonal injury, there may also be a reversible metabolic component *(19)*. This notion is supported by the DCCT findings; 51% of patients in the combined study cohort with confirmed clinical neuropathy at study baseline had no evidence of neuropathy after 5 yr of treatment. Although this suggests that improved glucose control might reverse clinical neuropathy, it is important to note, that many of these patients had no improvement in objective measures of neuropathy, such as nerve conduction studies and autonomic nervous system tests. Given the relatively small number of patients with neuropathy at baseline ($n = 92$), further research is needed to better define the effect of glycemic control on the reversibility of diabetic neuropathy.

A key finding of the DCCT was that no glycemic threshold was identified. This suggests that for patients with IDDM, improving glycemic control should always result in a lower risk of developing microvascular complications until $HbA_{Ic}$ falls below 6.05%. However, the benefits of tighter glucose control must be weighed against the risk of potential side effects associated with intensive insulin management. Most important is the risk of hypoglycemia that can lead to seizures or coma. Because of this it has been suggested that intensive therapy be avoided or initiated cautiously in patients with a previous history of hypoglycemic episodes *(52)*.

What are the implications of DCCT with regard to patient age? Although the trial evaluated patients from 13–39 yr old, there is certainly no reason to think that the results would not apply to older patients, provided the risks of intensive therapy are considered on an individual basis. A subanalysis of DCCT data has been evaluated for adolescents, age 13–17. Reduction in risk of microvascular complications was similar to that for adults. The risk of side effects associated with intensive insulin therapy was also similar, but even more common in adolescents. Eighty-two percent of adolescents had at least one episode of hypoglycemia requiring assistance. In addition, adolescent patients treated with intensive therapy had twice the risk of being overweight compared to the conventional therapy group *(53)*. Given these findings the DCCT has recommended that adolescents with type I diabetes be treated with intensive insulin treatment, but that they be monitored closely for complications of therapy. Because severe hypoglycemia may affect brain development in children, it is recommended that intensive insulin therapy be avoided entirely in patients under the age of 13 *(53)*.

The implications of the DCCT results for patients with type II diabetes mellitus are uncertain. It has been demonstrated in a multicentered prospective trial of patients with type II diabetes that intensive insulin therapy can maintain near-normal glycemic control for over 2 yr without episodes of severe hypoglycemia, weight gain, hypertension, or lipid abnormalities *(53)*. Previous studies of patients with type II diabetes have also demonstrated a significant reduction in cardiovascular events because of tighter glucose control *(54,55)*. A recently concluded prospective study, with a protocol similar to the DCCT, evaluated 110 patients with type II diabetes for development of microvascular complications over a 6-yr period. Patients treated with intensive insulin therapy showed improvement in nerve conduction velocities and RR variation, whereas patients treated with conventional therapy showed deterioration in these measures *(56)*. Further studies evaluating larger sample populations are needed to more definitively address the issues of risks and benefits of intensive insulin therapy in patients with Type II diabetes *(57)*.

Despite the clearly demonstrated cost-effectiveness of intensive insulin therapy *(49)*, a major concern is whether the intensive therapy program recommended by the DCCT is one that can be reproduced in everyday clinical practice. Such a program requires frequent physician visits, intensive monitoring, and extensive education, which may be beyond the scope of what a typical office can provide. Also, patients chosen for participation in the DCCT were highly motivated and had excellent protocol compliance; it is unknown whether the average diabetic patient would be able to comply with such a rigorous protocol. Regardless, the DCCT has clearly demonstrated that improved glycemic control, to any extent, results in a lower risk of complications; therefore, benefit can be conferred by intensive insulin therapy, even if the DCCT methodology cannot be entirely reproduced.

## CONCLUSIONS

The DCCT was the first well-designed large multicenter trial to clearly demonstrate that intensive insulin therapy and improved glycemic control results in a reduced risk of the development and progression of retinopathy, nephropathy, and neuropathy in persons with IDDM. Given the significant reduction in the risk of complications, the improved quality and increased length of life, intensive therapy had been shown to be cost-effective, despite its higher cost than conventional treatment. Intensive therapy should be the treatment of choice and should be offered to all type I diabetic patients between the ages of 13–39, although it should be administered cautiously in patients with a history of severe hypoglycemic episodes. Further research is needed to assess the compliance of a DCCT-like protocol for physicians and patients in the community and to evaluate the benefits of intensive insulin therapy in patients with NIDDM.

## REFERENCES

1. Pirat J. Diabetes mellitus and its degenerative complications: a prospective study of 4,400 patients observed between 1947 and 1973. Diabetes Care 1978;1:168–188.
2. Committee on Health Care Issues, American Neurological Association. Does improved control of glycemia prevent or ameliorate diabetic neuropathy? Ann Neurol 1986;19:288–290.
3. The DCCT Research Group. The Diabetes Control and Complications Trial (DCCT): design and methodologic considerations for the feasibility phase. Diabetes 1986;35:530–545.
4. Raff MC, Sangalang V, Asbury AK. Ischemic mononeuropathy multiplex associated with diabetes mellitus. Arch Neurol 1968;18:487–499.
5. Yagihashi S, Matsunaga M. Ultrastructural pathology of peripheral nerves in patients with diabetic neuropathy. Tohoku J Exp Med 1979;129:357–366.
6. Greene DA, Pfeifer MA. Diabetic neuropathy. In: Olefsky JM, Sherwin RS, eds. Diabetes Mellitus Management and Complications, vol. 1. Churchill Livingston, New York, 1985, pp. 223–254.
7. Gelber DA, Pfeifer MA. Management of diabetic neuropathy. In: Marshall SM, Home PD, eds. The Diabetes Annual/8 Elsevier Science, Amsterdam, 1994, pp. 349–363.
8. Appenzeller O, Ogin G. Myelinated fibers in human paravertebral sympathetic chain: white rami communicantes in alcoholic and diabetic patients. J Neurol Neurosurg 1974;37:1155–1161.
9. Faerman I, Glocer L, Celener D, Jadzinsky M, Fox D, Maler M, Alvarez E. Autonomic nervous system and diabetes: histological and histochemical study of the autonomic nerve fibers of the urinary bladder in diabetic patients. Diabetes 1973;22:225–237.
10. Kristensson K, Nordborg C, Olsson Y, Sourander P. Changes in the vagus nerve in diabetes mellitus. Acta Pathol Microbiol Scand 1971;79:684–685.
11. Smith B. Neuropathology of the esophagus in diabetes mellitus. Diabetes 1974;37:1151–1154.
12. Greene DA, Sima AA, Albers JW, Pfeifer MA. Diabetic neuropathy. In: Rifken H, Porte D, eds. Diabetes Mellitus Elsevier, New York, 1990, pp. 710–755.
13. Low PA, Walsh JC, Huang CY, McLeod JG. The sympathetic nervous system in diabetic neuropathy—a clinical and pathological study. Brain 1975;98:341–356.
14. Dyck PJ, Sherman WR, Hallcher LM, Service FJ, O'Brien PC, Grina LA, Palumbo PJ, Swanson CJ. Human diabetic endoneurial sorbitol, fructose, and myo-inositol related to sural nerve morphometry. Ann Neurol 1980;8:590–596.
15. Kimura J, Yamada T, Stevland NP. Distal slowing of motor nerve conduction velocity in diabetic polyneuropathy. J Neurol Sci 1979;42:291–302.
16. Harati Y. Diabetic peripheral neuropathies. Ann Intern Med 1987;107:546–559.
17. Brownlee M. Glycation products and the pathogenesis of diabetic complications. Diabetes Care 1992;15:1835–1843.
18. Greene DA. A sodium-pump defect in diabetic peripheral nerve corrected by sorbinil administration: a relationship to myoinositol metabolism and nerve conduction slowing. Metabolism 1986;35:60–65.
19. Pfeifer MA, Schumer MP. Clinical trials of diabetic neuropathy: past, present, and future. Diabetes 1995;44:1355–1361.
20. Stevens MJ, Dananberg J, Feldman EL, Lattimer SA, Sima A, Greene D. The linked roles of nitric acid, aldose reductase and (Na+, K+)-ATPase in the slowing of nerve conduction in the streptozotocin-diabetic rat. J Clin Invest 1994;94:853–859.
21. Gabbay KH. Role of sorbitol pathway in neuropathy. Adv Metab Disord 1973;2(Suppl. 2):417–424.
22. Ward JD. The polyol pathway in the neuropathy of early diabetes. Adv Metab Disord 1973;2(Suppl. 2):425–429.
23. Clements RS, Reynertson R. Myoinositol metabolism in diabetes mellitus: effect of insulin treatment. Diabetes 1977;26:215–221.
24. Greene DA, DeJesus PV, Winegrad AL. Effects of insulin and dietary myoinositol on impaired peripheral motor nerve conduction velocity in acute streptozotocin diabetes. J Clin Invest 1975;55:1326–1336.
25. Tchobroysky G. Relation of diabetic control to development of microvascular complications. Diabetologia 1978;15:143–152.
26. Maser RD, Steenkiste AR, Dorman JS, Nielsen VK, Bass EB, Qurasha M, Drash AL, Becker DJ, Kuller LH, Greene DA, Orchard TJ. Epidemiological correlates of diabetic neuropathy. Report from Pittsburgh Epidemiology of Diabetes Complication Study. Diabetes 1989;8:1456–1461.
27. Gregerson G. Diabetic neuropathy: influence of age, sex, metabolic control, and duration of diabetes on motor conduction velocity. Neurology 1967;17:972–980.

28. Skillman TG, Johnson EW, Hamwi GJ, Driskill HJ. Motor nerve conduction velocity in diabetes mellitus. Diabetes 1961;10:46–51.
29. Graf RJ, Halter JB, Halar E, Porte D. Nerve conduction abnormalities in untreated maturity-onset diabetes: Relation to levels of fasting plasma glucose and glycosylated hemoglobin. Ann Intern Med 1979;90:298–303.
30. Ward JD, Barnes CG, Fisher FJ, Jessup JD, Baker RW. Improvement in nerve conduction following treatment in newly diagnosed diabetes. Lancet 1971;1:428–430.
31. Fraser DM, Campbell IW, Ewing DJ, Murray A, Neilson JM, Clerke BF. Peripheral and autonomic nerve function in newly diagnosed diabetes mellitus. Diabetes 1977;26:546–550.
32. Terkildesen AB, Christensen NJ. Reversible nervous abnormalities in juvenile diabetes with recently diagnosed diabetes. Diabetologia 1971;7:113–117.
33. Graf RJ, Halter JB, Pfeifer MA, Halar E, Brozovich F, Porte D. Glycemic control and nerve conduction abnormalities in non-insulin-dependent diabetic subjects. Ann Intern Med 1981;94:307–311.
34. Dahl-Jorgensen K, Brinchmann-Hansen O, Hanssen KF, Ganes T, Kierulf P, Smeland E, Sandvik L, Aaenaes O. Effect of mean normoglycemia for two years on progression of early diabetic retinopathy, nephropathy, and neuropathy: the Oslo study. Br Med J 1986;293:1195–1199.
35. Pietri A, Ehle AL, Raskin P. Changes in nerve conduction velocity after six weeks of glucoregulation with portable insulin infusion pumps. Diabetes 1980;29:668–671.
36. Service FJ, Rizza RA, Daube JR, O'Brien PC, Dyck PJ. Near normoglycemia improved nerve conduction and vibration sensation in diabetic neuropathy. Diabetologia 1985;28:722–727.
37. The Diabetes Control and Complications Trial Research Group. The effect of intensive treatment of diabetes on the development and progression of long-term complications in insulin-dependent diabetes mellitus. N Engl J Med 1993;329:977–986.
38. The DCCT Research Group. Diabetes Control and Complications Trial (DCCT): results of feasibility study. Diabetes Care 1987;10:1–19.
39. The Diabetes Control and Complications Trial (DCCT) Research Group. Effect of intensive diabetes management on macrovascular events and risk factors in the Diabetes Control and Complications Trial. Am J Cardiol 1995;75:894–903.
40. The DCCT Research Group. The Diabetes Control and Complications Trial (DCCT): design and methodologic considerations for the feasibility phase. Diabetes 1986;35:530–545.
41. The DCCT Research Group. Factors in development of diabetic neuropathy: baseline analysis of neuropathy in feasibility phase of Diabetes Control and Complications Trial (DCCT). Diabetes 1988;37:476–481.
42. Early Treatment Diabetic Retinopathy Study Research Group. Grading diabetic retinopathy from steroscopic color fundus photographs- an extension of the modified Airlie house classification: ETDRS report no. 10. Ophthalmology 1991;98:786–806.
43. Diabetes Control and Complications Research Group. Implementation of treatment protocols in the Diabetes Control and Complications Trial. Diabetes Care 1995;18:361–376.
44. The Diabetes Control and Complications Trial Research Group. The effect of intensive diabetes therapy on the development and progression of neuropathy. Ann Intern Med 1995;122:561–568.
45. Diabetes Control and Complications Trial (DCCT) Research Group. Effect of intensive diabetes treatment on nerve conduction in the Diabetes Control and Complications Trial. Ann Neurol 1995;38:869–880.
46. Pfeifer M, Cleary P, Kenny D, Schumer M, The Diabetes Control and Complications Trial Research Group. The effect of intensive diabetes therapy on measures of autonomic nervous system (ANS) function in the Diabetes Control and Complications Trial (DCCT) (abstract). Diabetes 1995;44:30A.
47. The Diabetes Control and Complications Trial Research Group. The absence of a glycemic threshold for the development of long-term complications: the perspective of the Diabetes Control and Complications Trial. Diabetes 1996;45:1289–1298.
48. The Diabetes Control and Complications Trial Research Group. Resource utilization and costs of care in the Diabetes Control and Complications Trial. Diabetes Care 1995;18:1468–1478.
49. The Diabetes Control and Complications Trial Research Group. Lifetime benefits and costs of intensive therapy as practiced in the Diabetes Control and Complications Trial. JAMA 1996;276: 1409–1415.
50. Wang PH, Lau J, Chalmers TC. Meta-analysis of effects of intensive blood-glucose control on late complications of type I diabetes. Lancet 1993;341:1306–1309.
51. Reichard P, Nillson BY, Rosenqvist U. The effect of long-term intensified insulin treatment on the development of microvascular complications of diabetes mellitus. N Engl J Med 1995;329:304–309.

52. Rubin RR, Peyrot M. Implications of the DCCT: looking beyond tight control. Diabetes Care 1994;17:235, 236.
53. Diabetes Control and Complications Trial Research Group. Effect of intensive diabetes treatment on the development and progression of long-term complications in adolescents with insulin-dependent diabetes mellitus: Diabetes Control and Complications Trial. J Pediatr 1994;125:177–188.
54. Abraira C, Colwell JA, Nuttall FQ, Sawain CT, Nagel NJ, Comstock JP, Emanuele NV, Levin SR, Henderson W, Lee HS, . Veterans Affairs Cooperative Study on glycemic control and complications in type II diabetes (VA CSDM Group): results of the feasibility study. Diabetes Care 1995; 18:1113–1123.
55. University Group Diabetes Program. A study of the effects of hypoglycemic agents on vascular complications in patients with adult-onset diabetes II: mortality results. Diabetes 1970;19(Suppl 2):785–830.
56. Ohkubo Y, Kishikawa H, Araki E, Miyata T, Isami S, Motoyoshi S, Kojima Y, Furuyoshi N, Shiohiri M. Intensive insulin therapy prevents the progression of diabetic microvascular complications in Japanese patients with non-insulin-dependent diabetes mellitus: a randomized prospective 6-year study. Diabetes Res Clin Pract 1995;28:103–117.
57. Prospective Diabetes Study Group. U.K. Prospective Diabetes Study. VIII. Study design, progress and performance. Diabetologia 1991;34:877–890.
58. Colwell JA. Intensive insulin therapy in type II diabetes. Rationale and collaborative clinical trial results. Diabetes 1996;45:887–890.

# 8 Aldose Reductase Inhibitors and Other Potential Therapeutic Agents for the Treatment of Diabetic Neuropathy

*Aristidis Veves,* MD

*CONTENTS*



## INTRODUCTION

It has been more than 20 yr since the first aldose reductase inhibitor was tested in diabetic and galactosemic rats and found to control polyol accumulation *(1)*. Since then, a considerable number of aldose reductase inhibitors have been tested in experimental and human diabetes and have considerably increased our knowledge in this field (Table 1). A thorough review of work on experimental diabetes would be outside the scope of this volume; however, the interested reader can find more information in recently published extensive reviews. The following chapter will focus on the results from clinical trials in diabetic neuropathy *(2,3)*.

## END-POINTS FOR CLINICAL TRIALS IN DIABETIC NEUROPATHY

Painful symptoms and foot ulcerations are the two most important clinical problems related to peripheral somatic diabetic neuropathy. The conduction of clinical trials that test the efficacy of new therapies for painful neuropathy is straightforward: Patients with this condition are provided trial medication and the primary endpoint is the reduction of the symptoms, which is expected to occur during a reasonable period after the treatment has been initiated. In contrast, foot ulcers develop long after the initiation of events that lead to nerve damage and, by this time, the possibility of restoring the nerve lesions, or halting their progression, is close to nonexistant. Therefore, if a study was to

From: *Contemporary Endocrinology: Clinical Management of Diabetic Neuropathy*
Edited by: A. Veves © Humana Press Inc., Totowa, NJ

Table 1
ARIs Trials in Human Neuropathy

| *Authors* | *Design* | *Duration of Active Treatment* | *Results* |
|---|---|---|---|
| 1. Alrestatin | | | |
| Culebras 1981 | Uncntr | 5 d | symptomatic improvement |
| Handelsman 1981 | sb, nonrmd, co | 4 mo | symptomatic improvement |
| Fagious 1981 | db, rmd | 12 wk | improvement of symptoms, VPT and ulnar mcv |
| 2. Sorbinil | | | |
| Judzewitsch 1983 | db, rmd | 9 wk | improvement of peroneal mcv and median mcv and scv |
| Jaspan 1983 | sb | 3–5 wk | symptomatic improvement |
| Young 1983 | db, rmd, co | 4 wk | improvement of symptoms and sural sap |
| Lewin 1984 | db, rmd, co | 4 wk | no improvement |
| Fagious 1985 | db, rmd | 6 mo | improvement of posterior tibial mcv and ulnar nerve F wl and dsl |
| O'Hare 1988 | db, rmd | 12 mo | no benefit |
| Guy 1988 | db, rmd | 12 mo | no benefit |
| Sima 1988 | db, rmd | 12 mo | improvement of symptoms, sural sap and mfd |
| 3. Ponalrestat | | | |
| Ziegler 1991 | db, rmd | 12 mo | no benefit |
| Krentz 1992 | db, rmd | 12 mo | no benefit |
| 4. Tolrestat | | | |
| Ryder 1986 | db, rmd | 8 wk | improvement of median mcv |
| Boulton 1990 | db, rmd | 12 mo | improvement of paresthetic symptoms and peroneal mcv |
| Macleod 1992 | db, rmd | 6 mo | improvement of VPT, median and ulnar mcv |
| Boulton 1992 | db, rmd withdrawal | 12 mo | improvement of symptoms, median and peroneal mcv |
| Giugliano 1993 | db, rmd | 12 mo | improvement of autonomic measurements and VPT |
| Giugliano 1995 | db, rmd | 12 mo | improvement of autonomic measurements and VPT |

Abbreviations: sb: single blind, db: double blind, uncntr: uncontrolled, nonrmd: nonrandomized, rmd: randomized, co: crossover, mcv: motor nerve conduction velocity, scv: sensory nerve conduction velocity, sap: sensory action potential, wl: wave latency, dsl: distal sensory latency, VPT: vibration perception threshold, mfd: myelinated fiber density.

be conducted having as primary endpoint the prevention of foot ulceration, it should involve patients who have diabetic neuropathy in the early stages and follow them until they reach the very late stages of the disease. This would mean that a large number of patients should be followed for prolonged periods of time, even decades, before any conclusion could be reached.

It is obvious from the above that more practical endpoints should be employed in order to conduct clinical therapeutic trials that will be financially supported by the pharmaceutical industry in which efficient development of new medications are of paramount importance. In addition, these endpoints should give an accurate and more detailed picture of the effects of the treatment on the progression of the disease, mainly to what extent it can restore the already established lesions.

As discussed in Chapter four and five, sural nerve biopsies are the best method in use today for evaluating new medications. However, as they are invasive, they should be employed very cautiously and there are cases in which they may be unavailable. In such cases, electrophysiological measurements should be employed as a surrogate endpoint (for more details, see Chapter 4). Based on epidemiological data, Dyck and O'Brian have suggested that a mean change of 2.9 m/s in the combined conduction velocities of the ulnar, median, and peroneal nerves, or a change of 2.2 m/s in the peroneal nerve alone should be achieved in order that the results can have meaningful clinical significance *(4)*. Additional measurements that should accompany the above endpoints include assessments of symptoms, signs, and quantitative sensory testing (Chapter 4).

## CLINICAL TRIALS WITH ALDOSE REDUCTASE INHIBITORS

### *Alrestatin*

Alrestatin was the first aldose reductase inhibitor (ARI) to be tried in human diabetic neuropathy. In the first, uncontrolled study conducted in 1981, 10 patients with symptomatic neuropathy were treated with iv infusions of alrestatin for 5 d *(5)*. Although symptomatic improvement was noticed in 7 patients, objective measurements failed to improve. Therefore, as the trial was not controlled, a placebo effect accounting for the symptomatic improvement cannot be excluded. No adverse effects of alrestatin were noticed in this trial.

The next trial included nine diabetic patients with severe symptomatic neuropathy that had necessitated at least one hospital admission before the study *(6)*. The trial was a single-blind, non-randomized, placebo crossover that lasted 4 mo. Each patient received the maximum tolerated oral dose for 2 mo and was on placebo for the other 2. Subjective improvement was noted by most of the patients (eight out of nine), but electrophysiological measurements remained virtually unchanged. The most notable side effects were nausea, and photosensitivity that was severe in two cases.

Around the same time, the most comprehensive trial of alrestatin was conducted. Thirty patients with long-standing diabetes and mild-to-moderate neuropathy were studied in a double-blind, randomized, placebo-controlled trial that lasted 12 wk *(7)*. Symptomatic improvement, reduction of the sensory impairment score, and improvement of vibration perception threshold and ulnar-nerve conduction velocity were noticed, but the rest of the electrophysiological measurements in the median, peroneal, and sural nerves did not show any significant difference.

The above studies-indicated that treatment with ARIs might be helpful in treating diabetic neuropathy and also highlighted the need for well-conducted, long-term trials in order to fully explore the potential of this new therapeutic approach. On the down side, the high incidence of side effects of alrestatin prohibited its further development. This led the way for employing some newly discovered compounds such as sorbinil and tolrestat.

### *Sorbinil*

Sorbinil was the second ARI to be tested in human diabetic neuropathy, and a considerable number of studies have been conducted during the last decade using this drug. An early study using sorbinil for the treatment of neuropathy was published in 1983 and included 39 patients with stable diabetes and no clinical symptoms of neuropathy *(8)*. The design of the study was randomized, double-blind cross-over, and each patient received active treatment for 9 wk. The results showed a small but statistically significant increase of the conduction velocity of the peroneal motor nerve (0.70 m/s), the median motor nerve (0.66 m/s), and the median sensory nerve (1.16 m/s) during the treatment with the active drug. Another important finding was that the increase declined rapidly after cessation of the treatment, so that the nerve conduction velocity was similar to pretreatment levels 3 wk later. Five patients were withdrawn from the study because of fever and rash attributed to sorbinil.

In contrast with the previous trial, the ones that followed included mainly diabetic patients with symptomatic neuropathy. The first studied 11 patients with severely painful neuropathy that failed to respond to conventional treatment with analgesics or tricyclic antidepressants *(10)*. In a single-blind design, the patients were treated with sorbinil for 3–5 wk and the pain relief was measured using a graphic scale. Marked-to-moderate pain relief was noted in eight patients, usually 3–4 d after being on treatment, whereas the pain returned to pretreatment levels in seven of the responders when they stopped taking the drug. The motor and sensory conduction velocities of the median nerve improved in four patients, whereas the peroneal motor conduction velocity improved in two patients. It is of interest, however, that in four patients who responded to the treatment, the pain was related to proximal motor neuropathy, a condition that is thought to be caused by mechanisms not related to polyol accumulation. No significant side effects were noted in the 11 patients who finished the study, whereas a twelfth patient who started the study was withdrawn because of rash.

The next study had a double-blind, randomized, placebo-controlled cross-over design and included 15 patients with painful symptoms that were present for more than 1 yr *(10)*. The patients were observed for 16 wk but were on active treatment for only 4 wk, either from wk 5–8 or 9–12. Painful symptoms were assessed using a standardized symptom score, whereas other measurements included neurologic findings on clinical examination, vibration perception threshold, motor and sensory nerve conduction velocities, and autonomic system function tests. A significant number of patients reported improvement of painful symptoms while on the active treatment, but when the pain score was calculated using their diaries, no difference was found between sorbinil and placebo treatment. Significant improvement was also noticed in the sural sensory potential action, and the rest of the electrophysiological measurements remained unchanged. The number of patients who withdrew because of side effects (mainly rash and fever) was increased compared to the previous study; four patients in total had an idiosyncratic reaction that resolved rapidly after the discontinuation of the drug.

The next trial used the same layout, i.e., double blind, placebo-controlled crossover, and included 13 diabetic patients with chronic symptomatic neuropathy (mean duration of symptoms 6 yr) *(11)*. The duration of treatment with sorbinil was the same as in the previous trial, 4 wk out of a total study period of 16 wk. The pain intensity was measured using a 100-mm visual analog scale, whereas other measurements included vibration perception threshold, motor and sensory conduction velocities, autonomic function tests, and duration of sleep. In contrast to the previous study, no difference was found in any parameter, including the severity of neuropathic symptoms and the objective measurements of peripheral nerve function. In one patient who took sorbinil, side effects were present in the form of a febrile rash, necessitating his withdrawal from the study.

The above, short-term trials were followed by long-term ones that examined the effects of aldose reductase inhibition for periods of 6–12 mo. The first long-term study included 55 diabetic male patients with symptomatic neuropathy for 6 mo in a double-blind, placebo-controlled, parallel-group design *(12)*. To avoid a possible long-term effect of the drug, the authors elected to randomize their patients to active and placebo treatment and to avoid the cross-over design. Patient assessment included clinical examination, neurophysiological measurements, thermal and vibration perception thresholds, and autonomic system function tests.

No significant improvement was found in the sorbinil treated group when it was compared to the placebo group, although three sorbinil-treated patients reported a marked overall improvement compared to none from the placebo group. Comparing these three patients to the whole sorbinil-treated group revealed that their ages were below the mean group age and their neuropathics, assessed by electrophysiology, were less severe. All three patients worsened to pretreatment levels when sorbinil was discontinued. No significant changes were found in the vibration and thermal discrimination threshold. From the electrophysiological measurements, improvement was noticed in the motor posterior tibial nerve conduction velocity (approx 1.5 m/s), F wave latency of the ulnar nerve, and the distal sensory latency of the ulnar nerve. From the autonomic tests, a significant improvement in the R R interval variation during deep breathing was found in the sorbinil-treated group. The number of patients with serious side effects was smaller in this study; only two patients had to be withdrawn from the study because of rash and lymphadenopathy.

The next long-term study included 31 patients with mild-to-moderate neuropathy and lasted for 14 mo (including a 2-mo run-in period) *(13)*. The study was designed as double-blind, randomized, placebo-controlled and two thirds of patients were treated with sorbinil and one third received placebo. Assessments of the patients' responses were performed every 3 mo and included the measurement of symptoms such as pain, tingling, and temperature insensitivity using a 100-mm visual analog scale, clinical examination, vibration perception thresholds, electrophysiology, and autonomic function tests. The results indicated no benefit for the sorbinil-treated patients in any of the measured parameters. In addition, as similar doses of the drug were used in this trial and the previous ones and was accompanied by serum sorbinil levels measurements, inadequate drug dosage or poor patient compliance could not be held responsible for the observed discrepancies. Hypersensitivity reactions with fever, rash, and myalgia occurred in two patients who recovered completely after the drug was discontinued.

No improvement was also found in another double-blind, randomized trial that lasted for 12 mo and included patients with severe neuropathy with or without symptoms *(14)*. Thirty-nine patients took part in this study and the severity of neuropathy is indicated by the fact that a history of foot ulceration was present in 21 patients. Efficacy assessments included clinical evaluation, vibration, and thermal perception thresholds, nerve conduction velocities in 12 nerves, and somatosensory-evoked potentials. The results showed no difference in any of the above measurements between sorbinil- and placebo-treated patients, both for the lower and upper extremities, despite the fact that the arms were less severely affected.

As can be seen from the above studies, the beneficial results that were initially reported, failed to be confirmed in subsequent, better-designed, long-term trials. In an effort to clear the confusion, the next trial employed sural-nerve biopsies, which allow more precise evaluation of the therapeutic efficacy *(15)*. This trial included 16 patients with established peripheral neuropathy and involved subjects undergoing fascicular sural-nerve biopsies of the same limb at the beginning and the end of the study *(16)*. The design of the trial was double-blind, randomized, placebo-controlled, and lasted 12 mo. Additional investigations included clinical neurologic assessments, thermal-perception thresholds, and electrophysiological measurements. Although both actively and placebo-treated groups showed some clinical improvement at the end of the study, this was more pronounced in the sorbinil-treated group. The nonbiopsied sural nerve of the sorbinil group showed an improvement of 1 μV in the action-potential amplitude and of 2 m/s in the sensory conduction velocity (2 m/s), results that were not found in the placebo group.

The analysis of the sural-nerve biopsies showed that the sorbitol levels in the sorbinil group were reduced, indicating a successful aldose reductase inhibition in the nerve tissue. The myelinated fiber density, the best single histopathologic criterion to quantify neuropathy, was similarly reduced at baseline by 50% in both the sorbinil and placebo groups when they were compared to age-matched nondiabetic subjects. After 12 mo of treatment, a significant increase of 33% was found in the sorbinil group, whereas no difference was noted in the placebo group. The regeneration and remyelination activity in the sorbinil group was also increased, whereas no change was noticed in the placebo group. Important changes were also noticed in the degree of paranodal demyelination, segmental demyelination, and myelin wrinkling. The main importance of this study lies in the fact that it was the first to demonstrate morphological improvements in nerve biopsies after long-term aldose reductase inhibition in humans and suggested that long-term treatment in properly selected patients may be the most beneficial.

A second clinical trial that employed repeated sural-nerve biopsies, assessed the changes in nerve concentrations of alcohol sugars after a 12-mo period with sorbinil treatment *(17)*. Six patients took part in this study and histochemical measurements showed a significant decrease in nerve sorbitol and fructose levels in the follow-up visit compared to baseline, whereas the levels of glucose and myo-inositol remained unchanged. The above findings were interpreted by the investigators as indicating that sorbinil is an effective inhibitor of aldose reductase, but raised doubts about the role of myo-inositol in the pathogenesis of diabetic neuropathy.

A common factor, present in virtually all the above studies that used sorbinil, was the relatively high rate of side effects. The main adverse reactions were rash, fever, and lymphadenopathy, which subsided when the drug was discontinued. Nevertheless, these adverse reactions would make the use of sorbinil for prolonged period of time in relatively asymptomatic patients unacceptable, and therefore, the compound was withdrawn.

### *Ponalrestat*

The main characteristic of ponalrestat compared to the previous two drugs was its safety profile: very few adverse reactions were reported during the preliminary safety trials, making it ideal for long-term usage. These early expectations were soon dashed as it became apparent that the nerve-tissue concentration levels were probably insufficient to inhibit aldose reductase. Therefore, it is hardly surprising that the few properly conducted trials with this compound reported negative results, despite some modest improvements that were reported in short, preliminary trials *(18,19)*.

An example of a published paper with ponalrestat was that by Ziegler et al. who reported a randomized, double-blind, placebo-controlled trial of 60 patients with chronic symptomatic peripheral diabetic neuropathy for 12 mo *(20)*. No difference in any peripheral nerve function measurements, including electrophysiology, were documented at the end of the study. As was expected, the drug was well-tolerated and no significant side effects were present during the study. Similar results were subsequently reported by Krentz et al. in a study with almost identical design *(21)*.

### *Tolrestat*

Tolrestat was the first ARI to be licensed for the treatment of diabetic neuropathy in certain countries all over the world including Italy, Mexico, and Ireland. Given orally, tolrestat is rapidly absorbed at a rate of 60–70%. Its plasma half life is 10 and, in clinical practice, a dose of 200 mg once a day is sufficient to provide satisfactory inhibition of the aldose reductase for 24 h. Excretion is mainly through the kidneys (70%), whereas a further 25% of the dose is excreted in the fees.

In a multicenter, double-blind, randomized, placebo-controlled trial that lasted for 12 mo, the efficacy of tolrestat on symptomatic neuropathy was studied in 556 patients with either type 1 or type 2 diabetes *(22)*. Inclusion criteria were stable or increasing severity of neuropathic symptoms, and abnormal motor or sensory-nerve electrophysiological measurements in at least three of six tested nerves. Patients were randomized to doses from 50 to 200 mg/d, and efficacy assessments included the response of the painful and paresthetic symptoms and electrophysiological measurements.

The painful symptoms improved in both the tolrestat and placebo-treated patients, but the paresthetic symptoms improved significantly in patients treated with 200 mg tolrestat daily over placebo. From the objective measurements, a significant improvement (up to 2 m/s) was noticed for the tibial and peroneal nerve conduction velocities when they were compared both to the baseline measurements and to the placebo-treated group. Improvement in both symptoms and electrophysiological measurements was found in 28% of tolrestat-treated patients, significantly higher when compared to the 5% of the placebo-treated patients who had a similar response. The adverse-reaction profile of the tolrestat was also satisfactory. The only symptom that occurred more frequently in the tolrestat group was dizziness. Elevation of transaminases was found in 13 (2.9%) diabetic patients treated with tolrestat on any dose, but the transaminases returned to normal levels within 8–16 wk after the drug was discontinued. There was no evidence of severe liver dysfunction in any of the patients. A small but significant drop of the blood pressure, up to 7 mmHg in the systolic and 3.4 mm in the diastolic was also noticed without any consequences. No hypersensitivity reactions similar to the ones that were present with other aldose reductase inhibitors were noticed.

The same design with the previous study was adopted by a multicenter European study that enrolled 190 patients with symptomatic diabetic neuropathy *(23)*. The study lasted for 6 mo and patients were randomized to take either placebo or tolrestat 200 mg once daily. The efficacy analysis included measurements of painful and paresthetic symptoms, vibration perception threshold in three sites, and nerve conduction velocities of four motor and two sensory nerves. No difference in the painful symptoms was found between the placebo and tolrestat group at the end of the study, although both groups improved compared to baseline measurements. In contrast, a significant improvement of paresthetic symptoms was noticed in the placebo group compared both to tolrestat group and to baseline measurements. Regarding the vibration perception threshold measurements, a significant change in favor of tolrestat-treated patients was found in one of the three sites it was measured (carpal site, which was located at the dorsum of the second metacarpal bone).

Significant increases in the motor conduction velocities in tolrestat-treated patients were recorded at the median nerve compared both to baseline (2 m/s) and to the placebo group, and in the ulnar nerve compared to baseline. When the changes of all motor conduction velocities were combined together, a significant improvement was found at the end of the study, compared to baseline measurements and to the placebo group. All the above changes were present only at the end of the study, after 24 wk of treatment. At the same time, 48% of the tolrestat-treated patients showed an improvement in three of the four motor-nerve conduction velocities, whereas in the placebo-treated patients, similar response was noticed in 28%. No changes in the two sensory-nerve function measurements were present at the end of the study, whereas the heart rate in the tolrestat group was slower compared to baseline measurements of the same group and to the placebo group. Six tolrestat-treated and two placebo-treated patients were discontinued from the study because of elevated liver enzymes.

A considerable number of patients who took part in the above studies continued to take the drug for several yr after the studies were completed and were the cohort of the subsequent trial that was designed as a randomized, double-blind, placebo-controlled withdrawal study *(24)*. Thus, 372 patients who had already received tolrestat for a mean period of 4.2 yr were randomly selected either to continue receiving tolrestat at a dose of 200 or 400 mg or to switch to placebo for 1 yr. Another interesting feature of the design of this trial was the fact that patients were given the option to change treatment on one occasion after the first 3 mo of the study without breaking the code and therefore, maintaining the double-blind design of the trial. The symptom score and the motor conduction velocities of four nerves were used as endpoints.

A significant deterioration of the symptom score was noticed at the 24th and 36th wk in the placebo group compared to the tolrestat group. However, at the end of the study, although a small difference still existed between the two groups, it failed to reach statistical significance. The conduction velocities of three out of the four motor nerves also deteriorated considerably in the patients who switched to placebo, whereas no change was noticed in the patients who continued on tolrestat. Thus, in the median nerve there was a drop of 0.9 m/s, in the ulnar 1.3 m/s, and in the peroneal 0.8 m/s, whereas the mean reduction of both nerves was 0.9 m/s. In addition, in patients who switched from tolrestat to placebo during the study there was a mean drop of 1.3 m/s for all four nerves, whereas in the patients who switched from placebo to tolrestat an improvement of 1 m/s was recorded. Therefore, a small but significant benefit of long-term treatment with tolrestat that can disappear when the treatment is discontinued, was the main finding of the above study.

In a parallel study, sural-nerve biopsies were obtained at the end of the above trial from 13 patients who continued to receive tolrestat and 14 patients who received placebo *(25)*. Morphometric analysis showed no difference between the above two groups but when compared to nerve biopsies from untreated neuropathic patients, both groups showed increased nerve-fiber regeneration. In addition, treatment with tolrestat was found to ameliorate the increase in the sorbitol and fructose levels in the nerve tissue, indicating that tolrestat can achieve satisfactory concentration levels in the peripheral nerves.

The following two trials with tolrestat were performed at the University of Naples and were both randomized, placebo-controlled, double-blind, parallel trials of 52 wk duration. The first one examined the effect of 200 mg/d tolrestat on patients with asymptomatic autonomic diabetic neuropathy, defined as at least one abnormal cardiovascular reflex *(26)*. At the end of the study, improvement in the tolrestat-treated group was found in all autonomic tests, which included deep breathing (E/I ratio), lying to standing (30/15) ratio, Valsalva (L/S ratio), and postural hypertension. In contrast to this improvement, a worsening in all the above parameters except the orthostatic hypotension was observed in the placebo-treated group. Similar results, namely an improvement in the tolrestat group and a worsening in the placebo group, were found in vibration perception threshold measurements, the only reported assessment of the peripheral somatic nerve function.

Similar results were reported in the second study that included patients with subclinical neuropathy, defined as abnormality in only one autonomic test, the squatting test *(27)*. Improvement was found in all the autonomic tests and the vibration perception thresholds in the tolrestat group, whereas a deterioration was observed in the placebo group in all but the orthostatic hypotension tests. Taken together, the above two studies emphasize the point that treatment of diabetic neuropathy with aldose reductase inhibitors may be most beneficial if it is initiated at the early stages of the disease, even before any symptoms are present. Despite the above promising results, tolrestat was subsequently withdrawn from clinical use in all countries in which it was licensed, and is no longer available.

### *Other Aldose Reductase Inhibitors*

Numerous other aldose reductase inhibitors are currently under investigation, either in preclinical or clinical trials. In particular, encouraging results have been reported in abstract form for two such compounds, zenarestat and zopolrestat *(28,29)*. Zenarestat was reported to improve nerve conduction velocities and nerve-fiber density in sural-nerve biopsies, whereas zopolrestat improved the nerve conduction velocities. It is hoped that more information will be available in the near future.

## GAMMA-LINOLENIC ACID

Gamma-linolenic acid (GLA) is produced from linolenic acid (LA) through the action of the delta-6-saturase enzyme in a rate-limited reaction. Further metabolism of the GLA leads to the production of prostagladins (such as thromboxane, PGE1, and prostacyclin), which regulate the blood flow and long-chain fatty acids that are essential components of the nerve axons and the myelin sheath. In diabetes, the conversion of LA to GLA is impaired and it has been suggested that the resulting deficiency of GLA and its metabolites play a role in the development of long-term diabetes complications including neuropathy *(30)*. Therefore, it was suggested that supplementation of GLA may be beneficial in treating diabetic neuropathy and the fact that no serious side effects should be expected, as GLA is a natural oil, made this option even more appealing.

The effect of supplementation of 360 mg of GLA daily, given as seed oil of evening primrose, was studied in a 6-mo, single-center, double-blind, randomized, placebo-controlled trial that included 22 diabetic neuropathic patients *(31)*. At the end of the study, significant improvement was found in a number of parameters, including the neuropathy symptoms score, the median-nerve conduction velocity (1.38 m/s), the peroneal-nerve conduction velocity (1.86 m/s), and the sural sensory-nerve action potential amplitude (0.42 V). As expected, no serious side effects were noticed during the study.

Similar results were reported in a subsequent multicenter, randomized, double-blind, placebo-controlled trial of GLA, also given as seed oil of evening primrose at a dose of 480 mg/d *(32)*. The duration of this study was 1 yr and included 111 diabetic patients with mild neuropathy. At the end of the study, significant improvement was found in 13 of the 16 studied parameters, including the median-nerve conduction velocity (2.37 m/s), the peroneal-nerve conduction velocity (2.23 m/s), and the sural-sensory-nerve action-potential amplitude (1.68 V). As there was a deterioration in the placebo group during the study, the difference between the GLA and placebo-treated groups was 4.51 m/s for the median-nerve conduction velocity, 4.09 m/s for the peroneal-nerve conduction velocity, and 2.64 V for the sural-sensory-nerve action potential amplitude. As with the previous study, no serious side effects were observed. A minor setback for this otherwise very successful trial was that patients in one center tended to do better than the rest and, if omitted from the analysis, the statistical significance was reduced or lost.

The results of another large multicenter, randomized, double-blind, placebo-controlled trial of GLA have recently been reported in abstract form *(32)*. According to these preliminary results, significant improvement after 1 yr of GLA treatment was present in 10 out of 28 clinical assessments, whereas differences between GLA and placebo-treated groups were in favor of GLA in 21 assessments.

In conclusion, GLA seems to combine efficacy and safety, which makes it a strong candidate for clinical use. Although it has not been approved for the treatment of diabetic neuropathy yet, these favorable results make it a strong candidate for acceptance in daily clinical practice.

## OTHER POTENTIAL TREATMENTS

A number of possible medications are currently under investigation for their possible role in treating diabetic neuropathy, including nerve growth factors, acetylcarnitine, omega-3 fatty acids, ACE inhibitors, and protein kinase C inhibitors. However, most of the currently available results come from experimental diabetes in animals and little is known about their efficacy in human diabetes. As the completion of clinical trials will require time and their use in clinical practice in the near future does not seem probable, a detailed discussion of these agents would be outside the scope of this work.

## CONCLUSIONS

Despite the initial encouraging results from trials conducted over the last 15 yr, aldose reductase inhibitors have not yet been established for the treatment of diabetic neuropathy. The main reasons for this are inconsistent results in subsequent trials and the unacceptable high rate of side effects associated with the initially tested compounds. The development of less toxic inhibitors and the results of large clinical trials, which are currently under way, with more focused selection criteria and more robust endpoints, such as sural-nerve biopsies, are expected to greatly enhance our knowledge about the efficacy of this strategy. Therefore, until this information is available, no final recommendation can be made about their daily use in clinical practice. Encouraging agents like the gamma-linolenic acid that are devoid of side effects may prove a successful alternative.

## REFERENCES

1. Dvornik D, Simard-Duquesne N, Krami M, Sestanj K, Gabbay KH, Kinoshita JH, Varma SD, Merola LO. Polyol accumulation in galactosemic and diabetic rats: control by an aldose reductase inhibitor. Science 1973;182:1146–1148.
2. Sarges R, Oates PJ. Aldose reductase inhibitors: recent developments. Prog Drug Res 1993;40:99–161.
3. Tomlinson DR, Willars GB, Carrington AL. Aldose reductase inhibitors and diabetic complications. Pharmacol Ther 1992;54:151–194.
4. Dyck PJ, O'Brian PC. Meaningful degrees of prevention or improvement of nerve conduction in controlled clinical trials of diabetic neuropathy. Diabetes Care 1989;12:649–652.
5. Culebras A, Alio J, Herrera JL, Lopez-Fraile IP. Effect of an aldose reductase inhibitor on diabetic peripheral neuropathy. Arch Neurol 1981;38:133,134.
6. Handelsman DJ, Turtle JR. Clinical trial of an aldose reductase inhibitor in diabetic neuropathy. Diabetes 1981;30:459–464.
7. Fagius J, Jameson S. Effects of aldose reductase inhibitor treatment in diabetic polyneuropathy a clinical and neurophysiological study. J Neurol Neurosurg Psychiatry 1981;44:991–1001.
8. Judzewitsch RG, Jaspan JB, Polonsky KS, Weinberg CR, Halter JB, Halar E, Pfeifer MA, Vukadinovic C, Bernstein L, Schneider M, Liang KY, Gabbay KH, Rubenstein AH, Porte D. Aldose reductase inhibition improves nerve conduction velocity in diabetic patients. N Engl J Med 1983;308:119–125.
9. Jaspan J, Maselli R, Herold K, Bartkus C. Treatment of severely painful diabetic neuropathy with an aldose reductase inhibitor: relief of pain and improved somatic and autonomic nerve function. Lancet 1983;ii:758–762.
10. Young RJ, Ewing DJ, Clarke BF. A controlled trial of sorbinil, an aldose reductase inhibitor, in chronic painful diabetic neuropathy. Diabetes 1983;32:938–942.
11. Lewin IG, O'Brien AD, Morgan MH, Corrall RJM. Clinical and neurophysiological studies with the aldose reductase inhibitor, sorbinil, in symptomatic diabetic neuropathy. Diabetologia 1984; 26:445–448.
12. Fagius J, Brattberg A, Jameson S, Berne C. Limited benefit of treatment of diabetic neuropathy with an aldose reductase inhibitor: a 24-week controlled trial. Diabetologia 1985;28:323–329.
13. O'Hare JP, Morgan MH, Alden P, Chissel S, O'Brien AD, Corrall RJM. Aldose reductase inhibition in diabetic neuropathy: clinical and neurophysiological studies of one year's treatment with sorbinil. Diabet Med 1988;5:537–542.
14. Guy RJC, Gilbey SG, Sheehy M, Asselman P, Watkins P. Diabetic neuropathy in the upper limb and the effect of twelve months sorbinil treatment. Diabetologia 1988;31:214–220.
15. Consensus Statement. Report and Recommendations of the San Antonio Conference on Diabetic Neuropathy. Diabetes 1988;37:1000–1004.
16. Sima AAF, Brill V, Nathaniel T, McEwen TA, Brown MB Lattimer SA, Greene DA. Regeneration and repair of myelinated fibres in sural nerve biopsy specimens from patients with diabetic neuropathy treated with sorbinil. N Engl J Med 1988;319:548–555.

17. Dyck PJ, Zimmerman BR, Vilen TH, Minnerath SR, Karnes JL, Yao JK, Poduslo JF. Nerve glucose, fructose, sorbitol, myo-inositol, and fiber degeneration and regeneration in diabetic neuropathy. N Engl J Med 1988;319:542–548.
18. Gill JS, Williams G, Ghatei MA, Hetreed AH, Mather HM, Bloom SR. Effect of the aldose reductase inhibitor, ponalrestat, on diabetic neuropathy. Diabetes Metab 1990;16:296–302.
19. Price DE, Alani SM, Wales JK. Effect of aldose reductase inhibition on resistance to ischemic conduction block in diabetic subjects. Diabetes Care 1991;14:411–413.
20. Ziegler D, Mayer P, Rathmann W, Gries FA. One-year treatment with the aldose reductase inhibitor, ponalrestat, in diabetic neuropathy. Diabetes Res Clin Pract 1991;14:63–73.
21. Krentz AJ, Honigsberger L, Ellis SH, Hardman M, Nattrass M. A 12-month randomized controlled study of the aldose reductase inhibitor ponalrestat in patients with chronic symptomatic diabetic neuropathy. Diabet Med 1992;9:463–468.
22. Boulton AJM, Levin S, Comstock J. A multicentre trial of the aldose reductase inhibitor, tolrestat, in patients with symptomatic diabetic neuropathy. Diabetologia 1990;33:431–437.
23. Macleod AF, Boulton AJM, Owens DR, Van Rooy P, Van Gerven JMA, MacRury S, Scarpello JHB, Segers O, Heller SR, Van der Veen EA. A multicentre trial of the aldose reductase inhibitor tolrestat in patients with symptomatic diabetic peripheral neuropathy. Diabete et Metab 1992;18:14–20.
24. Santiago JV, Sonksen PH, Boulton AJM, Macleod A, Beg M, Bochenek W, Graepel GJ, Conen B. Withdrawal of the aldose reductase inhibitor tolrestat in patients with diabetic neuropathy: Effect on nerve function. J Diab Comp 1993;7:170–178.
25. Sima AAF, Greene DA, Brown MB, Hohman TC, Hicks D, Graepel GJ, Bochenek WJ, Beg M, Gonen B. Effect of hyperglycemia and the aldose inhibitor tolrestat on sural nerve biochemistry and morphometry in advanced diabetic peripheral polyneuropathy. J Diab Comp 1993;7:157–169.
26. Giugliano D, Marfella R, Quatraro A, De Rosa N, Salvatore T, Cozzolino D, Ceriello A, Torella R. Tolrestat for mild diabetic neuropathy. A 52-week, randomized, placebo controlled trial. Ann Int Med 1993;118:7–11.
27. Giugliano D, Acampora R, Marfella R, Di Maro G, De Rosa N, Misso L, Ceriello A, Quatraro A, D'Onofrio F. Tolrestat in the primary prevention of diabetic neuropathy. Diabetes Care 1995;18: 536–541.
28. Greene DA, Arezzo J, Brown M. Dose-related effects of the aldose reductase inhibitor zenarestat on nerve sorbitol levels, nerve conduction velocity and nerve fiber density in human diabetic neuropathy. Diabetes 1996;45 (Suppl. 2):5A(abstract).
29. Greene DA, Arezzo JC, Klioze SS, Peterson MJ, Lakshminary MY. Results of phase II multicenter study of zopolrestat in patients with peripheral diabetic neuropathy. Diabetologia 1996;39 (Suppl. 1):A35(abstract).
30. Jamal GA. The use of gamma linolenic acid in the prevention and treatment of diabetic neuropathy. Diabetic Med 1994;11:145–149.
31. Jamal GA, Carmichael H. The effect of gamma-linolenic acid on human diabetic peripheral neuropathy: a double blind placebo controlled trial. Diabetic Med 1990;7:319–323.
32. Keen H, Payan J, Allawi J. Treatment of diabetic neuropathy with gamma-linolenic acid. Diabetes Care 1993;16:8–15.
33. Boulton AJM, Ziegler D, Scarpello J, Jamal GA, Keen H, Almer LO, Gamstedt A. A multicenter double-blind trial of gamolenic acid in diabetic peripheral sensorimotor neuropathy. Diabetologia 1997;40 (Suppl. 1):A32(abstract).

# 9 Painful Diabetic Neuropathy
## *Aetiology and Nonpharmacological Treatment*

*Solomon Tesfaye, MD, MRCP*

***Contents***



## INTRODUCTION

Pain is probably the most distressing symptom of diabetic neuropathy *(1)*. The features of pain in diabetic neuropathy were clearly documented by Pavy *(2)*, who observed, that it was of burning and unremitting quality often with a nocturnal exacerbation. Indeed the quality of neuropathic pain has been described as burning, shooting, lancinating, prickling, and aching in character, often with many of these symptoms manifesting in the same patient *(3)*. Some patients describe these symptoms as the feeling of walking barefoot on hot sand or pebbles. Others describe an odd sensation of their legs feeling swollen. The intensity of neuropathic pain is also variable among different individuals and often varies with time in the same individual. Some patients may have mild paresthesia in one or two toes; others may have intolerable unremitting pain involving both legs *(4)*. Most patients with chronic, painful neuropathy have a moderate background pain with relatively short intervals of peak neuropathic pain. Sleep is often disturbed because of the nocturnal exacerbation of these symptoms, in addition to allodynia (contact hypersensitivity to bed clothes) *(4)*. In some patients, neuropathic pain can be so disabling as to lead to loss of employment, reduction in exercise tolerance, and hence interference with daily activities, a reduction in recreational activities, and depression *(4,5)*.

Pain is not only a feature of acute and chronic symmetrical sensorimotor neuropathy occurring in a stocking distribution, but may also develop in relation to focal and multifocal neuropathy such as isolated lesions of cranial-nerve palsy, proximal lower-limb motor neuropathy affecting thighs, and truncal neuropathy *(6)*. Conventional treatment for painful diabetic neuropathy is largely symptomatic and frequently ineffective *(7)*. Although significant pain relief can be achieved in some patients by the use of tricyclic agents, the use of these compounds is frequently complicated by unacceptable side

From: *Contemporary Endocrinology: Clinical Management of Diabetic Neuropathy*
Edited by: A. Veves © Humana Press Inc., Totowa, NJ

effects *(7)*. In this chapter, we look at the possible mechanisms involved in the generation of neuropathic pain, and review the methods available for the assessment of pain in diabetic neuropathy. Finally, we discuss nonpharmacological treatments of painful diabetic neuropathy.

## MECHANISMS OF PAIN IN DIABETIC NEUROPATHY

Pain is an unpleasant, subjective sensory and emotional experience. Neuropathic pain is caused by dysfunction of the peripheral or central nervous system, that does not require any receptor stimulation. Painful symptoms are relayed by nociceptive, afferent small myelinated A-delta, and unmyelinated C fibers. Unmyelinated C fibers are thought to transmit the slower component of pain, whereas myelinated A-δ fibers relay the faster component.

The exact pathophysiological mechanisms underlying pain in diabetic neuropathy are not known *(8)*, although several workers have tried to provide a neuro-structural correlate for neuropathic pain *(9–11)*. Brown et al. *(12)*, found a predominant loss of small myelinated and unmyelinated fibers on nerve biopsy of patients with chronic painful diabetic neuropathy. Said et al. *(13)*, also found similar pathological changes in some of their patients with painful neuropathy. However, other workers have demonstrated degeneration of all nerve fiber sizes, both myelinated and unmyelinated, in subjects with painful neuropathy *(14–17)*. Some observers have suggested that a clear relationship between selective degeneration of fibers of certain size and the presence of neuropathic pain is unlikely by virtue of the fact that neuropathic pain is variable in intensity and may remit for variable periods *(18)*. This does imply that biochemical or vascular factors that are likely to vary with time, may be important in the generation of neuropathic pain, in the context of an already damaged nerve. As nerve biopsy studies do not give a dynamic view of nerve function, the author and colleagues have attempted to study human sural nerve in vivo, in subjects with relatively sudden-onset painful neuropathy *(18)*, by employing the techniques of nerve photography and fluorescein angiography. This study has suggested that vascular factors may be important contributing factors in the generation of neuropathic pain *(18)*. The following are some of the hypotheses put forward as possible mechanisms of neuropathic pain generation based on studies in humans and animal models with nerve injuries.

### *Ectopic Impulse Formation by Regenerative Sprouts*

Asbury and Fields *(19)* suggested that spontaneous ectopic impulse generation in regenerative sprouts (Fig. 1) could be the cause of neuropathic pain. The sprouting was thought to occur in small-diameter primary afferent fibers. Dandona et al. *(20)*, have also suggested that regenerative sprouts initiated by strict glycemic control may provide the explanation for treatment-induced painful neuropathy that occurs in previously poorly controlled diabetic subjects with asymptomatic small-fiber neuropathy. Fowler and Ochoa *(21)* demonstrated that when primary sensory afferents are damaged in rats, they develop axonal sprouts (Fig. 1). Animal experiments have shown that these regenerative sprouts have heightened mechano sensitivity *(22–24)*. This may be the explanation for Tinel's sign in which paresthesia in the distribution of peripheral nerve is elicited by a gentle tapping of a damaged regenerating nerve. Increased adrenergic chemosensitivity has also been found in axonal sprouts *(25)*. This may be secondary to the development to alpha receptors by neuroma sprouts *(25)*.

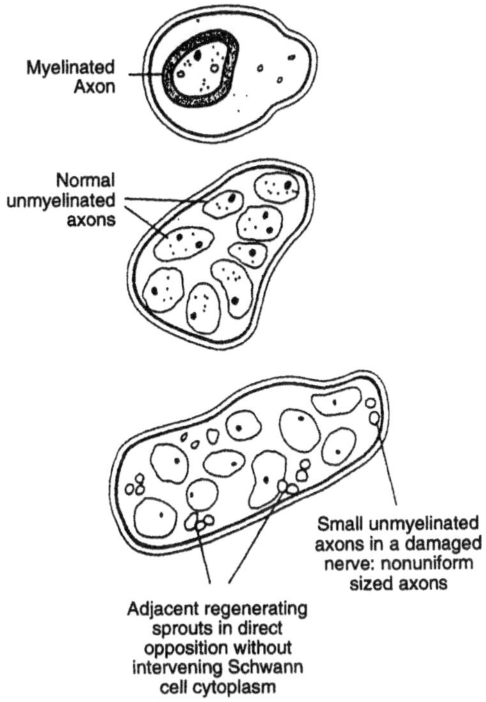


**Fig. 1.** Axon sprouting in an undamaged peripheral nerve. After Fowler and Ochoa (1975). (Reproduced from Diabetic Neuropathy, 1997, with permission).

However, recent studies in human diabetic neuropathy have not confirmed the ectopic impulse formation hypothesis of neuropathic pain generation, as degeneration of unmyelinated fibers was not confined to patients with neuropathic pain alone, but was also found in patients with painless neuropathy *(16)*.

### *Peripheral Nerve Ischemia*

Pain is usually caused by peripheral nerve ischemia, a feature of focal neuropathy such as cranial mono neuropathies, proximal-motor neuropathies, and truncal neuropathies *(26)*. The case for ischemia as cause of nerve damage is probably strongest in acute third-cranial-nerve palsy as the blood vessels supplying the nerve have been found to be diseased in association with a localized nerve pathology *(27)*. In addition, the rapid onset of the condition and the time course of recovery suggest an ischemic etiology.

Recent in vivo, human studies have shown the presence of active epineurial arterio-venous shunts in subjects with chronic painful neuropathy *(28)*. As pain usually accompanies acute ischemia, (e.g., claudication and angina) and in the absence of a clear structural correlate for neuropathic pain *(10,11,26)*, hemodynamic factors that are likely to change more rapidly may provide an explanation for neuropathic pain. Recently, patients with acute painful neuropathy of rapid glycemic control (insulin neuritis) in whom a transient severe painful neuropathy is precipitated with rapid improvement in metabolic control, have been studied *(18)*. These patients were found to have numerous epineurial arterio-venous shunts and a fine network of proliferating neural new vessels

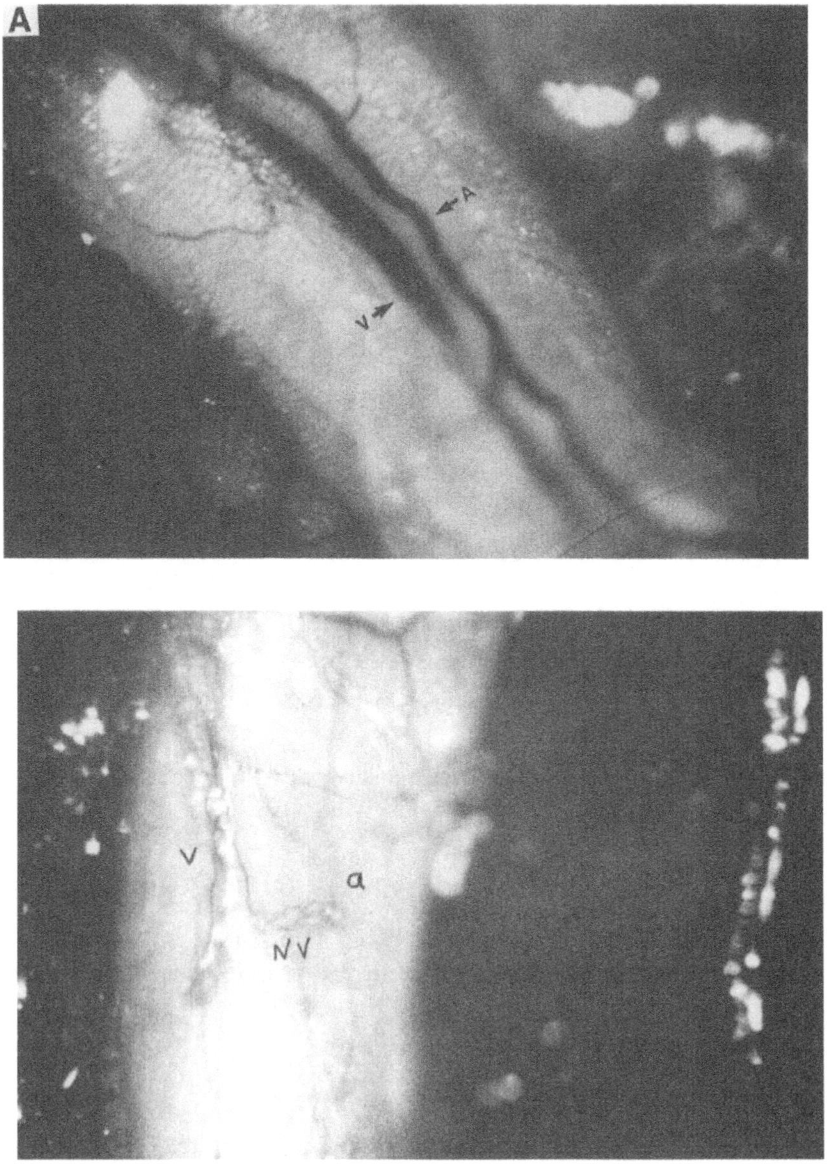


**Fig. 2.** (A) Sural-nerve epineurial arterial (A) and venous (V) anatomy in a normal subject. (B) A fine network of tortuous epineurial vessels resembling the new vessels (NV) of the retina in a subject with insulin neuritis who also developed retinal microinfarcts with rapid improvement in glycemic control.

that resembled those of the eye *(18)* (Fig. 2B). Excessive epineurial shunt flow that may render the endoneurium ischemic was suggested as a possible contributing factor for the generation of neuropathic pain *(18)*. As the neuropathic pain improves within 10 mo in this patients, it remains to be established whether these arterio-venous shunts close when the pain resolves.

### *The Role of Dorsal-Horn Neurons and Dorsal-Root Ganglia*

The gate control theory forwarded by Melzack and Wall *(29)* proposed that large-diameter myelinated-fiber activity (e.g., vibration sense) inhibits the activity of dorsal-horn neurons, gating the transmission of pain via C fibers. However, there is as yet no definitive evidence for a selective loss of large myelinated fibers in diabetic peripheral neuropathy *(16)*. The observation that loss of afferent input can increase activity of dorsal-horn cells leading to high frequency discharge *(30)* has prompted some observers to speculate whether this could provide an explanation for neuropathic pain. The observation that normal dorsal-root ganglia have marked mechanosensitivity *(31)*, and their spontaneous hyperactivity with damage to peripheral axons *(32)* have also led some to speculate that dorsal-root ganglia may be important in the generation of pain.

### *Blood Flow in the Neuropathic Leg*

It is now well-established that the neuropathic foot is warm because of an increase in peripheral blood flow associated with arterio-venous shunting *(33–36)*. The observations that neuropathic pain appears to be exacerbated by the increase in peripheral blood flow associated with poor metabolic control *(37)*, and the reduction in painful neuropathic symptoms via cooling of a limb and measures that reduce peripheral blood flow *(34)*, suggest that peripheral blood flow may be linked to painful neuropathic symptoms. Thus, one can speculate that raised lower-limb skin temperature may have an influence on the sensitivity of nociceptive sensory afferents.

A recent study has demonstrated that some subjects with severe diabetic neuropathy have limitation of exercise tolerance, principally as a result of painful symptoms on walking *(5)*. This is likened to "walking on pebbles" and appears to be distinct from spontaneous neuropathic pain *(5)*. This suggests that part of the neuropathic pain experienced from exertion may be caused by "neuro-claudication," which may be caused by blood being shunted away from peripheral nerve to surrounding tissue. This is supported by the observation that some neuropathic patients have a paradoxical fall in nerve conduction velocity following exercise, in contrast to nonneuropathic diabetic subjects, who have an increase in their nerve conduction velocity of 4 m/s *(38)*.

### *Chronic Hyperglycemia and Acute Glycemic Fluxes*

The glycemic state in which the damaged peripheral nerve functions may be important in the modulation of neuropathic pain for the following reasons:

1. Boulton et al. *(39)* reported that patients with symptomatic neuropathy have higher glycated hemoglobin at presentation compared to nonneuropathic diabetic subjects. This observation is supported by other cross-sectional epidemiological studies *(40)*.
2. Some patients present with acute painful neuropathy associated with poor metabolic control and precipitous weight loss *(15)*. This syndrome occurs in patients with variable duration of diabetes who present with burning pain, allodynia, and nocturnal exacerbation of symptoms (Table 1). Ellenberg described the condition as 'neuropathic cachexia' *(41)*. There is complete resolution of symptoms and weight gain within approx 10 mo, with sustained improvement in glycemic control achieved with insulin *(15)*. Steel et al. *(42)* also reported painful neuropathy in young anorexic women with poorly controlled insulin-dependent diabetes, which raised the possibility of whether nutritional deficiencies could account for the neuropathy. However, there is no convincing evidence for this

Table 1
Clinical Features of Acute Painful Neuropathies Associated with Rapid and Poor Glycemic Control

| *Acute Painful Neuropathy of Rapid Glycemic Control* | *Acute Painful Neuropathy of Poor Glycemic Control* |
|---|---|
| Occurs in IDDM and NIDDM | Occurs in IDDM and NIDDM |
| Burning pain, paresthesia, allodynia, nocturnal exacerbation of symptoms, depression | Burning pain, allodynia, impotence, nocturnal exacerbation of symptoms, depression |
| No weight loss | Severe and precipitous weight loss |
| Sensory loss mild or absent | Sensory loss mild or absent |
| No motor signs | No motor signs |
| Normal nerve conduction studies; impaired exercise-induced conduction velocity increment | Normal or mildly abnormal nerve conduction studies |
| Complete resolution of symptoms within 10 mo | Complete resolution of symptoms within 10 mo and weight gain with continued insulin treatment |
| Nerve biopsy: changes of chronic neuropathy with active regeneration | Nerve biopsy: degeneration of myelinated and unmyelinated fibers |

as vitamin supplements do not have any significant effect in diabetic neuropathy. Remission of pain occurred as weight was gained.

3. Painful neuropathic symptoms often improve with an improvement in metabolic control, sometimes achieved by the use of continuous subcutaneous insulin infusion *(43)*.
4. Morley et al. *(44)*, made the observation that glucose infusion led to a reduction in pain threshold in nondiabetic subjects, and also found a lower pain threshold and pain tolerance in diabetic compared to nondiabetic subjects. However, this assertion, has been challenged by a recent observation that acute hyperglycemia does not alter sensitivity to thermally induced pain *(45)*.
5. Sudden improvements in glycemic control, often with the use of insulin, in previously poorly controlled patients, can also lead to acute painful neuropathy within a few weeks *(18,46–49)* (Table 1). This syndrome was initially described by Caravati *(50)* who used the term 'insulin neuritis,' but as 'neuritis' implies an inflammatory process, a more appropriate term would be acute painful neuropathy of rapid glycaemic control *(18)*. Painful symptoms resolve with continued improved glycemic control within 10 mo in the same way as patients with acute painful neuropathy of poor glycaemic control (Table 1). The etiology of this condition is still undertermined, and although on face value, it would seem reasonable that it may be purely metabolic in origin, recent work showing the presence of neural new vessels (Fig. 2) similar to those found in the retina that can also result with rapid metabolic control *(51)*, suggest that hemodynamic factors may be important in the pathogenesis of this syndrome *(18)*. Table 1 shows clinical features of acute painful neuropathies associated with rapid and poor glycemic control.

## ASSESSMENT OF NEUROPATHIC PAIN

Chan et al. *(52)* reported that approx 7.5% of unselected adults attending hospital diabetic clinics have painful neuropathic symptoms, mainly in their lower limbs. In clinical practice, a careful history detailing the features of the pain is usually sufficient to ascertain the presence and severity of neuropathic pain. This should be accompanied with full neurological and vascular examination. Differential diagnoses such as lumbar-root pain, pain caused by spinal stenosis, pain caused by peripheral vascular disease, and musculoskeletal pain should be excluded. It is important to appreciate that neuropathic pain could rarely be from causes other than diabetes in the diabetic patient, and particularly excessive alcohol intake and neuropathies associated with malignancies and vitamin deficiencies need to be kept in mind. It is also important to remember that some patients may present with neuropathic pain in the absence of objective clinical or electrophysiological evidence of neuropathy, in contrast to some patients with advanced neuropathy who have neuropathic pain in association with numb feet—the so called "painful-painless foot" (53).

The fact that pain is a subjective experience has made it very difficult to quantify. The following methods are recommended for the assessment of the severity of pain in diabetic neuropathy, mainly for research purposes.

### *Visual-Analog and Verbal-Descriptive Scales*

The intensity of neuropathic pain can be assessed by visual-analog scale (VAS). The patient is asked to indicate pain intensity on a scale from 0–100, 0 indicating "no pain present" and 100 indicating "worst pain ever." The VAS score has been found to correlate with other measures of pain *(54)*. The VAS scoring method makes an assumption that equal intervals along the scale correspond to equal degrees of pain. The verbal-descriptive scale may also be used, the patient being asked to describe pain intensity with a series of descriptive statements (absent, slight, mild, moderate, intense, very intense, and so on).

### *McGill Pain Questionnaire*

The McGill Pain Questionnaire (MPQ) *(55)* was devised to assess both the quality and emotional aspects of pain (Table 2). The MPQ comprises four major categories and 20 subgroups: sensory (subgroups 1–10); affective (subgroups 11–15); evaluative (subgroup 16); and miscellaneous (subgroups 17–20). Table 2 shows the words in each of the 20 subgroups that are of similar quality and are also ranked by intensity (the word at the top has a value of 1, and the next word has a value of 2, and so on). The pain rating index (PRI) score is the sum of individual rank values and can be calculated for each category of the MPQ (e.g., sensory PRI, affective PRI).

### *Dyck's Neuropathy Staging*

Controversies exist as to what exactly constitutes diabetic neuropathy. Dyck *(56)* suggested that a number of factors that include symptoms (such as neuropathic pain, numbness, ataxia, paresthesae, motor and autonomic symptoms), physical signs on neurological examination, autonomic function tests, quantitative sensory tests, and electrophysiology need to be considered for a more accurate detection and characterization of diabetic neuropathy. The presence and extent of neuropathic pain is an important determining factor for staging of neuropathy *(56)*. Pain was graded as being "disabling" when the patient had previously attended a physician for pain relief, work and recreational activities had been curtailed by at least 25% because of pain, and medication for pain relief had been taken on a continuing basis (i.e., for more than 50% of the day) for at least 6 wk. Disabling pain would place the patient in Dyck's neuropathy score stage 3 as compared to stage 2 (pain of less severity).

Table 2
The McGill Pain Questionnaire

| | | | |
|---|---|---|---|
| 1. Flickering<br>Quivering<br>Pulsing<br>Throbbing<br>Beating<br>Pounding | 2. Jumping<br>Flashing<br>Shooting | 3. Pricking<br>Boring<br>Drilling<br>Stabbing<br>Lancinating | 4. Sharp<br>Cutting<br>Lacerating |
| 5. Pinching<br>Pressing<br>Gnawing<br>Cramping<br>Crushing | 6. Tugging<br>Pulling<br>Wrenching | 7. Hot<br>Burning<br>Scalding<br>Searing | 8. Tingling<br>Itching<br>Smarting<br>Stinging |
| 9. Dull<br>Sore<br>Hurting<br>Aching<br>Heavy | 10. Tender<br>Taut<br>Rasping<br>Splitting | 11. Tiring<br>Exhausting | 12. Sickening<br>Suffocating |
| 13. Fearful<br>Frightful<br>Terrifying | 14. Punishing<br>Gruelling<br>Cruel<br>Vicious<br>Killing | 15. Wretched<br>Blinding | 16. Annoying<br>Troublesome<br>Miserable<br>Intense<br>Unbearable |
| 17. Spreading<br>Radiating<br>Penetrating<br>Piercing | 18. Tight<br>Numb<br>Drawing<br>Squeezing<br>Tearing | 19. Cool<br>Cold<br>Freezing | 20. Nagging<br>Nauseating<br>Agonising<br>Dreadful<br>Torture |

Patients are asked to look carefully at each of the 20 groups of words and to circle one work in each group that most closely applies to their pain (if no word is appropriate, then none is circled).

## NONPHARMACOLOGICAL TREATMENTS OF PAINFUL DIABETIC NEUROPATHY

It has to be appreciated that there is no totally satisfactory treatment for pain in diabetic neuropathy *(5,7)*. This stems from our inadequate understanding of the pathogenesis of diabetic neuropathy *(8)*, although extensive research has implicated metabolic *(57)* and vascular mechanisms *(58–60)*. Whereas the search for potential therapeutic agents to halt or reverse the neuropathic process continues *(61,62)*, current treatment is largely aimed at relieving painful symptoms *(7)*. In this section, we will look at nonpharmacological treatment of painful diabetic neuropathy. Conventional drug treatment of painful diabetic neuropathy is usually necessary and, currently, tricyclic compounds are the most effective *(7)*, but many patients fail to respond to these agents and side effects are frequent. Other drugs include anticonvulsants *(63)*, mexiletine *(64)*, iv lignocaine *(65)*, and topical capsaicin *(66)*. Pharmacological treatment of painful diabetic neuropathy is covered in detail in the following chapter.

### *Psychological Support*

There is usually a psychological component to pain and psychological support and explanation of the condition to the patient in an empathetic way is, therefore, essential *(3,4)*. Some patients may have unnecessary worries that can be allayed by simple explanation of the condition in that even severe symptoms may remit, as is the case in those with acute painful neuropathies associated with poor glycemic control, or in those with rapid glycemic control who were previously poorly controlled (Table 1). Many experienced physicians have observed that psychological support of the patient may be sufficient to enable the patient to cope with mild neuropathic pain, and indeed researchers have also experienced that the intensity of neuropathic pain does sometimes improve when patients are seen regularly and examined and investigated in research projects, as patients feel that somebody has taken interest in their predicament. Moreover, several studies have shown that the placebo effect is quite marked in painful neuropathy *(66)*. Thus, the empathic approach that addresses the concerns, feelings, and anxieties of patients with neuropathic pain is essential for their successful management. Future research needs to address the impact of various models of counselling on the successful management of painful neuropathic symptoms as there are relatively few studies looking specifically into this.

### *Physical Measures*

Physical measures are often adopted by patients in order to relieve pain. These include measures designed to reduce lower limb temperature as the neuropathic leg is often warm because of arterio-venous shunting *(33–36)*. Cooling may reduce the abnormally increased shunt flow and thereby improve neuropathic pain. Patients often immerse their feet in cold water or sleep with their feet uncovered by bed clothes. Contact pain (allodynia) may be improved by wearing silk pyjamas, the use of a bed cradle, or covering painful areas with an adhesive film such as Opsite (Smith and Nephew Medical, Hull, UK) *(67)*. Some patients with moderate-to-severe neuropathic pain describe unpleasant sensory symptoms on walking likened to walking barefoot on pebbles. These patients may also benefit from the use of protective and comfortable shoes.

### *Glycemic control*

The Diabetes Control and Complications Trial *(68)* demonstrated that meticulous blood-sugar control delays the onset or prevents diabetic neuropathy. In addition, painful neuropathic symptoms can also be improved by tightening in metabolic control *(43)*, although these studies have been criticized on the basis of being unblinded. Nevertheless, as poor glycemic control is associated with acute painful neuropathy, it is generally felt that the first step in the management of painful neuropathic symptoms is to try to improve blood-glucose control, with the use of insulin in subjects with non-insulin-dependent diabetes if necessary. Support for this assertion comes from the work of Morley *(44)* who demonstrated that hyperglycemia does lower pain threshold, but this has subsequently been questioned by Chan et al. *(45)*.

### *Electrical Spinal-Cord Stimulation*

A significant proportion of patients with chronic neuropathic pain fail to respond to conventional drug treatment and indeed, some patients may not tolerate tricyclic agents and anticonvulsants, as these drugs may result in unacceptable side effects *(7)*. A recent study looked at the use of electrical spinal-cord stimulation (ESCS) for the treatment of

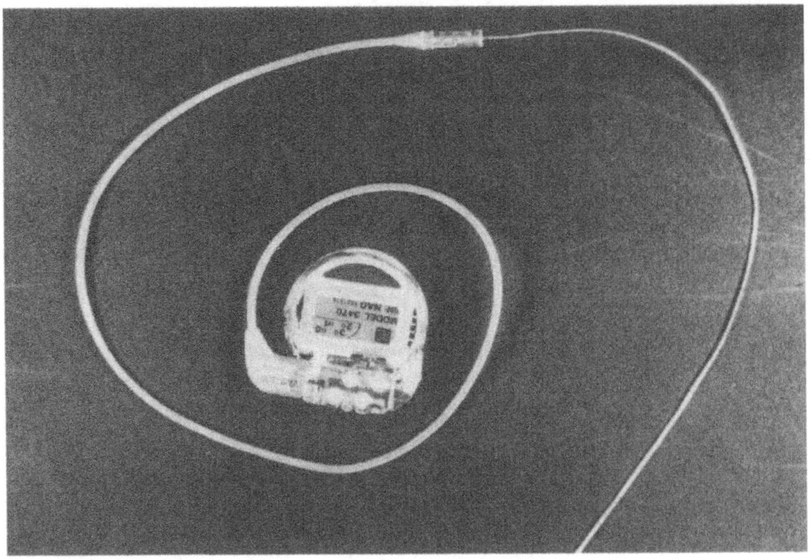

**Fig. 3.** Electrical spinal cord stimulator wire (PICES-Quad lead) that has four electrodes connected to an X-Trel receiver (permanent system) that is implanted in the anterior abdominal wall.

chronic diabetic neuropathic pain that does not respond to conventional drugs *(5)*. ESCS has been used for several painful conditions including back pain, phantom-limb pain, peripheral vascular disease, and severe angina, but this was the first study that specifically looked at its use in painful diabetic neuropathy. The study reported significant relief of both background and peak neuropathic pain over a period of 14 mo *(5)*. At the end of the study, 75% of patients fitted with the permanent system benefited from ESCS and used it as a sole treatment for their neuropathic pain, all pain-relieving drugs having been stopped. In addition to spontaneous dysesthetic pain, all the patients that took part in the study had unpleasant sensory symptoms on walking and half the patients could only manage 30 or less on a treadmill. The worst affected patients were more or less confined to home, unable to cope even with, for instance shopping, whereas others could not garden or dance. With ESCS, all the patients had an increase in exercise threshold with a median increase of over 150% at 6 mo *(5)*. Figure 3 depicts an ESCS wire connected to the X-Trel receiver (Medtronic, Watford, Herts, UK) and Fig. 4 shows an X-ray of a patient fitted with the permanent ESCS system.

Patient's selection is important and one has to be careful in assessing both the presence and severity of neuropathic pain. Psychological assessment of patients is also essential as ESCS seems to be more effective in those without major psychological overlay *(69,70)*. The best results from ESCS appear to be in those with well-localized pain, and those whose area of pain is covered with ESCS-induced paresthesiae *(71)*. Although fully blind studies are impossible, as the user feels a "buzzing" sensation over the area of pain, a placebo response is unlikely because of the sustained benefit obtained in some patients *(72)*. Also the need for accurate positioning of the electrode above the level of pain with the projection of paresthesiae over the whole area of pain to achieve pain relief, and observation that pain relief is lost immediately when there is lead displacement argues against the placebo response *(73)*.

The gate-control theory of pain has been suggested as an explanation *(29)* for the mechanisms of ESCS. Nocicepetive C fibers that carry painful stimuli relay at the sub-

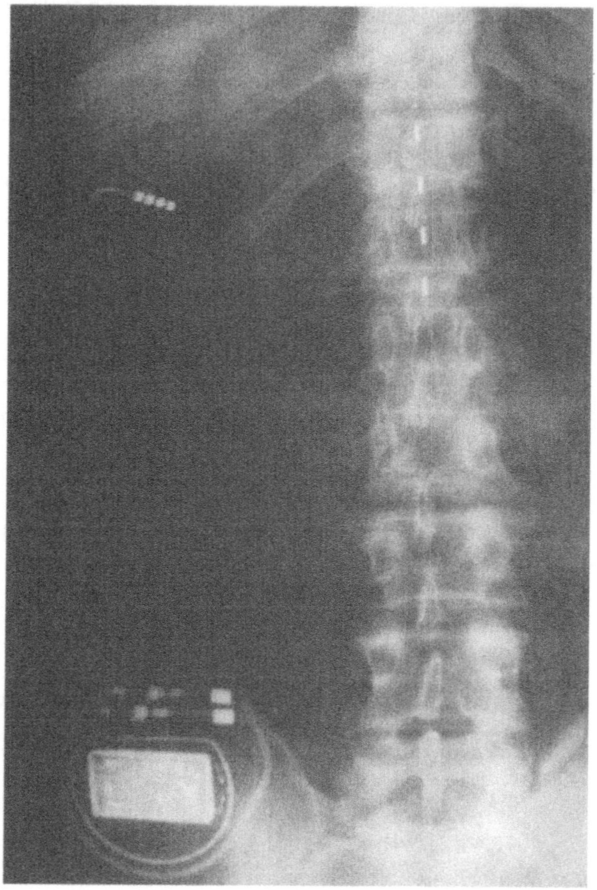

**Fig. 4.** An X-ray of a man fitted with electrical spinal cord stimulator wire that is situated midline in the epidural space, with the electrodes at the level of T11–T12. Under local anesthetic, the wire is introduced into the epidurial space at L1–L2, and using an image intensifier, the lead is manipulated so that the electrode lies exactly midline on the dorsal aspect of the spinal cord. The lead is connected to the X-Trel receiver implanted in the subcutaneous tissue in the right lower abdominal wall. The antenna of an external transmitter is placed over the X-Trel receiver and when patients have pain they switch on the transmitter, which uses a radio frequency signal that is converted by the X-Trel receiver into electrical current, leading to induced paresthesia over the area of pain.

stantia gelatinosa of the spinal cord to travel in the ascending contralateral anterior spinothalamic tract. ESCS is thought to stimulate the dorsal columns (A-beta fibers) that inhibit the C fibers and thus gating/interrupting the pain input *(29)*. With loss or gross dysfunction of the inhibitory A-beta fibers, ESCS is unlikely to work. This was the case in the two patients who failed to respond in the initial trial stimulation *(5)*. Thus elevation of vibration perception threshold to unrecordable range (or complete absence of vibration and joint position sense on clinical examination) may characterize patients who are unlikely to respond to ESCS. Although this initial study is very encouraging, larger studies conducted over longer periods are now required to firmly establish ESCS as the treatment of choice for painful diabetic neuropathy that does not respond to conventional therapy.

Transcutaneous electrical nerve stimulation has also been recommended in diabetic neuropathy *(73)*. In the author's opinion it is rarely effective, mainly because diabetic neuropathic pain is symmetrical and affects many nerves and thus is unlikely to respond to single-nerve stimulation.

## REFERENCES


1. Tesfaye S, Price DE. Therapeutic approaches in diabetic neuropathy and neuropathic pain. In: Boulton AJM, ed. Diabetic Neuropathy. Marius Press, Carnforth, Lanceshire, UK, 1997, pp. 159–181.
2. Pavy FW. Introductory address to the discussion on the clinical aspect of glycosuria. Lancet 1885;ii:1085–1087.
3. Young RJ. The management of diabetic neuropathy. In: Pickup J, Williams G, eds. Textbook of Diabetes, vol 2. Blackwell Science, Oxford, UK, 1997, pp. 51.1–51.13.
4. Watkins PJ. Pain and diabetic neuropathy. Br Med J 1984;288:168–169.
5. Tesfaye S, Watt J, Benbow SJ, Pang KA, Miles J, MacFarlane IA. Electrical spinal-cord stimulation for painful diabetic peripheral neuropathy. Lancet 1996;348:1696–1701.
6. Watkins PJ, Edmunds ME. Clinical features of diabetic neuropathy. In: Pickup J, Williams G, eds. Textbook of Diabetes, Vol 2. Blackwell Sciences, Oxford, UK, 1997, pp. 50.1–50.19.
7. Tesfaye S. Diabetic neuropathy: current treatment and potential therapeutic approaches. Diab Nutr Metab 1994;7:375–379.
8. Ward JD, Tesfaye S. Pathogenesis of human diabetic neuropathy. In: Pickup J, Williams G, eds. Textbook of Diabetes, Vol 2. Blackwell Sciences, Oxford, UK, 1997, pp. 49.1–49.19.
9. Editorial. Pain perception in diabetic neuropathy. Lancet 1985;i:83, 84.
10. Boulton AJM. Causes of neuropathic pain. Diabetic Med 1993;10(Suppl 2):87S–88S.
11. Young RJ. Structural functional interactions in the natural history of diabetic polyneuropathy: a key to the understanding of neuropathic pain? Diabetic Med 1993;10(Suppl 2):89S–90S.
12. Brown MJ, Martin JR, Asbury AK. Painful diabetic neuropathy: a morphometric study. Arch Neurol 1976;33:164–171.
13. Said G. Progressive centipetal degeneration of axons in small fibre diabetic neuropathy. Brain 1983;106:791–807.
14. Behse F, Buchthal F, Carlsen F. Nerve biopsy and conduction studies in diabetic neuropathy. J Neurol Neurosurg Psychiatry 1977;40:1072–1082.
15. Archer AG, Watkins PJ, Thomas PK, Sharma AK, Payan J. The natural history of acute painful neuropathy in diabetes mellitus. J Neurol Neurosurg Psychiatr 1983;26:491–499.
16. Britland ST, Young RJ, Sharma AK, Clarke BF. Association of painful and painless diabetic polyneuropathy with different patterns of nerve fibre degeneration and regeneration. Diabetes 1990;39:898–907.
17. Townsend CA, Malik RA, Thompson SD, Tesfaye S, Veves A, Sharma AK, Boulton AJM, Ward JD. Do neurophysiological and pathological abnormalities discriminate painful from painless human diabetic neuropathy? Diabetologia 1992; 35:A157.
18. Tesfaye S, Malik R, Harris N, Jakubowski JJ, Mody C, Rennie IG, Ward JD. Arterio-venous shunting and proliferating new vessels in acute painful neuropathy of rapid glycaemic control (insulin neuritis). Diabetologia 1996;39:329–335.
19. Asbury AK, Fields HL. Pain due to peripheral nerve damage: an hypothesis. Neurology 1984;34:1587–1590.
20. Dandona P, Fonseca V, Thomas PK, Llewelyn G, Bolger JP. Painful diabetic neuropathy. Lancet 1985;1:697.
21. Fowler TJ, Ochoa J. Unmyelinated fibres in normal and compressed peripheral nerves of the baboon: a quantitative electronmicroscopic study. Neuropathol Appl Neurobiol. 1975;1:247–265.
22. Scadding JW. Development of on going activity, mechanosensitivity and adrenaline sensitivity in severed peripheral nerve axons. Exp Neurol 1981;73:345–364.
23. Wall PD, Gutnick M. Ongoing activity in peripheral nerves: the physiology and pharmacology of impulses originating from a neuroma. Exp Neurol 1974;43:580–593.
24. Govrin-Lippman R, Devor M. Ongoing activity in severed nerves. Sources and variation with time. Brain Res 1978;159:406–410.
25. Korenman EMD, Devor M. Ectopic adrenergic sensitivity in damaged peripheral nerve axons in the rat. Exp Neurol 1981;72:63.
26. Thomas PK, Scadding JW. Treatment of pain in diabetic neuropathy. In: Dyck PJ, Thomas PK, Asbury AK, Winegrad AI, Porte D, eds. Diabetic Neuropathy. Saunders, Philadelphia, 1987, pp. 216–222.

27. Asbury AK. Focal and multifocal neuropathies of diabetes. In: Dyck PJ, Thomas PK, Asbury AK, Winegrad AI, Porte D, eds. Diabetic Neuropathy. Saunders, Philadelphia 1987, pp. 45–55.
28. Tesfaye S, Harris N, Jakubowski JJ, Mody C, Wilson RM, Rennie IG, Ward JD. Impaired blood flow and arterio-venous shunting in human diabetic neuropathy: a novel technique of nerve photography and fluorescein angiography. Diabetologia 1993;36:1266–1274.
29. Melzack R, Wall PD. Pain mechanisms: a new theory. Science 1965;150:971–979.
30. Loeser JD, Ward AA. Some effects of deafferentiation on neurons of the cat spinal cord. Arch Neurol 1967;17:629–636.
31. Howe JF, Loeser JD, Calvin WH. Mechanosensitivity of dorsal root ganglia and chronically injured axons: a physiological basis for the radicular pain of nerve root compression. Pain 1977;3:25–41.
32. Wall PD, Devor M. Sensory afferent impulses originate from dorsal root ganglia as well as from the periphery in normal and nerve injured rats. Pain 1983;17:321–339.
33. Boulton AJM, Scarpello JHB, Ward JD. Venous oxygenation in the diabetic neuropathic foot: evidence of arterio-venous shunting? Diabetologia 1982;22:6–8.
34. Edmunds ME, Roberts VC, Watkins PJ. Blood flow in the diabetic neuropathic foot. Diabetologia 1982;22:9–15.
35. Ward JD, Simms JM, Knight G, Boulton AJM, Sandler DA. Venous distension in the diabetic neuropathic foot (physical sign of arterio-venous shunting). J Roy Soc Med 1983;76:1011–1014.
36. Archer AG, Roberts VC, Watkins PJ. Blood flow patterns in painful diabetic neuropathy. Diabetologia 1984;27:563–567.
37. Mathiesen ER, Hilsted J, Feldt-Rasmussen B, Bonde-Petersen F, Christensen NJ, Parving H-H. The effect of metabolic control on haemodynamics in short-term insulin-dependent diabetic patients. Diabetes 1985;34:1301–1305.
38. Tesfaye S, Harris N, Wilson RM, Ward JD. Exercise induced conduction velocity increment: a marker of impaired nerve blood flow in diabetic neuropathy. Diabetologia 1992;35:155–159.
39. Boulton AJM, Hardisty CA, Worth RC, Drury J, Ward JD. Elevated glycosylated haemoglobin in diabetic neuropathy. Acta Diabet Lat 1982;19:345–349.
40. Tesfaye S, Stevens L, Stephenson J, Fuller JH, Plater M, Ionescu-Tirgovigtec, Nuber A, Pozza G, Ward JD. The prevalence of diabetic peripheral neuropathy and its relation to glycaemic control and potential risk factors: the EURODIAB IDDM Complications Study. Diabetologia 1996;39:1377–1384.
41. Ellenberg M. Diabetic neuropathic cachexia. Diabetes 1974;23:418–423.
42. Steel JM, Young RJ, Lloyd CG, Clark BF. Clinically apparent eating disorders in young diabetic women: associations with painful neuropathy and other complications. BMJ 1987;294:859–862.
43. Boulton AJM, Drury, Clarke B, Ward JD. Continuous subcutaneous insulin infusion in the management of painful diabetic neuropathy. Diabetes Care 1982;5:386–390.
44. Morley GK, Mooradian AD, Levine AL, Morley JE. Mechanisms of pain in diabetic peripheral neuropathy: effect of glucose on pain perception in humans. Am J Med 1984;77:79–82.
45. Chan AW, MacFarlane IA, Bowsher DR, Wells JCD. Does acute hyperglycaemia influence heat pain thresholds? J Neurol Neurosurg Psychiatr 1988;51:688–690.
46. Jordan WR. Neuritic manifestations in diabetes mellitus. Arch Intern Med 1936;57:308–366.
47. Martin MM. Diabetic neuropathy. Brain 1953;76:594–624.
48. Ellenberg M. Diabetic neuropathy precipitating after institution of diabetic control. Am J Med Sci 1958;236:466–471.
49. Llewelyn JG, Thomas PK, Fonseca V, King RHM, Dandona P. Acute painful diabetic neuropathy precipitated by strict glycaemic control. Acta Neuropathol (Berl) 1986;72:157–163.
50. Caravati CM. Insulin neuritis: a case report. Va Med Mon 1933;59:745–746.
51. Dandona P, Bolger J, Boag F, Abrams JD. Rapidly progressive retinopathy following strict diabetic control. B Med J 1985;290:845–896.
52. Chan AW, MacFarlane IA, Bowsher DR, Wells JC, Bessex C, Griffiths K. Chronic pain in patients with diabetes mellitus; comparison with non-diabetic population. Pain Clinic 1990;3:147–159.
53. Ward JD. The diabetic leg. Diabetologia 1982;22:141–147.
54. Scott J, Huskisson EC. Graphic representation of pain. Pain 1976;2:175–184.
55. The McGill Pain Questionnaire: major properties and scoring methods. Pain 1975;1:277–299.
56. Dyck PJ. Detection, characterisation, and staging of polyneuropathy. Muscle Nerve 1988;11:21–32.
57. Tomlinson DR. The pharmacology of diabetic neuropathy. Diab Metab Rev. 1992;8:67–84.
58. Tesfaye S, Malik R, Ward JD. Vascular factors in diabetic neuropathy. Diabetologia 1994;37:847–854.
59. Cameron NE, Cotter MA. The relationship of vascular changes and metabolic factors in diabetes mellitus and their role in the development of peripheral nerve complications. Diab Metab Rev 1994;10:189–224.

60. Malik RA, Tesfaye S, Thompson SD, Veves A, Hunter A, Sharma A, Ward JD, Boulton A. Transperineurial capillary abnormalities in the sural nerve of patients with diabetic neuropathy. Microvascular Res 1994;48:236–245.
61. Cameron NE, Cotter MA. Potential therapeutic approaches to the treatment or prevention of diabetic neuropathy. Diabetic Med 1993;10:593–605.
62. Reja A, Tesfaye S, Harris N, Ward JD. Improvement in nerve conduction and quantitative sensory tests after treatment with lisinopril. Diabetic Med 1995;12:307–309.
63. Wilton TD. Tegretol in the treatment of diabetic neuropathy. S Afr Med J 1974;48:869–872.
64. Dejgard A, Petersen P, Kastrup J. Mexiletine for the treatment of chronic painful diabetic neuropathy. Lancet 1988;ii:9–11.
65. Kastrup J, Angelo H, Petersen P, Dejgard A, Hilsted J. Treatment of chronic painful neuropathy with intravenous lidocaine infusion. B Med J 1986;292:173.
66. Capsaicin Study Group. The effect of treatment with capsaicin on daily activities of patients with painful diabetic neuropathy. Diabetes Care 1992;15:159–165.
67. Foster AV, Eaton C, McConville DO, Edmonds ME. Application of opsite film: a new and effective treatment for painful diabetic neuropathy. Diabetic Med 1994;11:768–772.
68. The Diabetes Control and Complications Trial Research Group. The effect of intensive treatment of diabetes on the development and progression of long-term complications in insulin dependent diabetes mellitus. N Engl J Med 1993;329:977–986.
69. Long DM, Erickson D, Campbell J, North R. Electrical stimulation of the spinal cord and peripheral nerves for pain control—10 years' experience. Applied Neurophysiology 1981;44:207–217.
70. Ray CHD. Implantation of spinal cord stimulators for relief of chronic and severe pain. In: Cauthen JC, ed. Lumbar Spine Surgery. Indications, Techniques, Failures and Alternatives, 2nd ed. William and Wilkins, Baltimore, 1988, pp. x–x.
71. Long DM, Erickson DE. Stimulation of the posterior columns of the spinal cord for the relief of intractable pain. Surgical Neurology 1975;4:134–141.
72. Simpson BA. Spinal cord stimulation in 60 cases of intractable pain. J Neurol Neurosurg Psychiatr 1991;54:196–199.
73. Watkins ES, Koeze TH. Spinal cord stimulation and pain relief. Br Med J 1993;307:462.
74. Thorsteinsson G. Management of painful diabetic neuropathy. JAMA 1977;238:2697.

# 10 Pharmacological Treatment of Painful Diabetic Neuropathy

*Dan Ziegler*, MD

*CONTENTS*



## INTRODUCTION

Pain is a subjective symptom of major clinical importance as it is often this complaint that motivates patients to seek healthcare. Pain is often associated with disability and is suggested as an important factor in affecting quality of life *(1)*. About 11% of the adult population has persistent pain and additional 5% experience temporary pain *(1)*. Neurogenic pain is defined as pain caused by dysfunction of the peripheral or central nervous system, in the absence of nociceptor (nerve terminal) stimulation by trauma or disease. Other terms used to describe some forms of neurogenic pain include neuropathic pain and deafferentation pain, and central pain. Neurogenic pain is common, accounting for at least 25% of the patients attending most pain clinics. When all categories of neurogenic pain syndromes are taken into account, there are probably >550,000 cases in the UK population at any one time, giving a prevalence of approx 1%. The incidence of neurogenic pain increases with age, accounting for one third of all pain-clinic patients aged >65 and one half of those aged >70 *(2)*.

People with diabetes experience more chronic pain than the nondiabetic population. It has been found that 25% of diabetic patients had chronic pain compared to 15% of nondiabetic subjects *(3)*. This difference is largely attributable to pain associated with neuropathy. Diabetic neuropathy has been defined as a demonstrable disorder, either clinically evident or subclinical, that occurs in the setting of diabetes without other causes for peripheral neuropathy and includes manifestations in the somatic and/or autonomic parts of the peripheral nervous system *(4)*. Diabetic peripheral neuropathy is encountered in at least one third of the patients with diabetes mellitus *(5)*. Neuropathic symptoms are present in 15 to 20% of the patients *(6,7)*, 7.5% of whom experience chronic neuropathic pain *(3)*.

From: *Contemporary Endocrinology: Clinical Management of Diabetic Neuropathy*
Edited by: A. Veves © Humana Press Inc., Totowa, NJ

## NEUROPATHIC PAIN

According to Asbury and Fields *(8)*, neuropathic pain may be subdivided into two types. The superficial *dysesthetic or deafferentation pain* is described as burning, tingling, raw, searing, crawling, drawing, and electric of variable constancy, i.e., intermittent, jabbing, lancinating, or shooting. It has been attributed to a cutaneous or subcutaneous distribution and may be linked to increased firing of damaged or abnormally excitable nociceptive fibers, particularly sprouting, regenerating fibers *(8)*. Dysesthetic pain is a common manifestation in diabetic polyneuropathy, particularly in those patients whose small-fiber modalities (cutaneous pin prick and temperature sensation and autonomic function) are disproportionately affected *(8)*. For the deep *nerve trunk pain* descriptors such as aching, occasionally knifelike, and tender have been used. It is usually continuous, but waxes and wanes. Its hypothetical basis includes increased firing caused by physiologic stimulation of endings of nociceptive afferents that innervate the nerve sheaths themselves (nervi nervorum) *(8)*. In addition, several other mechanisms have been proposed: spontaneous activity and increased mechanosensitivity near the cell body of damaged afferents in the dorsal root ganglion; loss of segmental inhibition of large myelinated fibers and small unmyelinated C-fibers (modified gate control hypothesis); and ectopic impulses generated from demyelinated patches of myelinated axons *(9)*. Examples for nerve-trunk pain include spinal-root compression, brachial neuritis, and neuritis of leprosy reactions. Asbury and Fields *(8)* emphasized that either type of pain rarely occurs in pure form and that most neuropathies associated with pain will manifest some mixture of these two types of painful experience.

In a model for the treatment of chronic painful diabetic neuropathy Pfeifer et al. *(9)* suggested *muscular pain* as a third type of pain that is described as a cramping, aching, muscle tenderness, or a drawing sensation. The muscle cramping and spasms may be secondary to injury to motor nerves or attributable to a reflex loop (Livingston's vicious circle), where a nociceptive input activates the motor neuron within the spinal cord leading to muscle spasm that in turn activates the muscle nociceptors and feed back to the spinal cord to sustain the spasm *(9)*.

According to Thomas and Scadding *(10)*, the putative mechanisms of pain in diabetic neuropathy include the following: nerve-trunk pain, sensitization of nociceptor endings, active axonal degeneration, damage to A-delta and C-fibers, neuroma properties (ectopic impulse generation from regenerating axon sprouts, ephaptic transmission), fiber shrinkage, ectopic impulse generation from dorsal-root ganglion cells after interruption of axons signaling pain, changes in peripheral blood flow, modulation of pain threshold by the glycemic state (hyperglycemic neuropathy), changes in the central nervous system secondary to peripheral nerve damage (reduced surround and presynaptic inhibition, deafferentation of dorsal horn neurons). This variety of possible underlying mechanisms of pain implies that different approaches to treatment may be required.

## PAINFUL DIABETIC NEUROPATHY

Since a classification of diabetic neuropathy based on pathogenetic grounds is not possible, the various manifestations have to be classified along clinical criteria. However, because of the variety of the clinical syndromes with possible overlaps not even a generally accepted classification exists. The most widely used approach has been proposed by Thomas *(11)* who uses a subdivision into diffuse symmetric polyneuropathies on the one hand and focal and multifocal neuropathies on the other. Pain may develop in both of these forms in which it can become one of the most unpleasant features of variable nature and distribution.

### *Diabetic Polyneuropathy*

The term "hyperglycemic neuropathy" has been used to describe sensory symptoms in poorly controlled diabetic patients that are rapidly reversible following institution of near-normoglycemia *(11)*. The most frequent form is the distal sensory symmetric polyneuropathy, commonly associated with autonomic involvement. The onset is insidious, and, in the absence of intervention, the course is chronic and progressive *(12)*. Persistent or episodic pain may be present in these patients usually in the feet or more diffusely in the legs, showing a characteristic nocturnal exacerbation. The pain is often described as a deep-seated aching, but there may be superimposed lancinating stabs or it may have a burning thermal quality *(11)*. Allodynia (pain caused by a stimulus that does not normally cause pain, e.g., stroking) may occur. The symptoms may be accompanied by sensory loss in a glove-and-stocking distribution, but patients with severe pain may have few clinical signs.

Pain may persist over several years *(13)* causing considerable disability and impaired quality of life in some patients *(14)*, whereas it remits partially or completely in others *(15,16)*, despite further deterioration in small-fiber function *(16)*. Pain remission tends to be associated with sudden metabolic change, short duration of pain or diabetes, preceding weight loss, and less severe sensory loss *(15,16)*.

### *Acute Painful Neuropathy*

Acute painful neuropathy has been described as a separate clinical entity *(17)*. The onset is associated with and preceded by precipitous and severe weight loss. The pain is of a continuous burning quality and experienced predominantly in the distal parts of the legs. Cutaneous contact discomfort (hyperalgesia) is often a troublesome feature, whereas motor function is preserved and sensory loss may be only slight, being greater for thermal than for vibration sensation. Depression and impotence are constant features. The weight loss has been shown to respond to adequate glycemic control, and the severe manifestations subsided within 10 mo in all cases. No recurrences were observed after follow-up periods of up to 6 yr *(17)*.

The syndrome of acute painful neuropathy seems to be equivalent to diabetic cachexia as described by Ellenberg *(18)*. It has also been described in girls with anorexia nervosa and diabetes in association with weight loss *(19)*.

The term insulin neuritis was used by Caravati *(20)* to describe a case with precipitation of acute painful neuropathy several weeks following the institution of insulin treatment (treatment-induced neuropathy). Sural-nerve biopsy shows signs of chronic neuropathy with prominent regenerative activity *(21)* as well as epineurial arteriovenous shunting and a fine network of vessels, resembling the new vessels of the retina, which may lead to a steal effect rendering the endoneurium ischemic *(22)*. This may happen in analogy to the transient deterioration of a pre-existing retinopathy following rapid improvement in glycemic control. Painful symptoms recover slowly with continued near-normoglycemic control. An association of the treatment-induced neuropathy with mitochondrial tRNA (Leu) mutation has been reported in five Japanese diabetic patients, but the underlying mechanisms are unknown *(23)*.

Short-term changes in blood glucose do not appear to play a major role in neuropathic pain. Marked fluctuations in spontaneous neuropathic pain within several hours were not associated with significant changes in blood glucose concentrations. Furthermore, the induction of acute hyperglycemia for 1 hour did not alter the heat-pain threshold in diabetic patients without symptomatic neuropathy *(24)*.

### *Focal and Multifocal Neuropathies*

Most of the focal and multifocal neuropathies tend to occur in long-term diabetic patients of middle age or older. The outlook for most of them is for recovery, either partial or complete, and for eventual resolution of the pain. With this in mind, physicians should always maintain an optimistic outlook in dealing with patients with these afflictions *(25)*.

Focal lesions of the third cranial nerve (diabetic ophthalmoplegia) are painful in approx 50% of the cases *(26)*. The onset is usually abrupt. The pain is felt behind and above the eye, and at times precedes the ptosis and diplopia (with sparing of pupillary function) by several days *(11)*. Oculomotor findings reach their nadir within a day or at most a few days, persist for several weeks, and then begin gradually to improve. Full resolution is the rule and generally takes place within 3–5 mo *(25)*.

Focal lesions affecting the limb nerves, most commonly the ulnar, median, radial, and peroneal may be painful, particularly if of acute onset, as may entrapment neuropathies such as the carpal tunnel syndrome that is associated with painful paresthesias *(11)*.

Pain is nearly universal in the syndrome of asymmetric lower-limb proximal-motor neuropathy (synonyms: Bruns-Garland syndrome, diabetic amyotrophy, proximal diabetic neuropathy, diabetic lumbosacral plexopathy, ischemic mononeuropathy multiplex, femoral-sciatic neuropathy, femoral neuropathy). Characteristically, it is deep, aching, constant, and severe, invariably worse at night, and may have a burning, raw quality. It is usually not frankly dysesthetic and cutaneous. Frequently, pain is first experienced in the lower back or buttock on the affected side, or may be felt as extending from hip to knee. Although severe and tenacious, the pain of proximal-motor neuropathy has a good prognosis. Concurrent distal sensory polyneuropathy is frequently present. Weight loss is also a frequently associated feature and may be as much as 35–40 lb. The weight is generally regained during the recovery phase *(25)*.

Patients with proximal or multifocal diabetic neuropathy show marked ischemic nerve lesions with vasculitis and inflammatory infiltration of mononuclear cells *(27,28)* and T-cells of the CD8+ cell type *(29)*. Activated endoneurial lymphocytes express immunoreactive cytokines and major histocompatibility class II antigens *(29)*. To classify these changes, Krendel *(30)* coined the term "diabetic inflammatory vasculopathy," which he describes as a "multifocal axonal neuropathy" caused by inflammatory vasculopathy, predominantly encountered in type 2 diabetic patients, indistinguishable from diabetic proximal neuropathy or mononeuritis multiplex. Separated from this form is the demyelinating neuropathy without vascular inflammation, predominantly encountered in type 1 diabetic patients, indistinguishable from chronic inflammatory demyelinating polyneuropathy (CIDP) *(31)*. These findings suggest that immunological mechanisms may be implicated in the pathogenesis of these neuropathies.

Diabetic truncal neuropathy (thoraco-abdominal neuropathy or radiculopathy) presents with an abrupt onset, with pain or dysesthesias being the heralding feature. Pain has been described as deep, aching, or boring, but also the descriptors of jabbing, burning, sensitive skin, or tearing have been used. The neuropathy is almost always unilateral or predominantly so. As a result, the pain felt in the chest or the abdomen may be confused with pain of pulmonary, cardiac, or gastrointestinal origin. Sometimes it may have a radicular or girdling quality, half encircling the trunk in a root-like distribution. Pain may be felt in one or several dermatomal distributions, and, almost universally, it is worst at night. Rarely, abdominal muscle herniation may occur predominantly in middle-aged men, involving 3–5 adjacent nerve roots between T6 and T12 *(32)*. The time from first symptom to the peak of the pain syndrome is often just a few days, although occasionally spread of the pain to adjacent dermatomes may continue for weeks or even months. Weight loss of 15–40 lb. occurs in >50% of the cases. The course of truncal neuropathy is favorable, and pain subsides within months with a maximum of 1.5–2 yr *(25)*.

## ASSESSMENT OF NEUROPATHIC PAIN

Quantitative assessment of pain is a challenging problem. This is exemplified by a statement of R. Melzack *(33)*. "Because pain is a private personal experience, it is impossible for us to know precisely what someone else's pain feels like." An important consequence of this simple statement is that there is no objective unit and no external gold standard for clinical pain, which instead constitutes the basis of any measuring method in use. In fact, pain is the result of a complex process involving neurophysiological and psychological mechanisms *(34)*. It has been shown that factors, such as cultural variables, can affect the perception of pain and its expression. Individual psychological attitudes and communication factors can influence the description of pain and the rating of its intensity by the patient *(34)*. During the last 20 yr, a number of reliable and valid measures for assessing chronic pain syndromes and evaluating treatment have been proposed and tested. Because of the multidisciplinary nature of the field, these measures have been derived from physiological, psychological (emotional, cognitive, and behavioral), sociocultural, and economic studies *(35)*. The following methods are being used in trials evaluating treatment effects on neuropathic pain in diabetic patients.

### *Visual-Analog Scale*

A visual-analog scale (VAS) is a straight line, the ends of which are defined as the extreme limits of the sensation or response to be measured. It has been shown that the VAS is a satisfactory method for measuring pain or pain relief. When assessing the response to treatment, it is better to use a pain-relief scale than to measure pain. With a pain-relief scale, all patients start at the same baseline and all have the same amount of potential response *(36)*.

### *Verbal-Descriptor Scale*

A verbal-descriptor scale (VDS) is a visual-analog scale with descriptive terms placed at intervals along the line. The descriptors may assist the patient in deciding the position of his score (especially if he has no experience of pain measurement) and make different patients more likely to record the same degree of severity in the same position *(36)*. Among different types of VDSs, a horizontal type with the words spread out along the whole length of the line performed best. The failure rate was slightly lower with the VDS than with the VAS *(36)*.

One way to ensure adequate sensitivity for analgesic trials is to test the intervention in patients who have pain of moderate-to-severe intensity. A recent study has shown that 85% of the patients reporting moderate pain scored >30 mm (mean: 49 mm) on a 100-mm VAS and 85% of those reporting severe pain scored >54 mm (mean: 75 mm). Thus, if a patient records >30 mm on a VAS score, he would probably have recorded at least moderate pain on a four-point VDS (no, mild, moderate, severe pain) *(37)*.

### *McGill Pain Questionnaire*

The McGill Pain Questionnaire (MPQ) consists of three major classes of word descriptors: *sensory* qualities (subclasses 1–10: temporal, spatial, pressure, thermal, brightness, dullness, and miscellaneous); *affective* qualities (subclasses 11–15: tension, autonomic, fear, punishment, and miscellaneous) that are part of the pain experience: *evaluative* words (subclass 16) that describe the subjective overall intensity of the total pain experience; and supplementary qualities (subclasses 17–20). The MPQ was designed to provide quantitative measures of clinical pain that can be treated statistically. The three major measures are (1) the *pain rating index* based on the rank values of the words that are then added up to obtain a score for each category, and a total score for each categories; the *number of words chosen*; and the *present pain intensity* based on a 1–5 intensity scale *(38)*. It has been shown that the MPQ is a useful aid to the differential diagnosis of the painful diabetic leg *(39)*.

### *Hamburg Pain Adjective List*

The Hamburg Pain Adjective List (HPAL) is another multidimensional, specific pain questionnaire that was introduced by Hoppe *(40)*. It includes 37 adjectives to describe pain "as it is usually." These adjectives are rated in seven steps ranging from "absolutely incorrect" (0 points) to "absolutely correct" (6 points). The items are summarized to four primary scales and three additional scales, respectively. Primary scales describe pain *suffering* by 12 items; *fear* of pain by 9 items; pain *acuity* by 9 items; and pain *rhythm* by 7 items. Pain suffering and fear of pain are allocated to the affective component (21 items), whereas pain acuity and pain rhythm are allocated to the sensory component (16 items). Affective and sensory components represent additional scales. The third additional scale is the total scale (37 items) that provides a measure of the general pain intensity.

### *Neuropathic Pain Scale*

Galer and Jensen *(41)* have recently argued that although VASs and VDSs have proven to be reliable and valid as measures of pain intensity and pain unpleasantness, these two pain dimensions do not adequately cover the domain of the neuropathic pain experience. A strength of the MPQ is that it does assess a variety of pain qualities, but although it can be scored to obtain global measures of the sensory, affective, and evaluative dimensions, it does not provide quantitation of each distinct pain quality. Another drawback of existing pain measures is that they do not identify potential subgroups of neuropathic pain that may benefit from specific therapies *(41)*. The Neuropathic Pain Scale (NPS) has been designed to assess distinct pain qualities associated with neuropathic pain. The NPS includes two items that assess the global dimensions of pain intensity and pain unpleasantness as well as eight items that assess specific qualities of neuropathic pain: sharp, hot, dull, cold, sensitive, itchy, deep, and surface pain. In addition, each item includes a description and other similar descriptive words for that item. Each of the 10 items has a 0 to 10 numerical score (0 = no, 10 = most). An eleventh item assess the temporal sequence of pain as constant with intermittent increases, intermittent, or constant with fluctuation. Preliminary validation of the NPS suggested discriminant and predictive validity, and all but one of the NPS items were sensitive to open-label treatment *(41)*. However, the NPS has not yet been used in randomized clinical trials on painful diabetic neuropathy.

## NONSPECIFIC EFFECTS OF PAIN TREATMENT

A number of nonspecific effects have to be considered in the interpretation of studies that deal with the treatment of pain. Two important nonspecific effects in this context are described below.

Patients with chronic regression to the mean conditions such as diabetic neuropathy seek medical care and enroll in research studies when symptoms are at their worst. Thus, the next change is likely to be an improvement. This tendency of extreme symptoms or findings to return toward the individual's more typical state is known as regression to the mean *(42,43)*.

### *Placebo Effects*

Placebo responses vary greatly and are frequently much higher than the often-cited one third. Individuals are not consistent in their placebo responses, and a placebo-responder personality has not been identified *(42)*. The true placebo effect has to be differentiated from the perceived placebo effect. The latter is a function of several factors including the true placebo effect and nonspecific effects including the natural history, regression towards the mean, and other time effects (e.g., increase of skill of the investigator) and unidentified parallel interventions (e.g., sensitization of the patient to the problem after inclusion in a trial). In order to obtain the true placebo effect in clinical trials, the nonspecific effects can be identified by including an untreated control group *(44)*.

Placebo effects on pain have repeatedly been shown to be greater than those on other symptoms *(45)*. However, placebo effects may not only affect subjective variables, but also objectively quantifiable ones *(44)*. Placebo effects in conjunction with the natural history of the disease and regression to the mean can result in high rates of good outcomes, which may be misattributed to specific treatment effects *(42,44)*.

Recently, some authors argued that placebo-controlled trials should no longer be part of the gold standard for assessing the efficacy of a new drug. As medical knowledge accumulates, these trials should become infrequent, because when an efficacious treatment already exists, it is unethical to assign placebo treatment to patients *(46)*. In such situations, one solution is to use an existing drug for the same disease as an active comparison in an equivalence trial *(46,47)*. Such trials generally need to be larger than placebo-controlled trials, their standard of conduct needs to be especially high, the handling of withdrawals, losses, and protocol deviations needs more care than usual, and different approaches to analysis and interpretation are appropriate. For example, analysis strategies to deal with unavoidable problems should not center on an intention-to-treat (as randomized) analysis but should seek to show the similarity from a range of approaches *(47)*.

## NUMBER NEEDED TO TREAT

The relative benefit of an active treatment over a control is usually expressed as the relative risk, the relative-risk reduction, or the odds ratio *(48)*. However, to estimate the extent of a therapeutic effect (i.e., pain relief) that can be translated into clinical practice, it is useful to apply a simple number measure that serves the physician to select the appropriate treatment for the individual patient. Such a practical measure is the number "needed to treat" (NNT), i.e., the number of patients that need to be treated with a particular therapy to observe a clinically relevant effect or adverse event in one patient *(48–50)*. This measure is expressed as the reciprocal of the absolute risk reduction, i.e., the difference between the proportion of events in the control group (Pc) and the proportion of events in the intervention group (Pi): NNT = 1/(Pc-Pi). The NNT for several classes of drugs used in the treatment of painful diabetic neuropathy has been calculated in recent meta-analyses *(51)*.

## TREATMENT OF PAINFUL DIABETIC NEUROPATHY

Painful symptoms in distal sensory neuropathy may constitute a considerable management problem. The efficacy of a single therapeutic agent is not the rule, and simple analgesics are usually inadequate to control the pain. Therefore, various therapeutic schemes have been previously proposed *(9,52,53)*. A six-step rational therapeutic algorithm based on the current evidence is shown in Table 1.

### *Causal Treatment Aimed at Near-Normoglycemia*

Three long-term prospective glycemic control studies including type 1 diabetic patients and one including type 2 diabetic patients either with mild retinopathy or without evidence of diabetic complications have recently been published *(54–59)*. However, these studies were neither primarily designed to establish the effects of near-normoglycemia on diabetic neuropathy, nor did they include sufficient numbers of patients with painful neuropathy. The Diabetes Control and Complications Trial (DCCT) conducted over approx 5 yr *(54,55)*, the Stockholm Diabetes Intervention Study (SDIS) over 7.5 and 10 yr *(56,57)*, the Oslo Study over 8 yr *(58)*, and the Kumamoto Study over 6 yr *(59)* have demonstrated that long-term near-normoglycemia prevents the development of neuropathy and retards the deterioration in motor and sensory nerve conduction velocity (NCV). However, a certain degree of neuropathy was also observed in the well-controlled groups, suggesting that by using the current methods of intensive insulin therapy, complete prevention of this complication is difficult to achieve. Other studies have shown that symptoms of diabetic neuropathy including pain may be improved and prevented by long-term near-normal glycemic control *(60,61)*, but pain was not used as a primary inclusion criterion.

Pancreas transplantation is the most effective method in achieveing long-term normoglycemia in type 1 diabetic patients, but is usually limited to patients with end-stage diabetic nephropathy in combination with a renal graft. Other indications have been questioned *(62)*. Four long-term studies in type 1 diabetic patients with established diabetic polyneuropathy who underwent successful pancreatic transplantation have recently been published. Kennedy et al. *(63)* have shown that 42 mo after transplantation the neuropathy was only slightly improved, but a significant difference was seen in the mean motor and sensory index in the transplanted group compared with a control

Table 1
Six-Step Algorithm for Treatment of Painful Diabetic Neuropathy

| *Step* | *Compound/ Measure* | *Dose Per Day* | *Remarks* |
|---|---|---|---|
| I: Near-normoglycemia | Diet, insulin, OAA | Individual adaptation | Aim: $HbA_{1c}$ <6.5 |
| II: Pathogenetically oriented treatment | α-Lipoic acid (thioctic acid) | 600 mg iv infusion | Duration: 3 wk<br>Rarely AE |
| III: ST, minor AE | Capsaicin (0,075%) cream | 4× topically | Duration: 8 wk |
| IV: ST, major AE | *Tricyclic antidepressants (TA)* | | |
| | Amitriptyline | (10–)25–150 mg | TA of 1st choice |
| | Desipramine | (10–)25–150 mg | Less AE |
| | Imipramine | (10–)25–150 mg | Variable effect |
| | Clomipramine | (10–)25–150 mg | Few data |
| IV: ST, alternatively if TA cause AE | *SSRI* | | |
| | Citalopram | 40 mg | Few data |
| | Paroxetine | 40 mg | Effect < than TA |
| IV: ST, alternatively if TA cause AE | *Anticonvulsants* | | |
| | Carbamazepine | 200–800 mg | Many AE |
| V: ST, medical last choice | Mexiletine | 450 mg | ECG monitoring |
| | Tramadol | 50–400 mg | Many AE |
| VI: ST, pain resistant to treatment | Electrical spinal cord stimulation (ESCS) | | Invasive, complications |
| Complementary: Physical therapy | TENS, medical | No AE | |
| | gymnastics, | No AE | |
| | Balneotherapy, | No AE | |
| | relaxation therapy | No AE | |
| | Acupuncture | Uncontrolled study | |

OAA: oral antidiabetic agents; TENS: transcutaneous electrical nerve stimulation; AE: adverse events; SSRI: selective serotonin reuptake inhibitors; ST: symptomatic treatment.

group that did not have a functioning graft after 42 mo. Improvement was more pronounced when only mild dysfunction was present initially. Solders et al. *(64)* found beneficial effects of combined pancreatic and renal transplantation on NCV after 4 yr of normoglycemia. The initial improvement in motor NCV observed in these patients was also noted in diabetic patients receiving a renal transplant only, and was most likely caused by the elimination of uremia. However, further improvement was seen only in the euglycemic pancreas-graft recipients. None of the beneficial effects on NCV described in these studies were demonstrable after 2 yr. Thus, periods of normoglycemia of up to about 2 yr are too short to influence established nerve conduction deficits, but longer-term normoglycemia may retard their further progression.

Pancreas-graft failure is associated with a deterioration in NCV to the pretransplant levels after 2 yr *(65)*. In contrast, controversial results have been reported regarding neuropathic symptoms. Müller-Felber et al. *(66)* observed a significant improvement in the neuropathic symptom score (NSS) from 1.7 to 0.6 after 3 yr in patients who underwent successful pancreas and kidney transplantation, whereas NSS did not change in those with early pancreas rejection and functioning kidney graft. However, Allen et al. *(67)* recently reported a nonsignificant decrease in the NSS from 0.43 to 0.39 in patients with combined pancreas-kidney transplants after up to 8 yr. Thus, unequivocal evidence from appropriately designed long-term studies to support the finding from earlier uncontrolled short-term studies that intensive insulin therapy is associated with a significant reduction in neuropathic pain *(68)* is still lacking. Nonetheless, intensive diabetes therapy aimed at near-normoglycemia is considered the first step in the treatment of any form and stage of diabetic neuropathy (Table 1).

### *Treatment Based on Pathogenetic Considerations*

A variety of experimental studies have provided new insights in the putative mechanisms implicated in the pathogenesis of diabetic neuropathy *(69,70)*. The following pharmacological treatment approaches have been developed to correct the underlying abnormality in the diabetic nerve (Table 2):

1. Aldose reductase inhibitors (ARIs) to reduce the enhanced flux through the polyol pathway *(71,72)*.
2. *myo*-Inositol to correct *myo*-inositol depletion *(73)*.
3. Gamma-linolenic acid (GLA) contained in evening primrose oil to prevent abnormalities in essential fatty acid and prostanoid metabolism *(74,75)*.
4. Antioxidants (α-lipoic acid) to reduce free-radical-mediated oxidative stress *(76,77)*.
5. Vasodilators (ACE inhibitors, prostacyclin analogs) to increase nerve blood flow and prevent hypoxia *(78,79)*.
6. Nerve growth factor (NGF) to prevent deficits in neurotrophism and axonal transport *(80,81)*.
7. Immunosuppresants, corticosteroids, and iv immunoglobulins to treat the inflammatory components associated with proximal diabetic neuropathy *(29–31)*.
8. Aminoguanidine to inhibit nonenzymatic advanced glycation end product (AGE) formation *(82)*.

Since in the near future the majority of diabetic patients presumably will not achieve near-normoglycemia, the advantage of the aforementioned treatments is that they may be effective despite the presence of hyperglycemia.

### *Gamma-Linolenic Acid*

Two multicenter trials of gamma-linolenic acid (GLA) have demonstrated improvement in neuropathic deficits and NCV after 1 yr of treatment in diabetic peripheral neuropathy *(75)*. However, in these studies, neuropathic pain has not been assessed. In one center participating in the second trial, the three major symptoms (pain, paresthesias, and numbness) were evaluated using VASs. Paresthesias and numbness but not pain

Table 2
Treatment of Diabetic Neuropathy Based on Putative Pathogenetic Mechanisms

| *Abnormality* | *Compound* | *Aim of Treatment* | *Status of RCTs* |
|---|---|---|---|
| Polyol pathway ↑ | Aldose reductase inhibitors: | Nerve sorbitol ↓ | |
| | sorbinil, tolrestat | | Withdrawn (AE!) |
| | ponalrestat | | Ineffective |
| | zopolrestat, | | Continuing |
| | zenarestat | | Continuing |
| | epalrestat | | Equivocal |
| *myo*-Inositol ↑ | *myo*-Inositol | Nerve *myo*-inositol ↑ | Equivocal |
| GLA synthesis ↓ | Gamma-linolenic acid (GLA) | EFA metabolism ↑ | Effective (deficits) |
| Oxidative stress ↑ | α-Lipoic acid | Oxygen free radicals ↓ | Effective (symptoms) |
| Nerve hypoxia ↑ | Vasodilators (ACE-Inhib., $PGE_2$) | Endoneurial blood flow ↑ | Continuing |
| ↑ | | | |
| Neurotrophism ↓ | Nerve growth factor (NGF) | Nerve regeneration, growth ↑ | Continuing |
| NEG ↑ | Aminoguanidine | AGE accumulation ↓ | Withdrawn |

NEG: nonenzymatic glycation; AGE: advanced glycation end products; EFA: essential fatty acids; AE: adverse events; RCTs: randomized clinical trials.

were significantly reduced after 1 yr in the group treated with GLA, but not in the placebo group *(83)*. Since no studies are available that examined the effects of GLA in diabetic patients with neuropathic pain as the primary inclusion criterion, it is not known whether the drug is useful in these patients.

### *α-Lipoic Acid (Thioctic Acid)*

There is accumulating evidence suggesting that free-radical-mediated oxidative stress is implicated in the pathogenesis of diabetic neuropathy by inducing neurovascular defects that result in endoneurial hypoxia and subsequent nerve dysfunction *(69)*. Antioxidant treatment with α-lipoic acid has been shown to prevent these abnormalities in experimental diabetes *(84)*, thus providing a rationale for a potential therapeutic value in diabetic patients. In Germany, α-lipoic acid has been licensed and used for treatment of symptomatic diabetic neuropathy for more than 25 yr. A 3-wk multicenter, randomized, double-blind placebo-controlled trial (**A**lpha-**L**ipoic **A**cid in **D**iabetic **N**europathy: ALADIN) has demonstrated that the infusion of α-lipoic acid (600 mg iv per day) over 3 wk (5-5-4 d) results in a significant reduction of the individual neuropathic symptoms (pain, burning, paresthesiae, and numbness) and the total symptom score (TSS) as compared with infusions containing placebo or 100 mg α-lipoic acid, without causing significant adverse reactions. The pain intensity in both the affective and sensory scales of the HPAL declined significantly by $-1.6 \pm 0.3$ and $-1.1 \pm 0.2$ points in patients treated with 600 mg α-lipoic acid as compared with $-0.5 \pm 0.1$ and $-0.4 \pm 0.1$ points in those on placebo, but the reduction by $-0.6 \pm 0.1$ and $-0.6 \pm 0.1$ points in those given 100 mg α-lipoic acid was similar to the placebo response *(76)*.

Table 3
Meta-Analyses of Medical Treatments for Painful Diabetic Neuropathy

| | *Antidepressants* | *Carbamazepine* | *Topical Capsaicin* | *α-Lipoic Acid* |
|---|---|---|---|---|
| Number of RCTs Study | 13 | 2 | 4 | ALADIN |
| Number of patients | 465 | 70 | 309 | 326 |
| Outcome measure | >50% pain relief | pain relief | analgesic efficacy | >30% symptom relief (TSS) |
| Number needed to treat (NNT) | 2.9 | 3.3/1.8 | 4.2 | 4.0 |
| NNT for minor adverse events | 2.8 | 1.9 | | ∞ |
| NNT for major adverse events | 19 | 15 | | ∞ |

Modified after McQuay and Moore *(51)*.
TSS: Total Symptom Score (pain, burning, paresthesia, numbness); RCTs: randomized clinical trials.

In the ALADIN study, the NNT was 4.0 for a ≤30% reduction in the TSS after 3 wk of iv infusion of 600 mg α-lipoic acid as compared with placebo (Table 3). This is comparable with the NNT estimated for the effective drugs in the symptomatic treatment of painful neuropathy. Since the infusion of α-lipoic acid (600 mg iv, for 30 min over 3 wk) is not accompanied by significant adverse reactions, this remedy can be recommended for the initial treatment of painful symptoms in diabetic neuropathy (Table 1).

Favorable effects of α-lipoic acid (800 mg/d orally) given for 4 mo on reduced HRV in diabetic patients with cardiac autonomic neuropathy have been shown in another randomized controlled trial (DEKAN Study) *(77)*. An ongoing multicenter trial in Germany is currently evaluating the efficacy of sequential treatment with α-lipoic acid (3 wk iv followed by 6 mo oral treatment) on neuropathic symptoms and deficits. Two large international multicenter trials have been recently started to confirm the results of the ALADIN Study (NATHAN 2 Study) and to evaluate the efficacy and safety of long-term treatment with α-lipoic acid over 4 yr on neuropathic deficits (NATHAN 1 Study) *(85)*.

## *Symptomatic Treatment*

### Topical Capsaicin

Since α-lipoic acid is currently licensed only in Germany, elsewhere capsaicin cream (0.075%) can be employed at step III (symptomatic treatment; Table 1) if painful symptoms persist despite near-normal glycemic control, or if the latter is not achievable. Capsaicin (trans-8-methyl-*N*-vanillyl-6-nonenamide) is an alkaloid and the most pungent ingredient in the red pepper. It depletes tissues of substance P and reduces neurogenic plasma extravasation, the flare response, and chemically induced pain. Substance P is present in afferent neurons innervating skin, mainly in polymodal nociceptors, and is considered the primary neurotransmitter of painful stimuli from the periphery to the

Table 4
Effects of Topical Capsaicin (0.075%) in Painful Diabetic Neuropathy

| *Reference* | *n* | *Duration (weeks)* | *Pain Relief (%)* | *Improvement in QOL* | *QST* |
|---|---|---|---|---|---|
| Chad et al. 1990 *(87)* | 58 | 4 | 71 vs 41%[a] | n.d. | n.d. |
| Scheffler et al. 1991 *(88)* | 54 | 8 | 89 vs 50%[a] | n.d. | n.d. |
| Basha et al. 1991 *(89)* | 15 | 8 | 100 vs 57% | n.d. | n.d. |
| Capsaicin Study Group, 1992 *(90)* | 277 | 8 | 60 vs 45%[a] | n.d. | n.d. |
| Capsaicin Study Group, 1992 *(91)* | 277 | 8 | n.d. | 18–30 vs 11–20%[b] | n.d. |
| Tandan et al. 1992 *(92)* | 22 | 8 | 64 vs 18% | n.d. | T/VPT= |
| Biesbroeck et al. 1995 *(93)*[c] | 235 | 8 | 76 vs 76% | 57 vs 59%[d] | n.d. |
| Low et al. 1995 *(86)*[e] | 40 | 12 | 59 vs 67% | n.d. | T/VPT= |

[a] $p < 0.05$ vs vehicle cream.
[b] ability to work (18 vs 11%), sleep (30 vs 20%), walk (27 vs 15%; all $p < 0.05$).
[c] capsaicin vs amitriptyline.
[d] improvement of sleep.
[e] different causes of neuropathy (idiopathic: $n = 20$; diabetic: $n = 7$).
QST: quantitative sensory testing, T/VPT: thermal/vibration perception threshold, n.d.: not determined; = no change; QOL: quality of life.

central nervous system *(86)*. Several recent studies have demonstrated significant pain reduction and improvement in quality of life in diabetic patients with painful neuropathy after 8 wk of treatment *(87–93)* (Table 4). On the basis of a meta-analysis of four controlled trials *(94)* the NNT for capsaicin is 4.2 for analgesic effectiveness as ascertained by the physician *(51)* (Table 3). However, it has been criticized that a double-blind design is not feasible for topical capsaicin because of the transient local hyperalgesia (usually mild burning sensation in >50% of the cases) it may produce as a typical adverse event *(11,94)*. Treatment should be restricted to a maximum of 8 wk, as during this period no adverse effects on sensory function (because of the mechanism of action) were noted in diabetic patients *(92)*. Appropriate studies are needed to evaluate the safety of capsaicin before it can be recommended for long-term treatment.

### Tricyclic Antidepressants

If the pain does not respond to capsaicin, tricyclic antidepressants are used at step IV (Table 1). Psychotropic agents, among which antidepressants are evaluated most extensively, have constituted an important component in the treatment of chronic pain syndromes for more than 30 yr *(95)*. Putative mechanisms of pain relief by antidepressants include the inhibition of norepinephrine and/or serotonin reuptake at synapses of central descending pain-control systems and the antagonism of N-methyl-D-aspartate receptor that mediates hyperalgesia and allodynia *(96)*. The following NNTs have been calculated for a pain reduction of ≥50%: amitriptyline: 2.1, imipramine: 3.7, desipramine:

3.2, clomipramine: 4.5 *(97)*. The NNTs for efficacy and adverse events of antidepressants on the basis of 13 studies *(51)* are shown in Table 3. Among 100 diabetic patients with neuropathic pain who are treated with antidepressants, 30 will experience pain relief by ≥50%, 30 will have mild adverse events, and four will discontinue treatment because of severe adverse events *(97)*. The most frequent adverse events of tricyclic antidepressants include tiredness and dry mouth *(98)*. The starting dose should be 25 mg (10 mg in frail patients) and taken as a single night-time dose 1 h before sleep. It should be increased by 25 mg at weekly intervals until pain relief is achieved or adverse events occur. The maximum dose is usually 150 mg per day *(99)*. Amitriptyline is frequently the drug of first choice, since it has been studied most extensively and the mean effect size was relatively high when compared with other antidepressants *(100)*. Alternatively, desipramine may be chosen because of its less-pronounced sedative and anticholinergic effects *(101)*. The median dose for amitriptyline is 75 mg/d, and there is a clear dose-response relationship *(102)*. The effect is comparable in patients with and without depression and is independent of a concomitant improvement in mood *(103)*. The onset of efficacy is much more rapid (1–7 d) than in the treatment of depression *(101)*.

The notion that the character of the neuropathic pain is predictive of response, so that burning pain should be treated with antidepressants and shooting pain with anticonvulsants is obviously incorrect *(99)*, since both pain qualities respond to tricyclic antidepressants *(101)*.

#### Selective Serotonin-Reuptake Inhibitors (SSRI)

Patients who do not tolerate tricyclic antidepressants because of adverse events should be alternatively treated with the selective serotonin-reuptake inhibitors (SSRIs) paroxetine (40 mg/d orally) or citalopram (40 mg/d orally) *(93,94)* (step IV; Table 1). The following NNTs have been calculated for the SSRIs: fluoxetine: 15.3, paroxetine: 5, citalopram: 3 *(97)*. Thus, on the basis of the present evidence, citalopram and paroxetine (20–40 mg/d orally) should be given preference over fluoxetine, *(101)*. Beside the relatively low rates of adverse events, the advantage of the SSRI compared to the tricyclic compounds is the markedly lower risk of mortality caused by overdose *(104)*. Most evidence of efficacy of antidepressants comes from studies that have been conducted over only several weeks. However, many patients continue to achieve pain relief for months to years *(99)*.

#### Anticonvulsants and Antiarrhythmic Agents

**Carbamazepine** The successful treatment of trigeminal neuralgia with carbamazepine resulted in a more extensive use of this anticonvulsant in painful neuropathies. There are three controlled clinical trials of carbamazepine (1–3 × 200 mg/d orally) in 30–40 patients that showed superiority over placebo treatment *(105–107)*. In the study by Rull et al. *(105)*, the NNT was 3.3 for pain reduction, 1.9 for mild (somnolence, dizziness), and 15 for severe (allergic skin reactions) adverse events *(108)* (Table 3). These relatively high rates of adverse events and the relative paucity of clinical trials somewhat limit the value of this remedy, so that it should find its place after the aforementioned drugs have been unsuccessful (step IV; Table 1). Whether patients with certain pain qualities (shooting or stabbing pain) respond preferentially is not known. A recent, small, 4-wk controlled study revealed no differences in pain relief between carbamazepine and a combination of nortriptyline-fluphenazine *(109)*. The pain relief by carbamazepine is mediated presumably by stabilizing neuronal membranes through an effect on sodium conductance *(11)*.

**Phenytoin (Diphenylhydantoin)** In the past, phenytoin (3 × 100 mg/d orally) has been frequently advocated on the basis of an open study. However, controlled trials have yielded controversial results *(105,106)*. Since efficacy has not been demonstrated unequivocally for this compound, it cannot be recommended.

**Mexiletine** Mexiletine, a class Ib antiarrhythmic agent, has been shown to be effective in a small 10-wk study including 16 patients using an increasing dose from 150 mg/d to 10 mg/kg/d orally. The NNT for a pain reduction of >35% was 1.6 and for mild adverse events (nausea, tremor) it was 5.3 *(112)*. In a 5-wk multicenter trial, using 3 × 75–225 mg/d orally, a beneficial effect has been demonstrated on burning and stabbing pain *(113)*. The NNT was 5.6 for pain relief in the MPQ. An oral dose of 3 × 150 mg/d, which is well below that required for antiarrhythmic therapy (600–800 mg/d), was sufficient and did not produce any adverse events or ECG abnormalities. Thus, short-term treatment with mexiletine can be recommended as a drug treatment of the last choice in patients with persistent severe pain, but regular ECG monitoring is mandatory (step V; Table 1).

**Lidocaine** In a controlled study in 15 diabetic patients with chronic painful neuropathy, a single iv infusion of lidocaine (5 mg/kg over 30 min during continuous ECG monitoring) resulted in a significant pain relief after 1 and 8 d *(114)*. The individual effect was sustained for 3–21 d. The NNT for a pain reduction of >30% after 3 d was 2.2. Since lidocaine resulted in an increase in the threshold for the nociceptive flexion reflex (M. biceps femoris) in diabetic patients with painful neuropathy, it is conceivable that this compound mediates its pain relieving effect via spinal or supraspinal mechanisms *(115)*. Thermal and pain thresholds are not influenced *(115,116)*. The onset of the analgesic effect during the iv infusion (500 mg in 60 min) is abrupt over a narrow dosage and concentration range *(117)*.

**Clonidine** A controlled 6-wk study using a transdermal clonidine patch (dose titration from 0.1 to 0.3 mg/d) in 24 diabetic patients has shown a nonsignificant trend towards pain relief *(118)*. The NNT for a moderate or marked pain reduction was 5.3, whereas the NNT for adverse events was relatively low, being 3.4 for dry mouth and drowsiness, respectively *(118)*. Likewise, in a 3-wk trial in 41 patients no significant difference between clonidine and placebo regarding pain relief could be observed *(119)*. However, 12 responders were identified, who experienced moderate-to-complete pain relief on clonidine compared to placebo patch. These patients were included in a second study using an "enriched enrollment" design (in which only patients who had been screened as responders are entered). In this study a significant 20% pain reduction compared with placebo was noted. The NNT for adverse events (dry mouth, sedation, orthostatic symptoms) was 2.0 in the responders. Thus, on the basis of these data, transdermal clonidine cannot be generally recommended. The potential mechanisms for the analgesic effect of clonidine include actions at $\alpha_2$ adrenergic or imidazoline receptors to cause postsynaptic inhibition of spinal cord neurons, presynaptic inhibition of nociceptive afferents, facilitation of brain-stem pain-modulating systems, or peripheral or central suppression of sympathetic transmitter release *(118)*.

**Opioids** There are two extreme positions on opioid sensitivity in pain. One suggests that opioid sensitivity is a relative phenomenon and therefore that any pain can be controlled by opioids, provided that there is an adequate dose escalation and control of adverse events *(120)*. The other extreme insists that some pains are intrinsically insensitive to opioids and that this insensitivity can be predicted from the clinical characteristics of the pain *(121)*. Nociceptive pain is thought to be sensitive to opioids, whereas neuropathic pain is regarded as insensitive. However, the latter view has been challenged by recent studies showing that the administration of morphine was associated with pain relief in 50% of patients with neuropathic pain of various origin *(122)*. Furthermore, an infusion of fentanyl induced a pain reduction by 66% compared with 23% by diazepam independent of the pain characteristics *(123)*. This analgesic effect is intrinsic and independent of the degree of sedation and change in mood *(122–124)*. Long-term studies using oral or transdermal application of opioids should evaluate the risk-to-benefit ratio of these drugs in patients with pain caused by diabetic neuropathy.

In painful diabetic neuropathy, tramadol (up to 400 mg/d orally, mean dose: 210 mg/d orally) has been studied in a 6-wk multicenter trial including 127 patients *(125)*. Pain relief was 44% on tramadol vs 12% on placebo. The most frequent adverse events were nausea and constipation. The NNT for drop-outs because of adverse events was relatively low (7.9), indicating significant toxicity. Its use as drug treatment of the last choice appears justified on the basis of these data (step V; Table 1). Trials to assess equivalence (e.g., vs antidepressants) should clarify the relative potency and toxicity of tramadol in painful neuropathy.

**B Vitamins** Since the neurotrophic B vitamins exhibit antinociceptive properties when given in high doses experimentally, they are being discussed in the treatment of various pain conditions *(126)*. Since there is usually no evidence of depletion of vitamin B1 (thiamine), B6 (pyridoxine), and B12 (cyanocobalamine) in diabetic patients, *(127)*, the putative analgesic effect rather than a substitution would appear relevant. However, the evidence for this assumption is not sufficient on the basis of the available controlled studies. Trials using vitamin B6 for 4 and 3 mo reported negative results *(128,129)*. Moreover, it is alarming that the intake of mega doses of vitamin B6 (up to a maximum of 2–6 g/d orally) may lead to a severe sensory neuropathy with ataxia *(130)*. The combination of vitamin B1, B6, and B12 (300/600/0.6 mg/Tag orally) administered for 18 wk in 33 diabetic patients was not associated with an appreciable effect on painful symptoms but resulted in an improvement in the warm and cold thresholds in the hands but not the feet *(131)*. Since the bioavailability of the water-soluble B vitamins is low, two recent studies have employed benfotiamine, a lipid-soluble thiamine derivative *(132,133)*, which has an approx 3.6-fold higher maximal bioavailability than the water-soluble thiamine *(134)*. In the first study, a combination of benfotiamine, vitamin B6 and B12 (120/270/0.75 mg/d orally) or placebo was administered to 24 patients over 12 wk. A beneficial effect could be demonstrated only in 1 out of 4 nerve function parameters tested *(132)*. In the second study, 40 patients were treated with 400 mg benfotiamine or placebo for 3 wk. A modest, albeit statistically significant, improvement was noted on a score for symptoms and deficits by 19% with benfotiamine vs 6% with placebo *(133)*. Because of these altogether marginal effects, a multicenter study to clarify the role of benfotiamine in the treatment of symptomatic polyneuropathy has been initiated in Germany.

**Rheologic Agents** Microvascular changes of the vasa nervorum and reduced endoneurial blood flow resulting in hypoxia are thought to be important factors in the pathogenesis of diabetic neuropathy *(69)*. Thus, there is solid theoretical background to support treatment with vasodilating drugs (*see* Chapter 7). However, regarding rheologic compounds, controlled studies have shown no effect on pentoxifylline (3 × 400 mg/d orally) over 4 wk on pain in 16 patients *(135)* and over 6 mo in 40 patients on symptoms *(136)* associated with diabetic neuropathy. The same applies to cyclandelate (1600 mg/d orally) *(137,138)*, ginkgo biloba special extract EGb 761 *(139)*, and sabeluzole *(140)*. Thus, there is no evidence to support favorable effects of rheologic remedies on symptomatic diabetic neuropathy.

**Other Treatment Approaches** In a controlled, 2-wk study of calcitonin (100 IU/d by intranasal spray) 3 and 1 out of 10 patients had complete and 50% pain relief, respectively *(141)*.

Based on the idea that nucleotides may enhance nerve regeneration, uridine (3 × 300 mg/d orally) has been evaluated in a controlled trial including 40 diabetic patients with peripheral neuropathy. After 6 mo, a positive effect on NCV and action potentials was noted *(142)*. It is unclear whether this improvement can be translated into favorable effects on clinical symptoms and deficits. Cerebrolysin, a peptidergic solution containing free aminoacids and biologically active peptides, has been infused iv over 10 d in 20 type 2 diabetic patients with painful neuropathy. Pain was relieved by 33% on cerebrolysin and by 12% on placebo after 6 wk, and no significant adverse events were observed *(143)*.

The administration of the nonsteroidal antirheumatic agents ibuprofen (4 × 600 mg/d orally) and sulindac (2 × 200 mg/d orally) in an 8-wk single-blind study including 18 diabetic patients was associated with an improvement in pain scores *(144)*.

In a 4-wk study, OpSite, an adherent polyurethane film that is waterproof and permeable to water vapor and oxygen, has been applied to painful sites of the leg in 33 diabetic patients. OpSite dressing alleviated pain and improved patients' quality of life when compared with no treatment *(145)*.

Regarding the role of traditional Asian medicine, only open-label studies are available. Traditional Chinese acupuncture (6 sessions in 1–2-wk intervals) resulted in pain relief in 12/15 (80%) of the patients *(146)*. Placebo acupuncture (needles inserted in wrong locations) helps in 33 to 50% of the cases *(147)*, indicating that a marked effect of acupuncture is conceivable but has yet to be verified in controlled studies. In Japan, goshajinkigan (herbal medicine; 3 × 2.5 g/d orally) has long been used to treat symptomatic diabetic neuropathy. However, possible effects on neuropathic symptoms and vibration perception threshold are rendered uninterpretable because of the uncontrolled study design *(148)*.

**Immunoglobulins, Immunosuppressants, and Glucocorticoids** Some patients with proximal or multifocal diabetic neuropathy show marked ischemic nerve lesions with vasculitis and inflammatory infiltration *(27–29)* termed *diabetic inflammatory vasculopathy (30)*, whereas in others a demyelinating neuropathy without vascular inflammation, indistinguishable from chronic inflammatory demyelinating polyneuropathy (CIDP) may be present *(31)*. Thus, it is thought that treatment with iv immunoglobulins, immunosuppressants, and glucocorticoids may be helpful in these patients *(28–31)*. However, there have been no controlled studies using these agents in proximal or multifocal diabetic neuropathy. This is a critical issue, since these forms frequently tend to resolve spontaneously, and the aforementioned drugs may produce significant adverse effects and are relatively expensive. In fact, some patients have been described recently who became free of pain shortly after nerve biopsy had been performed, so that additional treatment was not necessary *(28)*. It has been suggested that the interruption of a sensory branch of a nerve producing pain by stimulation of sensory fibers by mediators released by inflammatory cells may decrease painful afferents and give a feeling of relief to the patient *(28)*. Because of the self-limiting nature of the symptoms and the potential adverse effects, some authors are reluctant to use immunotherapy *(28,149)*, whereas others are not *(29,150)*. However, there is general agreement regarding the need for future controlled studies using these agents in proximal diabetic neuropathy *(28–31,149,150)*.

## REFERENCES

1. Crook J, Rideout E, Browne G. The prevalence of pain complaints in a general population. Pain 1994;18:299–314.
2. Bowsher D. Neurogenic pain syndromes and their management. Br Med Bull 1991;47:644–666.
3. Chan AW, MacFarlane IA, Bowsher DR, Wells JC, Bessex C, Griffiths K. Chronic pain in patients with diabetes mellitus: comparison with non-diabetic population. Pain Clinic 1990;3:147–159.
4. Consensus statement. Report and recommendations of the San Antonio conference on diabetic neuropathy. Diabetes Care 1988;11:592–597.
5. Ziegler D. Diagnosis, staging and epidemiology of diabetic peripheral neuropathy. Diab Nutr Metab 1994;7:342–348.
6. Dyck PJ, Kratz KM, Karnes JL, Litchy WJ, Klein R, Pach JM, Wilson DM, O'Brien PC, Melton III LJ. The prevalence by staged severity of various types of diabetic neuropathy, retinopathy, and nephropathy in a population-based cohort: the Rochester Diabetic Neuropathy Study. Neurology 1993;43:817–824.
7. Veglio M, Sivieri R, The Neuropathy Study Group of the Italian Society for the Study of Diabetes, Piemonte affiliate. Prevalence of neuropathy in IDDM patients in Piemonte, Italy. Diabetes Care 1993;16:456–461.
8. Asbury AK, Fields HL. Pain due to peripheral nerve damage: a hypothesis. Neurology 1984;34:1587–1590.
9. Pfeifer MA, Ross DR, Schrager JP, Gelber DA, Schumer MP, Crain GM, Markwell SJ, Jung S. A highly successful and novel model for treatment of chronic painful diabetic peripheral neuropathy. Diabetes Care 1993;16:1103–1115.
10. Thomas PK, Scadding JW. Treatment of pain in diabetic neuropathy. In: Dyck PJ, Thomas PK, Asbury AK, Winegrad AI, Porte D, eds. Diabetic Neuropathy. Saunders, Philadelphia, 1987, pp. 216–222.
11. Thomas PK. Painful diabetic neuropathy: mechanisms and treatment. Diab Nutr Metab 1994;7:359–368.
12. Watkins PJ. The natural history of the diabetic neuropathies. Q J Med 1990;77:1209–1218.
13. Boulton AJM, Scarpello JHB, Armstrong WD, Ward JD. The natural history of painful diabetic neuropathy—a 4-year study. Postgrad Med J 1985;59:556–559.
14. Chan AW, MacFarlane. The impact of chronic pain on quality of life in diabetes. Practical Diabetes 1989;6:249–253.
15. Young RJ, Ewing DJ, Clarke BF. Chronic and remitting painful diabetic neuropathy. Diabetes Care 1988;11:34–40.
16. Benbow SJ, Chan AW, Bowsher D, MacFarlene IA, Williams G. A prospective study of painful symptoms, small-fibre function and peripheral vascular disease in chronic painful diabetic neuropathy. Diabetic Med 1993;11:17–21.
17. Archer AG, Watkins PJ, Thomas PK, Sharma AK, Payan J. The natural history of acute painful neuropathy in diabetes mellitus. J Neurol Neurosurg Psychiat 1983;46:491–499.
18. Ellenberg M. Diabetic neuropathic cachexia. Diabetes 1974;23:418–423.
19. Steele JM, Young RJ, Lloyd GG, Clarke BF. Clinically apparent eating disorders in young diabetic women: associations with painful neuropathy and other complications. Br Med J 1987;294:859–866.
20. Caravati CM. Insulin neuritis: a case report. VA Med Mon 1933;59:745–746.
21. Llewelyn JG, Thomas PK, Fonseca V, King RHM, Dandona P. Acute painful diabetic neuropathy precipitated by strict glycaemic control. Acta Neuropathol 1986;72:157–163.

22. Tesfaye S, Malik R, Harris N, Jakubowski JJ, Mody C, Rennie IG, Ward JD. Arterio-venous shunting and proliferating new vessels in acute painful neuropathy of rapid glycaemic control (insulin neuritis). Diabetologia 1996;39:329–335.
23. Suzuki Y, Kadowaki H, Katagiri H, Suematsu M, Atsumi Y, Hosokawa K, Kadowaki T, Oka Y, Yazaki Y, Matsuoka K. Posttreatment neuropathy in diabetic subjects with mitochondrial tRNA (Leu) mutation. Diabetes Care 1994;17:777–778.
24. Chan AW, MacFarlene IA, Bowsher D. Short term fluctuations in blood glucose concentrations do not alter pain perception in diabetic patients with and without painful peripheral neuropathy. Diabetes Res 1990;14:15–19.
25. Asbury AK. Focal and multifocal neuropathies of diabetes. In: Dyck PJ, Thomas PK, Asbury AK, Winegard AI, Porte D, eds. Diabetic Neuropathy. Saunders, Philadelphia, 1987, pp. 45–55.
26. Zorilla E, Kozak GP. Ophthalmoplegia in diabetes mellitus. Ann Intern Med 1967;67:968–974.
27. Said G, Goulon-Goeau C, Lacroix C, Moulonguet A. Nerve biopsy findings in different patterns of proximal diabetic neuropathy. Ann Neurol 1994;35:559–569.
28. Said G, Elgrably F, Lacroix C, Plante V, Talamon C, Adams D, Tager M, Slama G, Goulon-Goeau C, Moulonguet A. Painful proximal diabetic neuropathy: inflammatory nerve lesions and spontaneous favorable outcome. Ann Neurol 1997;41:762–770.
29. Younger DS, Rosoklija G, Hays AP, Trojaborg W, Latov N. Diabetic peripheral neuropathy: a clinicopathologic and immunohistochemical analysis of sural nerve biopsies. Muscle Nerve 1996;19:722–727.
30. Krendel DA. Diabetic inflammatory vasculopathy. Muscle Nerve 1997;20:520.
31. Krendel DA, Costigan DA, Hopkins LC. Successful treatment of neuropathies in patients with diabetes mellitus. Arch Neurol 1992;52:1053–1061.
32. Chaudhuri KR, Wren DR, Werring D, Watkins PJ. Unilateral abdominal muscle herniation with pain: a distinctive variant of diabetic radiculopathy. Diabetic Med 1997;14:803–807.
33. Melzack R. Measurement of the dimensions of pain experience. In: B Bromm, ed. Pain Measurement in Man. Elsevier, Amsterdam, 1984, pp. 327–348.
34. De Conno F, Caraceni A, Gamba A, Mariani L, Abbattista A, Brunelli C, La Mura A, Ventafridda V. Pain measurement in cancer patients: a comparison of six methods. Pain 1994;57:161–166.
35. Williams RC. Toward a set of reliable and valid measures for chronic pain assessment and outcome research. Pain 1988;35:239–251.
36. Scott J, Huskisson EC. Graphic representation of pain. Pain 1976;2:175–184.
37. Collins SL, Moore RA, McQuay HJ. The visual analogue pain intensity scale: what is moderate pain in millimetres? Pain 1997;72:95–97.
38. Melzack R. The McGill Pain Questionnaire: major properties and scoring methods. Pain 1975;1:277–299.
39. Masson EA, Hunt L, Gem JM, Boulton AJM. A novel approach to the diagnosis and assessment of symptomatic diabetic neuropathy. Pain 1989;38:25–28.
40. Hoppe F. Hamburger Schmerz Adjektiv Liste (HSAL). Manual. Beltz-Verlag, Weinheim, 1991.
41. Galer BS, Jensen MP. Development and preliminary validation of a pain measure specific to neuropathic pain: the Neuropathic Pain Scale. Neurology 1997;48:332–338.
42. Turner JA, Deyo RA, Loeser JD, von Korff M, Foryce WE. The importance of placebo effects in pain treatment and research. JAMA 1994;271:1609–1614.
43. Whitney CW, von Korff M. Regression to the mean in treated versus untreated chronic pain. Pain 1992;50:281–285.
44. Ernst E, Resch KL. Concept of true and perceived placebo effects. Br Med J 1995;311:551–553.
45. Richardson PH. Placebo effects in pain management. Pain Rev 1994;1:15–32.
46. Rothman KJ. Placebo mania. Br Med J 1996;313:3–4.
47. Jones B, Jarvis P, Lewis JA, Ebbutt AF. Trials to assess equivalence: the importance of rigorous methods. Br Med J 1996;313:36–39.
48. Cook RJ, Sackett DL. The number needed to treat: a clinically useful measure of treatment effect. Br Med J 1995;310:452–454.
49. Chatellier G, Zapletal E, Lemaitre D, Menard J, Degoulet P. The number needed to treat: a clinically useful nomogram in its proper context. Br Med J 1996;312:426–429.
50. Laupacis A, Sackett DL, Roberts RS. An assessment of clinically useful measures of the consequences of treatment. N Engl J Med 1988;318:1728–1733.

51. McQuay HJ, Moore RA. Using numerial results from systematic reviews in clinical practice. Ann Intern Med 1997;126:712–720.
52. Young RJ, Clarke BF. Pain relief in diabetic neuropathy: the effectiveness of imipramine and related drugs. Diabetic Med 1985;2:363–366.
53. Vinik AI, Milicevic Z. Recent advances in the diagnosis and treatment of diabetic neuropathy. Endocrinologist 1996;6:443–461.
54. The Diabetes Control and Complications Trial Research Group. The effect of intensive diabetes therapy on the development and progression of neuropathy. Ann Intern Med 1995;122:561–568.
55. The Diabetes Control and Complications Trial (DCCT) Research Group. Effect of intensive diabetes treatment on nerve conduction in the Diabetes Control and Complications Trial. Ann Neurol 1995;38:869–880.
56. Reichard P, Nilsson B-Y, Rosenqvist U. The effect of long-term intensified insulin treatment on the development of microvascular complications of diabetes mellitus. N Engl J Med 1993;329:304–309.
57. Reichard P, Pihl M, Rosenqvist U, Sule J. Complications in IDDM are caused by elevated blood glucose level: the Stockholm Diabetes Intervention Study (SDIS) at 10-year follow up. Diabetologia 1996;39:1483–1488.
58. Amthor K-F, Dahl-Jorgensen K, Berg TJ, Skard Heier M, Sandvik L, Aagenaes O, Hanssen KF. The effect of 8 years of strict glycaemic control on peripheral nerve function in IDDM patients: the Oslo Study. Diabetologia 1994;37:579–584.
59. Ohkubo Y, Kishikawa H, Araki E, Miyata T, Isami S, Motoyoshi S, Kojima Y, Furuyoshi N, Shichiri M. Intensive insulin therapy prevents the progression of diabetic microvascular complications in Japanese patients with non-insulin-dependent diabetes mellitus: a randomized prospective 6-year study. Diabetes Res Clin Pract 1995;28:103–117.
60. Ziegler D, Dannehl K, Wiefels K, Gries FA. Differential effects of near-normoglycaemia for 4 years on somatic nerve dysfunction and heart rate variation in Type 1 diabetic patients. Diabetic Med 1992;9:622–629.
61. Ziegler D, Piolot R, Gries FA. The natural history of diabetic neuropathy is governed by the degree of glycaemic control. A 10-year prospective study in IDDM. Diabetologia 1996;39(Suppl 1):A34.
62. Tattersall R. Is pancreas transplantation for insulin-dependent diabetics worthwhile? N Engl J Med 1989;321:112–114.
63. Kennedy WR, Navarro X, Goetz FC, Sutherland DER, Najarian JS. Effects of pancreatic transplantation on diabetic neuropathy. N Engl J Med 1990;322:1031–1037.
64. Solders G, Tydén G, Persson A, Groth C-G. Improvement of nerve conduction in diabetic neuropathy. A follow-up study 4 yr after combined pancreatic and renal transplantation. Diabetes 1992;41:946–951.
65. Martinenghi S, Comi G, Galardi G, Di Carlo V, Pozza G, Secchi A. Amelioration of nerve conduction velocity following simultaneous kidney/pancreas transplantation is due to the glycaemic control provided by the pancreas. Diabetologia 1997;40:1110–1112.
66. Müller-Felber W, Landgraf R, Scheuer R, Wagner S, Reimers CD, Nusser J, Abendroth D, Illner W-D, Land W. Diabetic neuropathy 3 years after successful pancreas and kidney transplantation. Diabetes 1993;42:1482–1486.
67. Allen RDM, Al-Habri IS, Morris JGL, Clouston PD, O'Connell PJ, Chapman JR, Nankivell BJ. Diabetic neuropathy after pancreas transplantation: determinants of recovery. Transplantation 1997;63:830–838.
68. Boulton AJM, Drury J, Clarke B, Ward JD. Continuous subcutaneous insulin infusion in the management of painful diabetic neuropathy. Diabetes Care 1982;5:386–390.
69. Cameron NE, Cotter MA. The relationship of vascular changes to metabolic factors in diabetes mellitus and their role in the development of peripheral nerve complications. Diabetes/Metab Rev 1994;10:189–224.
70. Ziegler D. Diabetic cardiovascular autonomic neuropathy: prognosis, diagnosis, and treatment. Diabetes/Metab Rev 1994;10:339–383.
71. Nicolucci A, Carinci F, Graepel JG, Hohman TC, Ferris F, Lachin JM. The efficacy of tolrestat in the treatment of diabetic peripheral neuropathy. A meta-analysis of individual patient data. Diabetes Care 1996;19:1091–1096.
72. Nicolucci A, Carinci F, Cavaliere D, Scorpiglione N, Belfiglio M, Labbrozzi D, Mari E, Massi Benedetti M, Tognoni G, Liberati A. A meta-analysis of trials on aldose reductase inhibitors in diabetic peripheral neuropathy. Diabetic Med 1996;13:1017–1026.
73. Gregersen G. *myo*-Inositol supplementation. In: Dyck PJ, Thomas PK, Asbury AK, Winegrad AI, Porte D, eds. Diabetic Neuropathy. Saunders, Philadelphia, 1987, pp. 188–189.

74. The gamma-Linolenic Acid Multicenter Trial Group. Treatment of diabetic neuropathy with gamma-linolenic acid. Diabetes Care 1993;16:8–15.
75. Horrobin DF. Essential fatty acids in the management of impaired nerve function in diabetes. Diabetes 1997;46(Suppl 2):S90–S93.
76. Ziegler D, Hanefeld M, Ruhnau KJ, Meißner HP, Lobisch M, Schütte K, Nehrdich D, Dannehl K, Gries FA, The ALADIN Study Group. Treatment of symptomatic diabetic peripheral neuropathy with the antioxidant α-lipoic acid. A 3-week multicentre randomized controlled trial (ALADIN Study). Diabetologia 1995;38:1425–1433.
77. Ziegler D, Schatz H, Conrad F, Gries FA, Ulrich H, Reichel G, the DEKAN Study Group. Effects of treatment with the antioxidant α-lipoic acid on cardiac autonomic neuropathy in NIDDM patients. A 4-month randomized controlled multicenter trial (DEKAN Study). Diabetes Care 1997;20:369–373.
78. Malik RA, Abbott CA, Williamson S, Carrington AC, Schady W, Boulton AJM. ACE inhibition in human diabetic neuropathy: a double blind placebo controlled trial. J Peripher Nerv Syst 1997;2:284.
79. Shindo H, Tawata M, Aida K, Onaya T. Clinical efficacy of a stable prostacyclin analog, iloprost, in diabetic neuropathy. Prostaglandins 1991;41:85–96.
80. Yuen EC, Mobley WC. Therapeutic potential of neurotrophic factors for neurological disorders. Ann Neurol 1996;40:346–354.
81. Riaz SS, Tomlinson DR. Neurotrophic factors in peripheral neuropathies: pharmacological strategies. Prog Neurobiol 1996;49:125–143.
82. Yagihashi S, Kamijo S, Baba M, Yagihashi M, Nagai K. Effect of aminoguanidine on functional and structural abnormalities in peripheral nerve of STZ-induced diabetic rats. Diabetes 1992;41:47–52.
83. Ziegler D, Mühlen H, Rathmann W, Gries FA. Effects of one year's treatment with gamma-linolenic acid (EF4) on diabetic neuropathy. Diabetes 1993;42(Suppl. 1):99A.
84. Nagamatsu M, Nickander KK, Schmelzer JD, Raya A, Wittrock DA, Tritschler HT, Low PA. Lipoic acid improves nerve blood flow, reduces oxidative stress and improves distal nerve conduction in experimental diabetic neuropathy. Diabetes Care 1995;18:1160–1167.
85. Ziegler D. The design of clinical trials for treatment of diabetic neuropathy. Neurosci Res Commun 1997;21:83–91.
86. Low PA, Opfer-Gehrking TL, Dyck PJ, Litchy WJ, O'Brien PC. Double-blind, placebo-controlled study of the application of capsaicin cream in chronic distal painful polyneuropathy. Pain 1995;62:163–168.
87. Chad DA, Aronin N, Lundstrom R, McKeon P, Ross D, Molitch M, Schipper HM, Stall G, Dyess E, Tarsy D. Does capsaicin relieve the pain of diabetic neuropathy? Pain 1990;42:387–388.
88. Scheffler NM, Sheitel PL, Lipton MN. Treatment of painful diabetic neuropathy with capsaicin 0.075%. J Am Podiatr Med Assoc 1991;81:288–293.
89. Basha KM, Whitehouse FW. Capsaicin: a therapeutic option for painful diabetic neuropathy. Henry Ford Hosp Med J 1991;39:138–140.
90. The Capsaicin Study Group. Treatment of painful diabetic neuropathy with topical capsaicin. Arch Intern Med 1991;151:2225–2229.
91. The Capsaicin Study Group. Effect of treatment with capsaicin on daily activities of patients with painful diabetic neuropathy. Diabetes Care 1992;15:159–165.
92. Tandan R, Lewis GA, Badger GB, Fries TJ. Topical capsaicin in painful diabetic neuropathy. Diabetes Care 1992;15:15–18.
93. Biesbroeck R, Bril V, Hollander P, Kabadi U, Schwartz S, Singh SP, Ward WK, Bernstein JE. A double-blind comparison of topical capsaicin and oral amitriptyline in painful diabetic neuropathy. Advances in Therapy 1995;12:111–120.
94. Zhang WY, Li Wan Po A. The effectiveness of topically applied capsaicin. A meta-analysis. Eur J Clin Pharmacol 1994;46:517–522.
95. Philipp M, Fickinger M. Psychotropic drugs in the management of chronic pain syndromes. Pharmacopsychiatry 1993;26:221–234.
96. Eisenach JC, Hood DD, Curry R, Tong C. Alfentanil, but not amitriptyline, reduces pain, hyperalgesia, and allodynia from intradermal injection of capsaicin in humans. Anesthesiology 1997;86:1279–1287.
97. McQuay HJ, Tramer M, Nye BA, Carroll D, Wiffen PJ, Moore RA. A systematic review of antidepressants in neuropathic pain. Pain 1996;68:217–227.
98. Sindrup SH. Antidepressants in the treatment of diabetic neuropathy symptoms. Pharmacodynamic, -kinetic, and -genetic aspects. Dan Med Bull 1994;41:66–78.
99. McQuay HJ, Moore RA. Antidepressants and chronic pain. Br Med J 1997;314:763–764.

100. Onghena P, van Houdenhove B. Antidepressant-induced analgesia in chronic non-malignant pain: a meta-analysis of 39 placebo-controlled studies. Pain 1992;49:205–219.
101. Max MB, Lynch SA, Muir J, Shoaf SE, Smoller B, Dubner R. Effects of desipramine, amitrityline, and fluoxetine on pain in diabetic neuropathy. N Engl J Med 1992;326:1250–1256.
102. McQuay HJ, Carrol D, Glynn CJ. Dose-response for analgesic effect of amitriptyline in chronic pain. Anaesthesia 1993;48:281–285.
103. Max MB, Culnane M, Schafer SC, Gracely RH, Walther DJ, Smoller B, Dubner R. Amitriptyline relieves diabetic neuropathy pain in patients with normal or depressed mood. Neurology 1987;37:589–596.
104. Henry JA, Alexander CA, Sener EK. Relative mortality from overdose of antidepressants. Br Med J 1995;310:221–224.
105. Rull JA, Quibrera R, Gonzalez-Millan H, Castaneda LO. Symptomatic treatment of peripheral diabetic neuropathy with carbamazepine (Tegretol): double blind crossover trial. Diabetologia 1969;5:215–218.
106. Ocaranza Ochoa J, Cervantes Amezcua A, Macias Torres V, Casilas Ochoa O, Pere Becerra JL. La carbamazepina en el tratamiento de la neuropatia diabetica: informe preliminar. Prensa Med Mex 1968;33:132–135.
107. Wilton TD. Tegretol in the treatment of diabetic neuropathy. S Afr Med J 1974;48:869–872.
108. McQuay H, Carroll D, Jadad AR, Wiffen P, Moore A. Anticonvulsant drugs for management of pain: a systematic review. Br Med J 1995;311:1047–1052.
109. Gomez-Perez FJ, Choza R, Rios JM, Reza A, Huerta E, Aguilar CA, Rull JA. Nortriptyline-fluphenazine vs. carbamazepine in the symptomatic treatment of diabetic neuropathy. Arch Med Res 1996;27:525–529.
110. Saudek CD, Werns S, Reidenberg MM. Phenytoin in the treatment of diabetic symmetrical neuropathy. Clin Pharmacol Ther 1977;22:196–199.
111. Chadda VS, Mathur MS. Double blind study of the effects of diphenylhydantoin sodium on diabetic neuropathy. J Assoc Phys Ind 1978;26:403–406.
112. Dejgaard A, Petersen P, Kastrup J. Mexiletine for treatment of chronic painful diabetic neuropathy. Lancet 1988;2:9–11.
113. Stracke H, Meyer UE, Schumacher HE, Federlin K. Mexiletine in the treatment of diabetic neuropathy. Diabetes Care 1992;15:1550–1555.
114. Kastrup J, Petersen P, Dejgard A, Angelo HR, Hilsted J. Intravenous lidocaine infusion—a new treatment of chronic painful diabetic neuropathy? Pain 1987;28:69–75.
115. Bach FW, Jensen TS, Kastrup J, Stigsby B, Dejgard A. The effect of intravenous lidocaine on nociceptive processing in diabetic neuropathy. Pain 1990;40:29–34.
116. Wallace MS, Laitin S, Licht D, Yaksh TL. Concentration-effect relations for intravenous lidocaine infusions in human volunteers. Anesthesiology 1997;86:1262–1272.
117. Ferrante FM, Paggioli J, Cherukuri S, Arthur GR. The analgesic response to intravenous lidocaine in the treatment of neuropathic pain. Anesth Analg 1995;82:91–97.
118. Zeigler D, Lynch SA, Muir J, Benjamin J, Max MB. Transdermal clonidine versus placebo in painful diabetic neuropathy. Pain 1992;48:403–408.
119. Byas-Smith MG, Max MB, Muir J, Kingman A. Transdermal clonidine compared to placebo in painful diabetic neuropathy using a two-stage "enriched enrollment" design. Pain 1995;60:267–274.
120. McQuay HJ. Opioid use in chronic pain. Acta Anaesthesiol Scand 1997;41:175–183.
121. Arner S, Meyerson BA. Lack of analgesic effect of opioids on neuropathic and idiopathic forms of pain. Pain 1988;33:11–23.
122. Jadad AR, Carroll D, Glynn CJ, Moore RA, McQuay HJ. Morphine responsiveness of chronic pain: double-blind randomised crossover study with patient-controlled analgesia. Lancet 1992;339:1367–1371.
123. Dellemijn PL, Vanneste JAL. Randomised double-blind active-placebo-controlled crossover trial of intravenous fentanyl in neuropathic pain. Lancet 1997;349:753–758.
124. Moulin DE, Iezzi A, Amireh R, Sharpe WKJ, Boyd D, Merskey H. Randomised trial of oral morphine for chronic non-cancer pain. Lancet 1996;347:143–147.
125. Harati Y, Gooch C, Swenson M, Edelman S, Greene D, Raskin P, Donoforio P, Cornblatt D, Sachdeo R, the TPSDN study group. A double-blind placebo-controlled trial of tramadol for the pain of diabetic peripheral neuropathy. J Peripher Nerv Syst 1997;2:270.
126. Weber W, Walter-Sack I. Klinische Bedeutung von Vitamin B1, B6, B12 in der Schmerztherapie. Klin Wochenschr 1988;66:274–276.

127. Straub RH, Rokitzki L, Schumacher T, Hillmann C, Palitzsch K-D, Schölmerich J. No evidence of deficiency of vitamins A, E, β-carotene, B1, B2, B6, B12, and folate in neuropathic Type II diabetic women. Int J Vit Nutr Res 1993;63:239–240.
128. Levin ER, Hanscom TA, Fisher M, Lauvstad WA, Lui A, Ryan A, Glockner D, Levin SR. The influence of pyridoxine in diabetic peripheral neuropathy. Diabetes Care 1981;4:606–609.
129. McCann VJ, Davis RE. Pyridoxine and diabetic neuropathy: a double-blind controlled study. Diabetes Care 1983;6:102–103.
130. Schaumburg H, Kaplan J, Windebank A, Vick N, Rasmus S, Pleasure D, Browm MJ. Sensory neuropathy from pyridoxine abuse: a new megavitamin syndrome. N Engl J Med 1983;309:445–448.
131. Janka HU, Rietzel S, Mehnert H. Der Einfluβ von Neurobion auf die Temperatursensibilität bei Patienten mit diabetischer Neuropathie. In: N. Rietbrock, ed. Pharmakologie und klinische Anwendung hochdosierter B-Vitamine. Steinkopff, Darmstadt, 1991, pp. 87–97.
132. Stracke H, Lindemann A, Federlin K. A benfotiamine-vitamin B combination in treatment of diabetic polyneuropathy. Exp Clin Endocrinol Diabetes 1996;104:311–316.
133. Haupt E, Ledermann H, Köpcke W. Benfotiamine in treatment of diabetic polyneuropathy. J Peripher Nerv Syst 1997;2:270.
134. Loew D. Pharmacokinetics of thiamine derivatives especially of benfotiamine. Int J Clin Pharmacol Ther 1996;34:47–50.
135. Cohen KL, Lucibello FE, Chomiak MA. Lack of effect of clonidine and pentoxifylline in short-term therapy of diabetic peripheral neuropathy. Diabetes Care 1990;13:1074–1077.
136. Cohen SM, Mathews T. Pentoxifylline in the treatment of distal diabetic neuropathy. Angiology 1991;42:741–746.
137. De Leeuw IH, Van Roy P, Moeremans M, Driessens M. Clinical experience withy cyclandelate in insulin-dependent diabetic patients with neuropathy. Drugs 1987;33(Suppl 2):125–130.
138. Heimans JJ, Drukarch B, Matthaei I, Ijff GA, Bertelsmann FW, Strijers RL, Nauta J. Cyclandelate in diabetic neuropathy. A double-blind, placebo-controlled, randomized, cross-over study. Acta Neurol Scand 1991;84:483–486.
139. Janka HU, Schuh D, Nuber A, Mehnert H. Der Einfluβ von Ginkgo biloba Spezialextrakt EGb 761 auf die diabetische Neuropathie. Geriat Forsch 1992;2:173–179.
140. Hendriksen PH, Oey PL, Wieneke GH, Banga JD, van Dam PS. Antihypoxic treatment at an early stage of diabetic neuropathy: an electrophysiological study with sabeluzole. Acta Neurol Scand 1992;86:506–511.
141. Quatraro A, Minei A, De Rosa N, Giugliano D. Calcitonin in painful diabetic neuropathy. Lancet 1992;339:746–747.
142. Gallai V, Mazzotta G, Montesi S, Sarchielli P, Del Gatto F. Effect of uridine in the treatment of diabetic neuropathy: an electrophysiological study. Acta Neurol Scand 1992;86:3–7.
143. Biesenbach G, Grafinger P, Eichbauer-Sturm G, Zazgornik J. Cerebrolysin in der Behandlung der schmerzhaften diabetischen Neuropathie. Wien med Wschr 1997;147:63–66.
144. Cohen KL, Harris S. Efficacy and safety of nonsteroidal anti-inflammatory drugs in the therapy of diabetic neuropathy. Arch Intern Med 1987;147:1442–1444.
145. Foster AVM, Eaton C, McConville DO, Edmonds ME. Application of OpSite film: a new and effective treatment of painful diabetic neuropathy. Diabetic Med 1994;11:768–772.
146. Ewins DL, Vileikyte L, Borg-Costanzi J, Carrington A, Boulton AJM. Acupuncture: a novel treatment for painful diabetic neuropathy. In: Hotta N, Greene DA, Ward JD, Sima AAF, Boulton AJM, eds. Diabetic Neuropathy: New Concepts and Insights. Elsevier, Amsterdam, 1995, pp. 405–408.
147. Richardson PH, Vincent CA. Acupuncture for the treatment of pain: a view of evaluative research. Pain 1986;24:15–40.
148. Tawata M, Kurihara A, Nitta K, Iwase E, Gan N, Onaya T. The effects of goshajinkigan, a herbal medicine, on subjective symptoms and vibratory threshold in patients with diabetic neuropathy. Diabetes Res Clin Pract 1994;26:121–128.
149. Walk D. Immunotherapy of neuropathies in patients with diabetes mellitus requires closer scrutiny. Arch Neurol 1996;53:590–591.
150. Krendel DA. Immunotherapy of neuropathies in patients with diabetes mellitus requires closer scrutiny (in reply). Arch Neurol 1996;53:591–592.

# 11 Focal Diabetic Neuropathy

*Gérard Said, MD*

*CONTENTS*



## INTRODUCTION

Diabetic neuropathy is the most common neuropathy in industrialized countries, with a remarkable range of clinical manifestations. More than 80% of the patients with clinical diabetic neuropathy have a distal symmetrical form, with predominant or isolated sensory and autonomic manifestations *(1,2)*. In the others, and usually in association with symptomatic or latent distal symmetrical sensory polyneuropathy, diabetic patients may develop focal neuropathy that include cranial nerve involvement, limb and truncal neuropathies, and proximal diabetic neuropathy (PDN) of the lower limbs. In this group of neuropathies, the disorder tends to occur both in men and women over 50 yr of age, most with long-standing IDDM or NIDDM. The long-term prognosis of focal neuropathy is good in most cases, but sequelae occur in some patients with proximal diabetic neuropathy.

The occurrence of focal neuropathy in diabetic patients requires first exclusion of a nerve lesion from a superimposed cause by appropriate investigations, then consideration of the occurrence of nondiabetic neuropathies more common in diabetic patients, before concluding that the patient is suffering from a focal diabetic neuropathy and discussing which treatment, if any in addition to control of diabetes, is needed.

## CRANIAL DIABETIC NEUROPATHY

Oculomotor nerve palsies are the most common if not the only cranial neuropathy observed in diabetic patients.

### *Historical Background*

The first author to mention the occurrence of diabetic ophthalmoplegia is Ogle in 1866 (cited in ref. *3*). In 1905, Dieulafoy published a series of 58 personal cases in which he described most of the clinical characteristics of diabetic ophthalmoplegia *(4)*

From: *Contemporary Endocrinology: Clinical Management of Diabetic Neuropathy*
Edited by: A. Veves © Humana Press Inc., Totowa, NJ

and, in 1935, Waite and Beetham performed the first epidemiological study on the subject in which they compared the occurrence of oculomotor palsy in 2002 diabetic patients with 457 nondiabetic patients *(5)*. A series of other clinical reports have refined our knowledge on the subject, but pathological studies remain scanty with only a few autopsy cases studied *(6–8)* and the pathophysiology of oculomotor palsies in diabetic patients remains a matter of discussion.

## *Epidemiology*

Like focal neuropathy observed in other sites of the body, diabetic ophthalmoplegia is uncommon in diabetic patients. In 1933, Gray observed two patients with ophthalmoplegia among 500 diabetic patients examined *(9)* and Waite and Beetham estimated the incidence of oculomotor palsy among diabetics to be 0.8% *(5)* and to be 1.8% in ref. *10*. It is interesting to note that in this study, the frequency of oculomotor palsy was 0.8% in patients of less than 45 yr of age, vs 2.1% after 45 yr.

The sixth and the third cranial nerves are the most commonly affected oculomotor nerves. In a series of 58 cases of diabetic ophthalmoplegia, Dieulafoy (1906) reported 35 cases of sixth-nerve palsy, 12 cases of third-nerve palsy, five cases of fourth-nerve palsy, and six cases of external ophthalmoplegia *(4)*. The sixth cranial nerve was more often affected than the third one in two series *(11,5)*. Conversely, in another series, the third nerve is predominantly affected. The 14 patients reported by Weinstein and Dolger (1948) included seven cases of third-nerve palsy, six of sixth-nerve involvement, and one with simultaneous involvement of both nerves *(12)*. In an analysis of 811 cases of oculomotor palsies, diabetes accounted for 2.6% of third-nerve palsy, 1.9% of sixth-nerve palsy, and 0.6% of fourth-nerve palsy *(13)*. Finally, in Zorrilla and Kozak's series of 24 cases, 17 patients had an involvement of the third nerve, including two bilaterally, and seven cases of sixth-nerve palsy, but no fourth-nerve involvement *(14)*.

## *Clinical Manifestations*

In virtually all cases, diabetic ophthalmoplegia occurs in diabetic patients over 50 yr of age, both in insulin-dependent and in non-insulin-dependent diabetic patients. Rare cases have been reported in younger patients or even in children *(15)*. The onset is rapid, within a day or two. In many cases, the patient experiences pains during a few hours to a few days before noticing diplopia. Pain thus preceded the onset of diplopia in 14 out of the 25 patients reported by Green et al. *(16)* and in 18 out of the 22 episodes of oculomotor palsy that occurred in the 20 patients reported by Goldstein and Cogan *(17)*. Pain seems more common when the third cranial nerve is affected than when the sixth nerve is involved *(14)*. Pain is usually aching, behind or above the eye, and sometimes more diffuse but always homolateral to the oculomotor palsy. Pain is often attributed to the involvement of the first and second divisions of the trigeminal nerve within the cavernous sinus *(14)*, whereas others suggest a role for activation of pain-sensitive endings within the sheath of the third nerve as it traverses the cavernous sinus *(8,18)*. Pains does not persist after the onset of diplopia.

Oculomotor dysfunction is often incomplete—when the third nerve is involved one or two muscles only may be paralyzed. In their series of 22 episodes of ophthalmoplegia observed in 20 patients, Goldstein and Cogan mentioned 12 episodes of complete dysfunction, three episodes of nearly complete dysfunction, and three of partial paralysis *(17)*. Ptosis is marked, the eye is deviated outward when the internal rectus muscle is affected, and the patient is unable to move the eye medially, upward, or downward. Pupillary innervation is often spared, as in 75% of the cases in ref. *17*, whereas massive pupillar paralysis was observed in only two patients out of 20. In another study *(16)*, the pupillary function was spared in 68% of cases, whereas Rucker observed pupillary dysfunction in 3 out of 21 cases of third-nerve palsy *(13)*. Sparing of pupillary function permits one to differentiate third-nerve palsy of diabetic origin from third-nerve palsy resulting from compression of the nerve by an aneurysm of the posterior communicating artery, in which pupillary dilatation is very common. Centrofascicular lesion found by Asbury and coworkers at autopsy of a patient with third-nerve palsy accounts for sparing of pupillary function *(8)* because of the relative intactness of pupillomotor fibers that are peripherally placed in the third nerve *(18)*. However, it has been recently suggested that isolated third-nerve lesions in diabetic patients, with or without pupillary sparing, could result from mesencephalic infarcts *(19)*.

Spontaneous recovery invariably occurs within an average 2–3 mo, independently of the quality of control of hyperglycemia. Aberrant regeneration and synkinesia, which are common after facial-nerve palsy of different origin, do not disturb recovery of diabetic ophthalmoplegia.

### *Pathology*

Two serial sections studies performed in patients with third-cranial-nerve palsy demonstrated a centrofascicular lesion of the nerve in its intracavernous portion *(7,8)*. In the latter report, the axons were relatively spared on silver-stained sections. The myelin destructive lesion was 6–7 mm in length and the fibers placed at the periphery of the nerve trunk were relatively spared, which accounted for the pupillary sparing. The authors found no occluded vessel either intraneurally or in the nutrient vessels supplying the third nerve. In both reports, the authors agreed that the observed centrofascicular lesions of the third nerve were most likely ischemic in origin. It must be noted, however, that nerve ischemia usually induces axonal nerve lesions, not demyelinative ones. An inflammatory process of the type observed in biopsy specimens of the femoral nerve with partial ischemic lesions can also be considered.

## LIMB NEUROPATHY

Isolated involvement of peripheral nerve of the limbs including radial, median, and ulnar nerves in the upper limbs and of the peroneal nerve for the lower limbs, occurs in diabetic patient and it is sometimes difficult to know whether it is a manifestation of increased liability of nerves to pressure palsy in common sites of entrapment in diabetic patients, or a specific diabetic neuropathy. In other cases, development of sensorimotor deficit in the territory of one or several nerve trunks occur without evidence of superimposed cause for neuropathy. Such cases are extremely rare considering the frequency of distal symmetrical diabetic neuropathy and should always be investigated as in nondiabetic patients. In particular, it is necessary to perform electrophysiological testings to a more accurate localization of the lesions, and, when clinical and electrophysiological data point to spinal root lesions, to perform magnetic resonance imaging of the spine, or any other investigation needed to exclude another cause of neuropathy. When nerve trunks are clearly affected clinically and electrophysiologically, a nerve and muscle biopsy in an affected territory should be considered to exclude such causes as necrotizing arteritis, sarcoidosis, or leprosy. In some cases, however, no other cause than diabetes is found and the diagnosis of diabetic neuritis is likely. In the lower limbs, the most common pattern of focal neuropathy is characterized by proximal sensory and motor manifestations.

### *Proximal Diabetic Neuropathy (PDN) of the Lower Limbs*

Diabetic patients, usually over the age of 50, may also present proximal neuropathy of the lower limbs characterized by a variable degree of pain and sensory loss associated with uni- or bilateral proximal muscle weakness and atrophy. This syndrome, which was originally described by Bruns in 1890 *(20)*, has been subsequently reported under the terms of diabetic myelopathy *(21)*, diabetic amyotrophy *(22)*, femoral neuropathy *(23,24)*, proximal diabetic neuropathy *(25,26)*, femoral-sciatic neuropathy *(27)*, and the Bruns-Garland syndrome *(28,29)*. The neurological picture is limited to the lower limbs and is usually asymmetrical *(30)*. Clinically, the different patterns and the course of PDN strikingly differ from those of DSSP, suggesting different pathophysiologic features. In a recent study of 27 patients *(31)*, 24 had NIDDM and 3 had IDDM, and the mean age at diagnosis was 62 yr (range 46–71); the male:female ratio was 16:11.

The onset of the neuropathy is acute or subacute. The patient complains of numbness or pain of the anterior aspect of the thigh, often of the burning type, and it worsens at night. Difficulty in walking and climbing stairs occurs, because of weakness of the quadriceps and iliopsoas muscles. Muscle wasting is also an early and common phenomenon, which is often easier to palpate than to see in heavier patients. The patellar reflex is decreased or more often abolished. The syndrome progresses over weeks or months in most cases, then stabilizes and spontaneous pains decrease, sometimes rapidly. In many instances, as in those originally reported, there is no marked or any sensory loss, as emphasized by Garland who found inconstant extensor plantar response and increased CSF protein content, and felt that they resulted from a metabolic myelopathy in patients who were treated for diabetes but not under full diabetic control *(22)*. In approximately one third of the patients, there is a definite sensory loss over the anterior aspect of the thigh, and in the others a painful contact dysesthesia in the distribution of the cutaneous branches of the femoral nerve, without definite sensory loss.

Bruns who had described the condition, found that the disorder was reversible by dietetic restriction only *(20)*. Garland also noticed that in four of his five patients, there had been a striking recovery of power, with less obvious improvement of muscle wasting *(22)*. Most of the features identified by Garland were subsequently confirmed, including the usual good long-term prognosis, independently of the quality of diabetic control.

In most cases, the patient's condition improved after months, but sequelae including disabling weakness and amyotrophy, sensory loss, and patellar areflexia are common *(31,32)*. In a recent survey of long-term follow-up of up to 14 yr recovery began after a median interval of 3 mo (range 1–12 mo) *(31)*, pain was the first symptom to improve, resolution being comparatively rapid, beginning within a few weeks and being almost complete by 12 mo. Residual discomfort in the patients of Coppack and Watkins took up to 3 yr to subside. Motor recovery was satisfactory and none of their 27 cases showed disabling residual deficits, but seven complained of some persisting weakness and significant wasting of the thigh was evident in half of the cases *(31)*. Denervation atrophy found in the muscle samples fits well with the long-term, or permanent, weakness and amyotrophy that often affected distal muscles. Relapses on the other side are common, sometimes in spite of good diabetic control. In one fifth of the patients that we investigated for this syndrome, relapses occurred on the other side within a few months, the same proportion as in ref. *31*. Thus, the clinical features of PDN with frequent motor involvement, asymmetry of the deficit, and gradual yet often incomplete spontaneous recovery, markedly differ from those of DSSP in which the length-dependent symmetrical sensory deficit is associated with motor signs only in extreme cases, and which virtually never improves spontaneously. In the syndrome described by Garland as "diabetic amyotrophy," motor manifestations are more prominent and both sides are affected but the syndrome is a variant of proximal diabetic neuropathy, since lesions of the sensory branch of the femoral nerve are also present in patients who had no sensory signs or symptoms *(32)*.

### *Electrophysiological Studies*

Needle electromyography electrophysiological studies reveals signs of denervation in affected muscles with spontaneous fibrillation, usually bilaterally even in cases with weakness restricted to one side. In more severe cases, there may be evidence of widespread denervation affecting distal leg muscles as well and also those innervated by the lower thoracic spinal roots. In cases of long duration, motor-unit potentials are of increased amplitude, reflecting reinnervation by collateral sprouting from surviving motor axons. The motor action potentials may be polyphasic and of low amplitude, leading to the suspicion of myopathy *(33)*. Nerve-conduction studies indicate axonal loss rather than demyelination *(26)*, and the compound-muscle action potential in the quadriceps muscles on femoral nerve stimulation is reduced in amplitude. The F wave latencies to distal muscles *(34,35)* are difficult to interpret in view of the frequent coexistence of a distal polyneuropathy *(36,37,26)*.

### *Pathological Aspects of PDN*

In a recent pathological study of biopsy specimens of the intermediate cutaneous nerve of the thigh, a sensory branch of the femoral nerve that conveys sensation from the anterior aspect of the thigh, a territory commonly involved in PDN, we found that the pathology of proximal nerves varied with the clinical aspects of the neuropathy *(32)*. In the patients with the most severe sensory and motor deficit, examination of the biopsy specimen revealed lesions characteristic of severe nerve ischemia, including total axon loss in the two patients with the most severe deficit, and centrofascicular degeneration of fibers associated with a large number of regenerating fibers in one (Fig. 1), following a pattern of axonal loss observed in clinical and experimental nerve ischemia *(38,39)*. Lesions of nerve fibers coexisted with occlusion of a perineurial blood vessel in one of our patients, in keeping with the only detailed postmortem study of PDN available *(40)*, in which the authors found a small infiltration with mononuclear cells associated with the occlusion of an interfascicular artery of the obturator nerve in a patient with proximal and distal deficit of the left lower limb. In a patient who developed a rapid, asymmetrical, distal sensorimotor deficit shortly after the onset of the proximal deficit, recent occlusion of a perineurial blood vessel and perivascular, perineurial, and subperineurial inflammatory infiltration with mononuclear cells were demonstrated, along with axonal degeneration of the majority of nerve fibers of the superficial peroneal nerve. In the other patients, lesions of nerve fibers and of endoneurial capillaries were similar to those observed in the sural nerve in diabetic patients with

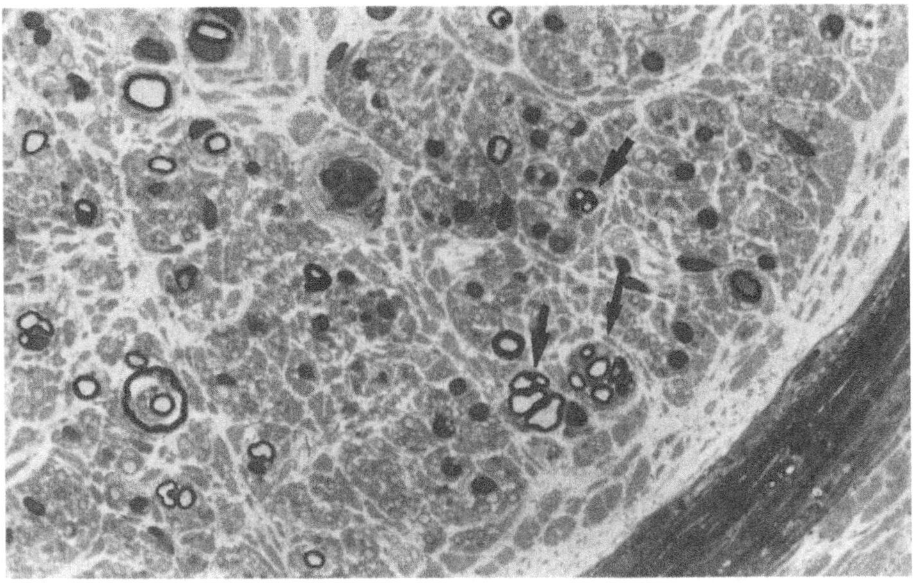

**Fig. 1.** One-micron thick cross-section of a biopsy specimen of the intermediate cutaneous nerve of the thigh from a patient with NIDDM who presented with proximal, purely motor, neuropathy of the lower limbs. There was no sensory loss upon examination. Note the striking reduction in the density of nerve fibers with several regenerating axons forming clusters (arrows). Thionin blue staining. Magnification: 1000X.

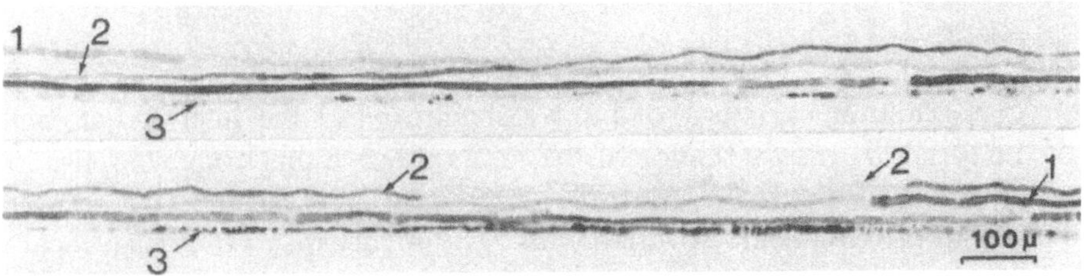


**Fig. 2.** Consecutive segments of groups of teased nerve fibers to illustrate the mixture of axonal degeneration (fiber 3) and segmental demyelination (fiber 2) and remyelination (fiber 1) observed in the intermediate cutaneous nerve of the thigh from a patient with clinically purely motor proximal diabetic neuropathy.

symptomatic DSSP. Mixed, axonal, and demyelinative nerve lesions were associated with increased endoneurial cellularity made of mononuclear cells that suggested the presence of a low-grade endoneurial inflammatory process in four of them (Fig. 2). In a recent study of patients with extremely painful PDN, we found similar inflammatory lesions with B- and T-lymphocytes mixed with macrophages *(41)*. The patients, who were already treated with insulin for weeks or months, became painless within days after performance of the biopsy, without additional treatment (Fig. 3). These observations show that the presence of inflammatory infiltrates does not preclude spontaneous recovery *(41)*.

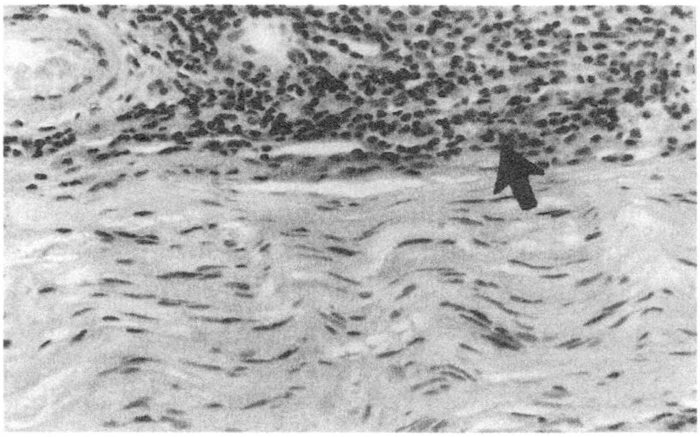

**Fig. 3.** Paraffin section of a nerve specimen from a patient with painful proximal diabetic neuropathy who recovered spontaneously after performance of the biopsy of the intermediate cutaneous nerve of the thigh. Note the conspicuous inflammatory infiltration of the epineurium and perineurium (arrow). Immunolabeling showed a mixture of B- and T-lymphocytes with a few macrophages. H & E staining. Magnification: 250X.

The relationship between the occurrence of inflammatory infiltrates, vasculitis, and diabetes is not clear. Small inflammatory infiltrates have been occasionally encountered in sural-nerve biopsy specimens of diabetic patients with neurological deficit *(42)* and in autonomic nerve bundles and ganglia *(43)*. Lesions of nerve fibers and of blood vessels caused by diabetes may trigger an inflammatory reaction and reactive vasculitis in some patients; alternatively diabetes may make the nerves more susceptible to intercurrent inflammatory or immune processes. In both cases, lesions of epi- or perineurial blood vessels can induce ischemic nerve lesions responsible for severe proximal sensory and motor deficits. Conversely, in milder forms, the lesions are more reminiscent of those observed in distal symmetrical polyneuropathy.

### *Focal Neuropathy of the Upper Limbs*

Focal nerve lesions of the upper limbs are very uncommon in diabetes, and another cause must always be looked for in this setting. During the past 25 yr, we saw only two patients with painful ulnar-nerve involvement, two patients with a radial-nerve palsy, and one patient who developed brachial neuritis after a proximal neuropathy of the lower limbs that could be attributed to diabetes. Proximal weakness of the upper limbs, as it appears in the lower limbs, is very uncommon, and seems to affect predominantly muscles supplied by the C5–C6 spinal roots *(44)*.

### *Truncal Neuropathy*

Trunk or thoraco-abdominal neuropathy affects almost exclusively older diabetic subjects *(45)*. It is unilateral or predominantly so. The onset is abrupt or rapid, with pains or dysesthesias as the main features. The pain may have a radicular distribution and is almost made worse by contact and at night. Weakness of abdominal muscles occurs *(46)*. Thoracic or truncal neuropathy should not be confused with sensory loss that affects the anterior aspect of the trunk in severe forms of length-dependent neuropathy, which is virtually never painful over the trunk *(47)*.

### *Nondiabetic Neuropathies more Common in Diabetic Patients*

In addition to specific neuropathies, diabetic patients seem more prone to develop some types of neuropathy than nondiabetic.

#### INCREASED LIABILITY TO PRESSURE PALSY

Pressure palsy is more common in diabetic individuals *(48)*. Carpal-tunnel syndrome occurs in 12% of diabetic patients *(49)* and the incidence of ulnar neuropathy caused by microlesions at the elbow level is high in diabetic patients also *(50)*.

#### ACQUIRED INFLAMMATORY DEMYELINATIVE POLYNEUROPATHY

Inflammatory, predominantly demyelinative neuropathy also must be differentiated from diabetic polyneuropathy, and may occur with a greater frequency in this population. This diagnosis must be suspected when an acute or subacute, often predominantly motor, demyelinative polyneuropathy occurs in a diabetic patient. Electrophysiological features are those of a demyelinative neuropathy *(51)*. The course and response to treatments are the same as in nondiabetic patients.

#### MUCORMYCOSIS

This rare condition is an acute disease that affects successively the air cavities of the face, the orbit, and the brain, in relation with proliferation of a fungus of the class *Phycomyceta (52)*. In 36% of the cases, it is associated with diabetes, especially diabetic acidosis. After an episode of rhinological involvement with epistaxis, a diabetic patient in acidosis manifests violent headaches and orbitonasal pains with swelling of the lids and ophthalmoplegia. The disease spreads to the meninges and to the brain through the arteries, inducing thrombosis of the ophthalmic, then of the internal carotid artery with subsequent hemiplegia. The prognosis is extremely poor. The diagnosis should be made very early by biopsy of the nasal lesions that allows identification of the causative phycomycete and beginning of treatment.

## DIFFERENTIAL DIAGNOSIS

In focal neuropathy occurring in diabetic patients, a neuropathy of another origin must always be excluded. In patients with ophthalmoplegia, preservation of pupillary motricity in a nearly complete third-nerve palsy strongly suggests a diabetic origin, however even in such cases, it is wiser to perform a noninvasive investigation of the area. Magnetic resonance angiogram, will permit one to rule out a compressive lesion of the third nerve by a large aneurysm of the carotid artery within the cavernous sinus, of the posterior communicating artery, or a fusiform aneurysm of the top of the basilar artery. Imaging will also permit exclusion of tumors occurring at the base of the brain or in the basal skull. In patients with progressive involvement of several cranial nerves without imaging abnormalities, examination of the CSF may detect malignant cells characteristic of a carcinomatous meningitis. In diabetic patients who develop a focal or multifocal neuropathy of the limbs, other causes than diabetes should also be considered. The first step in this context is to determine if the lesions are located in the spinal roots or in the peripheral nerves. A distinction that may be difficult clinically and electrophysiologically. In addition, the lesions may be mixed. A nerve and muscle biopsy may be considered, especially when another cause of focal or multifocal neuropathy is considered. When a diabetic patient develops proximal weakness without much pain, a superimposed cause of motor neuropathy or of motor neuron disease must be considered, and appropriate investigations undertaken.

## TREATMENT OF FOCAL DIABETIC NEUROPATHIES

Cranial-nerve palsies improve spontaneously and do not require specific treatment. Proximal diabetic neuropathy is often very painful and should be treated with paracetamol (acetaminophen) and codeine for example. Since some patients with disabling painful proximal neuropathy responded only to corticosteroids, this treatment should be considered in severe forms *(32)*. This will require adjustment of diabetic control with insulin in most cases. Others have suggested the use of immunosuppressives or immunomodulators, like iv, immunoglobulins *(42)*, but one should keep in mind that the overall spontaneous prognosis of focal diabetic neuropathies is good.

## REFERENCES


1. De Freitas MRG, Nascimento OJM, Chimelli L, et al. Neuropatia diabética. I-Conceito; Epidemiologia, Classificaçao, Quadro Clinico E Electroneuromiografico. Estudo De 210 Casos. Rev Bras Neurol 1992;28:69–73.
2. Thomas PK, Tomlinson DR. Diabetic and hypoglycemic neuropathy. In: PJ Dyck, PK Thomas, eds. Peripheral Neuropathy, Saunders, Philadelphia, 1993, pp. 1219–1250.
3. Man HX. Aspects neuro-ophtalmologiques du diabète sucré. In: Journées de Diabétologie de l'Hôtel Dieu. Editions Médicales Flammarion. Paris 1967, pp. 83–100.
4. Dieulafoy G. Clinique Médicale de l'Hotel-Dieu de Paris 1905–1906. Paris, Masson et Cie 1906, pp. 130–154.
5. Waite JH, Beetham VP. The visual mechanisms in diabetes mellitus (a comparative study of 2002 diabetics and 457 non diabetics). N Engl J Med 1935;212:429–443.
6. Weber RB, Daroff RB, Mackey EA. Pathology of oculomotor nerve palsy in diabetes. Neurology 1970;20:835–X
7. Dreyfus PM, Hakim S, Adams RD. Diabetic ophthalmoplegia. Arch Neurol Neurosurg Psychiat 1957;77:337–349.
8. Asbury AK, Aldredge H, Hershberg R, Fischer CM. Oculomotor palsy in diabetes mellitus: a clinicopathological study. Brain 1970;93:555–566.
9. Gray WA. (1933) Ocular conditions in diabetes mellitus. Br J Ophthal 1933;17:577–620.
10. Dollfus M. Examen ophtalmologique de 1300 diabétiques. XVII congrès international d'Ophtalmologie, Acta Concil 1954;119–127.
11. Collier J. Paralysis of the oculomotor nerve trunks in diabetes. Proc Roy Soc Med 1929;23:627–630.
12. Weinstein EA, Dolger H. External ocular muscle palsies occurring in diabetes mellitus. Arch Neurol Psychiat 1948;60:597–603.
13. Rucker CW. Paralysis of the third, fourth and sixth cranial nerves. Am J Ophthal 1958;46:787–794.
14. Zorrilla E, Kozak GP. Ophthalmoplegia in diabetes mellitus. Ann Intern Med 1967;5:968–977.
15. Jackson WPU. Ocular nerve palsy with severe headache in diabetes. Br Med J 1955;2:408,409.
16. Green WR, Hackett R, Schlezinger NS. Neuro-ophthalmologic evaluation of oculomotor nerve paralysis. Arch Ophthal 1964;72:154–167.
17. Goldstein JE, Cogan DG. Diabetic ophthalmoplegia with special reference to the pupil. Arch Ophthal 1960;64:592–600.
18. Sunderland S, Hughes ESR. The pupilloconstrictor pathway and the nerves to the ocular muscles in man. Brain 1946;69:301–309.
19. Hopf HC, Gutmann L. Diabetic third nerve palsy: evidence for a mesencephalic lesion. Neurology 1990;40:1041–1045.
20. Bruns L. Ueber neuritische Lähmungen beim diabetes mellitus. Berl Klin Wochenscher 1890;27:509–515.
21. Garland HT, Taverner D. Diabetic myelopathy. Br Med J 1953;1:1405–1408.
22. Garland HT. Diabetic amyotrophy. Br Med J 1955;2:1287–1290.
23. Goodman JI. Femoral neuropathy in relation to diabetes mellitus: report of 17 cases. Diabetes 1954;3:266–273.

24. Calverley JR, Mulder DW. Femoral neuropathy. Neurology 1960;10:963–967.
25. Asbury AK. Proximal diabetic neuropathy. Ann Neurol 1977;2:179.
26. Subramony SH, Wilbourn AJ. Diabetic proximal neuropathy. Clinical and electromyographic studies. J Neurol Sci 1982;53:293–304.
27. Skanse B, Gydell K. A rare type of femoral-sciatic neuropathy in diabetes mellitus. Acta Med Scand 1956;155:463–468.
28. Barohn RJ, Sahenk Z, Warmolts JR, Mendell JR. The Bruns-Garland syndrome (diabetic amyotrophy) revisited 100 years later. Arch Neurol 1991;48:1130–1135.
29. Chokroverty S, Reyes MG, Rubino FA. Bruns-Garland syndrome of diabetic amyotrophy. Trans Am Neurol Assoc 1977;102:1–4.
30. Asbury AK. Focal and multifocal neuropathies of diabetes. In: Dyck PJ, et al. eds. Diabetic Neuropathy. Saunders, Philadelphia, 1987, pp. 43–55.
31. Coppack SW, Watkins PJ. The natural history of diabetic femoral neuropathy. Q J Med 1991;79:307–313.
32. Said G, Goulon-Goeau C, Lacroix C, Moulonguet A. Nerve biopsy findings in different patterns of proximal diabetic neuropathy. Ann Neurol 1994;35:559–569.
33. Lamontagne A, Buchthal F. Electrophysiological studies in diabetic neuropathy. J Neurol Neurosurg Psychiatr 1970;33:442–52.
34. Williams IR, Mayer RF. Subacute proximal diabetic neuropathy. Neurology 1976;26:108–116.
35. Chokroverty S. Proximal nerve dysfunction in diabetic proximal amyotrophy. Arch Neurol 1982;39:403–407.
36. Isaacs H, Gilchrist G. Diabetic amyotrophy. S Afr Med J 1960;134:768–773.
37. Bastron JA, Thomas JE. Diabetic polyradiculopathy: clinical and electromyographic findings in 105 patients. Mayo Clin Proc 1981;56:725–732.
38. Fujimura H, Lacroix C, Said G. Vulnerability of nerve fibers to ischaemia. Brain 1991;114:1929–1942.
39. Nukada H, Dyck PJ. Microsphere embolization of nerve capillaries and fiber degeneration. Am J Path 1984;115:275–287.
40. Raff MC, Sangalang V, Asbury AK. Ischemic mononeuropathy and mononeuropathy multiplex in diabetes mellitus. Arch Neurol 1968;18:487–499.
41. Said G, Elgrably F, Lacroix C, Planté V, Talamon C, Adams D, Tager M, Slama G. Painful proximal diabetic neuropathy: inflammatory nerve lesions and spontaneous favourable outcome. Ann Neurol 1997, 41:762–770.
42. Krendel DA, Costigan DA, Hopkins LC. Successful treatment of neuropathies in patients with diabetes mellitus. Arch Neurol 1995;52:1053–1061.
43. Duchen LW, Anjorin A, Watkins PJ, Mackay JD. Pathology of autonomic neuropathy in diabetes mellitus. Ann Int Med 1980;92:301–303.
44. Wilbourn AJ. Diabetic neuropathies. In: Brown WF, Bolton CF, ed. Clinical Electromyography, 2nd ed. Butterworth-Heinemann, Boston, 1993, pp. 477–516.
45. Ellenberg M. Diabetic truncal mononeuropathy: a new clinical syndrome. Diabetes Care 1978;1:10–13.
46. Boulton AJM, Angus E, Ayyar DR, Weiss R. Diabetic thoracic polyradiculopathy presenting as an abdominal swelling. B Med J 1984;289:798–799.
47. Said G, Slama G, Selva J. Progressive centripetal degeneration of axons in small fibre type diabetic polyneuropathy. A clinical and pathological study. Brain 1983;106:791–807.
48. Mulder DW, Lambert EH, Bastron JA, Sprague RG. The neuropathies associated with diabetes: a clinical and electromyographic study of 103 unselected diabetic patients. Neurology 1961;11:275–284.
49. Palumbo PJ, Elveback LR, Whisnant JP. Neurologic complications of diabetic mellitus: transient ischemic attack, stroke and peripheral neuropathy. In: Schoenberg B.S., ed. Advances in Neurology, vol. 19. Raven, New York, 1978, pp. 593–598.
50. Fraser DM, Campbell IW, Ewing DJ, et al. Mononeuropathy in diabetes mellitus. Diabetes 1979;28:96.
51. Cornblath D, Drachman DB, Griffin JW. Demyelinating motor neuropathy in patients with diabetic polyneuropathy. Ann Neurol 1987;22:126–132.
52. Dhermy P. Phycomycosis (Mucormycosis). In: Vinken PJ, and Bruyn GW, eds. Handbook of Clinical Neurology, vol. 35. North Holland Publishing, Amsterdam 1978, pp. 541–555.

# 12 Diabetic Autonomic Neuropathy

*An Overview*

*Roy Freeman*, MD

*CONTENTS*



## INTRODUCTION

Diabetes is the most frequent cause of peripheral neuropathy in the developed world. A broad constellation of symptoms occur, affecting cardiovascular, urogenital, gastrointestinal, pupillomotor, thermoregulatory, and sudomotor function. Autonomic impairment is usually gradual and progressive. Estimates of the prevalence of diabetic autonomic neuropathy are dependent on the specific population under study and most reported studies have referral bias. A community-based population study in Oxford, UK showed the prevalence of autonomic neuropathy, defined by the presence of one or more abnormal heart-rate variability test result, was 16.7% *(1)*. Symptomatic autonomic neuropathy (excluding erectile failure) was present in 11.6% of type 1 and 0.5% of type 2 diabetic patients in this cohort. Erectile failure was present in 40.8% of the diabetic males *(1)*. Symptomatic visceral autonomic neuropathy had a prevalence of 5.5% in a population-based study of diabetic patients in Rochester, Minnesota *(2)*. The prevalence of erectile failure in this study was 13% of the insulin-dependent diabetic patients (IDDM) and 8% of the non-insulin-dependent (NIDDM) patients. Other autonomic symptoms were reported considerably less frequently. Gastroparesis was reported in 0% of IDDM patients and 1% of NIDDM patients; nocturnal diarrhea in 1% of IDDM patients and 0.4% of NIDDM patients; urinary incontinence in 1% of IDDM patients and 0% of NIDDM patients, and postural fainting in 1% of IDDM patients and 0% of NIDDM patients *(2)*.

From: *Contemporary Endocrinology: Clinical Management of Diabetic Neuropathy*
Edited by: A. Veves © Humana Press Inc., Totowa, NJ

## CARDIOVASCULAR AUTONOMIC NEUROPATHY

### *Clinical Features*

Severe symptomatic cardiovascular autonomic dysfunction occurs infrequently in community-based studies of diabetic autonomic neuropathy. In clinic-based studies, 15–40% of unselected diabetic patients display abnormalities in cardiovascular autonomic function *(3–8)*. Abnormalities are present in teenagers with IDDM and patients tested shortly after diagnosis, which suggests that, at least in some cases, autonomic nervous system dysfunction or damage occurs early in the course of diabetes *(9–11)*.

An increased resting heart rate is frequently observed in diabetic patients *(12,13)*. With disease progression, some patients display a fixed heart rate that, like the transplanted heart, responds only minimally to physiological stimuli. The heart-rate changes have a characteristic time course. Initially, there is a tachycardia, most likely because of the vagal cardiac neuropathy that results in unopposed cardiac sympathetic nerve activity. The tachycardia may be followed by a decrease in heart rate and, ultimately, a fixed heart rate caused by progressing cardiac sympathetic nervous system dysfunction *(14–16)*.

The normal autonomic nervous system displays circadian variability. Control subjects have a nocturnal increase in parasympathetic tone, whereas sympathetic tone increases in the first hours after awakening and is maintained throughout the day *(17)*. Thus, normal subjects have longer mean RR intervals and greater heart-rate variability at night *(18)*. Abnormal circadian rhythms because of decreased parasympathetic nervous system activity have been observed in diabetic patients. Twenty-four-h EKG recordings of diabetic patients have shown a reduced nocturnal fall of heart rate, higher mean hourly heart rate, and lower heart-rate variability compared to controls *(18–22)*.

Blood pressure also exhibits a circadian rhythm. In control subjects, blood pressure is lowest during sleep and highest during wakefulness. Several studies have demonstrated a loss, blunting, or reversal of the nocturnal blood pressure fall in diabetic patients. The disruption of the blood-pressure circadian rhythm has been associated with autonomic neuropathy *(22–24)*. A cardiomyopathy may be present in diabetic patients, even those without ischemic heart disease. The cardiomyopathy manifests as impaired myocardial contractility and a decreased left-ventricular diastolic filling observable by radionuclear ventriculography *(25,26)*. The causes of the cardiomyopathy include an autonomic neuropathy, microvascular myocardial disease, decreased cardiac-catecholamine responsivity, and myocellular hypertrophy with fibrosis. Silent or painless cardiac ischemia *(27,28)* attributed to damage to afferent fibers reaching the myocardium is also frequently reported.

Several authors have drawn attention to the increased frequency of sudden death in patients with autonomic neuropathy. Proposed etiologies have included cardiorespiratory arrest caused by cardiac arrhythmias, QT-interval dispersion, silent cardiac ischemia, sleep apnea, and an abnormal ventilatory response to hypoxia, particularly in association with pulmonary infection, surgery, and anesthesia *(29–32)*.

Numerous studies have identified a relationship between autonomic neuropathy and QT interval prolongation in diabetic subjects *(33–41)*. These observations may explain the sudden and unexpected death observed in some diabetic patients. The role of QT-interval prolongation in the complications of diabetes is not universally accepted. Furthermore, the association between autonomic neuropathy and QT prolongation is not present in all studies. Bazett's formula is the most widely used formula for adjusting the QT interval for heart rate. However, the use of this method to adjust the QT interval may overcorrect the interval at fast heart rates and undercorrect the interval at slow heart rate.

Orthostatic hypotension, defined as a fall in systolic blood pressure of 20 mmHg or a fall in diastolic blood pressure of 10 mmHg, *(42)* occurs in diabetic patients as a consequence of efferent sympathetic vasomotor denervation that causes reduced vasoconstriction of the splanchnic and other peripheral vascular beds *(43)*. Patients typically present with lightheadedness and presyncopal symptoms. Many patients, however, remain asymptomatic despite significant falls in blood pressure. There is a decrease in total, splanchnic, and cutaneous vascular resistance. The normal increase in plasma norepinephrine in response to postural change is typically reduced relative to the fall in blood pressure *(44)*. Diminished cardiac acceleration and cardiac output, particularly in association with exercise, may also play a role in the presentation of this disorder *(44,45)*. Less frequently, an increase in norepinephrine is observed that may be caused by low blood volume or decreased red-cell mass *(46,47)*. Fluctuations in the degree of orthostatic hypotension are frequently observed and may reflect postprandial blood pooling, the hypotensive role of insulin, and changing patterns of fluid retention because of renal failure or congestive heart failure *(48–50)*.

Treatment endeavors include nonpharmacological approaches such as a high sodium diet, raising the head of the bed during sleep, and supportive hose. These measures usually help only the mildly afflicted.

Pharmacological measures include mineralocorticoids, direct and indirect sympathomimetic agents and other pressors, prostaglandin-synthesis inhibitors, dopamine-blocking agents, and V-receptor agonists *(51,52)*. These medications may be used singly or in combination. Recent observations suggest that erythropoietin may increase standing blood pressure and improve orthostatic tolerance in patients with orthostatic hypotension *(53,54)*. Therapy should be initiated with 9-alpha-fludrocortisone. The usual starting dose is 0.1 mg. This agent can be gradually increased to a maximal daily dose of 0.5–1.0 mg. A pressor, sympathomimetic agent, erythropoietin, or prostaglandin-synthetase inhibitor can be added to the drug regimen of those patients who remain symptomatic (see Table 1). Most diabetic patients with orthostatic hypertension will respond to these interventions. Refractory patients may require a combination of several agents, although the orthostatic hypotension that is associated with diabetes only rarely demands such extensive therapy.

## *Laboratory Evaluation*

The heart receives reciprocal innervation by the sympathetic and parasympathetic nervous systems. Cardiac parasympathetic nerves originate in the dorsal motor nucleus and nucleus ambiguus of the medulla oblongata. The presynaptic vagus nerves synapse with postsynaptic epicardial and myocardial cells predominantly situated near the SA node and AV node. The right vagus predominantly innervates the SA node, whereas the left vagus predominantly innervates the AV node. Acetylcholine is the predominant neurotransmitter released at the postsynaptic parasympathetic nerve terminals. Vagal stimulation results in an abrupt bradycardia. The sympathetic preganglionic nerves originate in the intermediolateral column of spinal-cord segments C7–T6. These nerves

Table 1
Pharmacotherapy of Orthostatic Hypotension

| |
|---|
| Mineralocorticoids |
| 9 α-Fludrocortisone |
| Sympathomimetic agents |
| Ephedrine |
| Pseudoephedrine |
| Phenylpropanolamine |
| Midodrine |
| Nonspecific pressor agents |
| Ergot derivatives |
| Caffeine |
| Somatostatin analogs |
| β-Adrenergic blocking agents |
| Propranolol |
| Pindolol |
| Prostaglandin synthetase inhibitors |
| Indomethacin |
| Ibuprofen |
| Naproxen |
| Dopamine blocking agents |
| Metoclopramide |
| Domperidone |
| V1 and V2 receptor agonists |
| Desmopressin acetate (DDAVP) |
| Lysine-vasopressin |
| Erythropoietin |

synapse in the stellate and middle cervical ganglia and, upon reaching the heart, innervate the myocardium, atria, and conduction system. Norepinephrine is the neurotransmitter released by sympathetic nerves.

The autonomic nerves are usually subdivided under the classification proposed by Gasser *(55)*. Under this classification the unmyelinated C fibers and lightly myelinated Aδ fibers are responsible for autonomic-nerve transmission. The C fibers have a diameter of 0.25–1.35 mm and a conduction velocity of 0.5–2 m/s. These nerve fibers also convey innocuous warm and cold, noxious heat, and dull pain sensation. The Ad fibers have a larger diameter of 3–7 mm and a faster conduction velocity of 3–30 m/s. The Aδ nerve fibers also convey innocuous cold and sharp pain sensation. These nerves are not directly accessible and thus slow conduction velocities are not amenable to standard neurophysiological techniques (*see* Table 2).

A group of tests assessing autonomic function and dysfunction has been developed over the years that circumvent the problems created by the inaccessibility of the autonomic nerves and their slow conduction velocities. The most widely used of these tests are the measures of cardiovascular autonomic function. Combinations of these autonomic tests provide a sensitive measure of autonomic function and have been utilized by many investigators evaluating diabetic patients with autonomic failure *(56–58)*.

Table 2
Subdivision of Autonomic Fibers

| *Fiber type* | *Myelin* | *Diameter* | *C.V.* | *Other Functions* |
|---|---|---|---|---|
| Aδ fibers | lightly myelinated | 3–7 mm | 3–30 m/s | cold and sharp pain |
| C fibers pain | unmyelinated | 0.25–1.35 mm | 0.5–2 m/s | warm, cold, noxious heat and dull |

### *Cardiovascular Autonomic Function Testing*

In 1982, Ewing and Clarke advocated a battery of five tests, suitable for bedside autonomic function testing. These tests (the average inspiratory-expiratory heart-rate difference with six deep breaths, the Valsalva ratio, the 30:15 ratio, the diastolic blood pressure response to isometric exercise, and the systolic blood-pressure fall to standing), they suggested, provided an assessment of both sympathetic and parasympathetic nervous system function. With some modifications, this test battery still forms the core of the cardiovascular autonomic evaluation performed by many autonomic laboratories *(59)*.

Clinical studies using these noninvasive measures of cardiovascular function have demonstrated a strong correlation with the presence of symptoms *(60,61)*. Abnormal measures of cardiovascular autonomic function have also correlated with abnormal autonomic function in other organ systems including abnormal pupillomotor function, *(62,63)* gastrointestinal function *(64)* and norepinephrine production *(65)*. Although these cardiovascular tests are sensitive, abnormalities in lower-extremity sudomotor function and impotence may precede any detectable cardiovascular autonomic neuropathy *(60,66)*.

A pattern of initial parasympathetic cardiac dysfunction followed by sympathetic cardiovascular dysfunction has been observed. This observation may be a consequence of the nerve "length dependence" of the neuropathic process or a reflection of the sensitivity of the tests of cardiac autonomic function. Low et al. *(66)* addressed the latter possibility in a study comparing distal sweating (a cholinergic, sympathetic nervous system-mediated function) with heart-rate variation (a parasympathetic nervous system-mediated function) in patients with diabetic neuropathy. He demonstrated that distal abnormalities in sweating, occurred with equal frequency to abnormalities of heart rate variation.

#### The Evaluation of Cardiac Vagal Function

The laboratory evaluation of vagal function in patients with autonomic failure includes measures of heart rate variation at rest and in response to deep respiration, following a Valsalva maneuver, in response to postural change, and other physiological stimuli. These tests primarily provide an index of vagal cardiac (parasympathetic nervous system) function *(67)* (*see* Table 3).

**The Heart Rate Response to Respiration** The beat-to-beat variability of heart rate in response to respiration has been recognized since the mid-19th century. This variability, at normal respiratory rates, is predominantly mediated by the vagus nerve and is reduced or abolished by vagotomy and muscarinic blockade. The determinants of the respiratory fluctuations in heart rate include a stretch reflex from the lungs and thoracic

Table 3
Tests Assessing Cardiac Vagal (Parasympathetic Nervous System) Function

| |
|---|
| Time-domain measures of heart-rate variability (at rest and with deep respiration) |
| High frequency heart-rate spectral power |
| Heart-rate response to a Valsalva maneuver |
| Heart-rate response to postural change |

Table 4
Time-Domain Measures of HRV with Respiration

| |
|---|
| Maximum minus minimum HR difference |
| Maximum minus minimum RR interval difference |
| Maximum/minimum HR |
| Maximum/minimum RR interval |
| Standard deviation (SD) of RR intervals |
| SD of the HR |
| Histogram displays of RR intervals |
| Coefficient of variation of heart rate |
| Coefficient of variation of RR intervals |
| MSSD (mean square successive difference) |
| rMSSD (root mean square successive difference) |
| MSD (mean successive difference) |
| SDSD (SD of the successive differences in RR intervals) |
| Histogram displays of RR interval differences |
| Mean circular resultant |

wall, changes in cardiac filling, arterial baroreceptor responses to blood pressure changes, changes in baroreflex sensitivity with respiratory phase, and respiratory-center activity overflow to medullary vasomotor neurons. Wheeler and Watkins first suggested that the amplitude of the beat-to-beat variation with respiration could be used as a clinical measure of autonomic nervous system function *(12,13)*. In the ensuing years additional measures have been proposed including the standard deviation of the R R interval *(57)*, the mean square successive difference (MSSD) *(68)*, the mean successive difference (MSD) *(57)*, the expiratory-inspiratory ratio (E:I ratio) *(13)*, and the mean circular resultant *(69)* (*see* Table 4).

The mean circular resultant, a determination based on vector analysis, has been proposed as a method that is resistant to nonrespiratory sources of variability such as ectopic heart beats and slow trends in heart rate. In this method, RR intervals are recorded as time events plotted or wrapped on a circle with the periodicity of a single respiratory cycle. The distribution of the points on the circle is determined by vector analysis, giving a result in arbitrary units. Regular distribution of the events on the circle would result in a small vector and denote reduced heart rate variability. In contrast, clustering of the events on the circle would result in a large vector and suggest normal heart-rate variability. Five minutes of carefully controlled respiration is required *(69,70)*. Although this measure has not attained widespread use, it was the sole test of heart-rate variability with respiration in the DCCT study *(71)*.

Gundersen and Neubauer, 1977 proposed that a measure based on successive differences in the RR intervals, i.e., the actual differences between adjacent RR intervals, would be more sensitive than the standard deviation to short-term fluctuations in heart rate. The mean square successive difference (MSSD) is the average of the square of the differences between successive beats *(68)*, the rMSSD is its square root *(72)*, the mean successive difference (MSD) *(57)* is the average of the differences between successive beats, whereas the SDSD is the standard deviation of the successive differences *(21)*. Unlike the standard deviation of the RR intervals, these measures are dependent on the sequence of RR intervals. The measurements are theoretically robust against gradual trends in heart rate over time and are independent of mean heart rate *(73)* (although not in all studies) *(74)*. They are, however, sensitive to ectopic beats such as PVCs, i.e., a short interval followed by a long compensatory pause *(74)*.

The variables that influence heart-rate variation in response to deep breathing include the subject's age, and the rate and depth of respiration. If these variables are controlled, the maximum heart-rate variation in response to deep breathing is a sensitive and specific index of autonomic function. This test is the best noninvasive test to assess cardiac vagal innervation.

**The Heart-Rate Response to a Valsalva Maneuver** The Valsalva maneuver provides a measure of sympathetic, vagal, and baroreceptor function. The maneuver is typically performed by blowing through a mouthpiece connected to a mercury manometer for 15 or 20 s. The mercury column of the manometer is maintained at 40 mm. There should be a small air leak in the system to prevent closing of the glottis. The normal Valsalva maneuver has four phases. Phase 1 consists of a transient rise in arterial pressure and an associated decrease in heart rate. In phase 2, during the expiratory phase of the maneuver, there is a gradual fall in blood pressure followed by a recovery. An increase in heart rate accompanies this phase. Phase 3 consists of a sudden brief fall in blood pressure with an accompanying increase in heart rate occurring with the cessation of straining. In phase 4, there is an increase in blood pressure above the resting value (the "overshoot") that is accompanied by a bradycardia. Phases 1 and 3 most likely reflect mechanical factors, whereas phases 2 and 4 are a consequence of sympathetic, vagal, and baroreflex interactions *(75–80)* (see Fig. 1).

The Valsalva ratio (the ratio between the tachycardia during the maneuver and the postmaneuver bradycardia), provides an index of cardiac vagal function *(43,76,77,81)*. Variables that influence the Valsalva ratio include age *(82)* and the duration and magnitude of expiratory effort *(78)*. In addition, when sympathetic outflow is deficient, parasympathetic activity cannot be adequately assessed because blood pressure during phase 4 does not increase and thus there is no stimulus to increase vagal activity *(83)*.

**The Heart-Rate Response to Postural Change** Analysis of the heart-rate response to postural change also provides a measure of sympathetic nervous system, parasympathetic nervous system, and baroreceptor function. Active standing results in an abrupt increase in heart rate that peaks at approx 3 s followed by a more gradual increase that peaks at approx 12 s after standing. The initial increase in heart rate is mediated by the sudden inhibition of vagal tone, whereas the more gradual increase is caused by further vagal inhibition and increased sympathetic nervous system activity. The initial heart-rate increase is most likely an "exercise reflex" evoked by muscle contraction, whereas reduced baroreceptor stimulation because of transient hypotension is responsible for the later increase in heart rate *(84,85)*. The heart rate and blood pressure return to a new

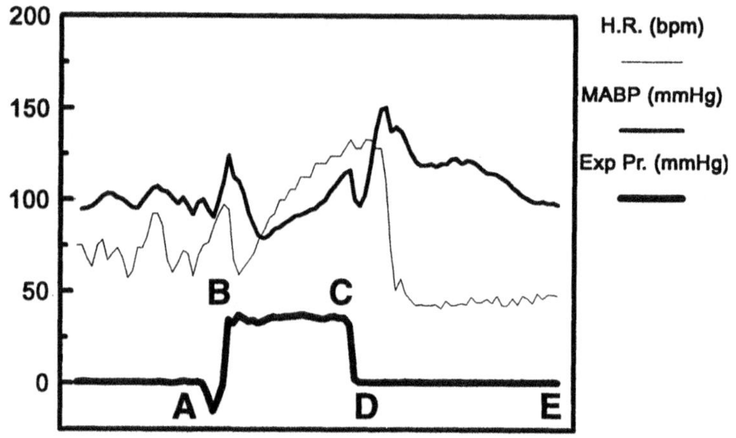


**Fig. 1.** A normal Valsalva maneuver. **(A–B)** Phase 1; **(B–C)** Phase II; **(C–D)** Phase III; and **(D–E)**: Phase IV. (HR indicates heart rate; bpm indicates beats per minute; MABP indicates mean arterial blood pressure, Exp. Pr. indicates expiratory pressure) (adapted with modifications from ref. *67*).

baseline after approx 30 s. The "30:15 ratio" assesses this physiological response by measuring the ratio of the heart rate increase that occurs at approx 15 s after standing to the relative bradycardia that occurs at approx 30 s after standing *(86,87)*. When cardiovagal function is deficient, the bradycardia does not occur. This ratio provides a measure of cardiac vagal function *(84)*.

Sundkvist et al. dissected the heart rate response to passive tilting by measuring the acceleration index (the shortest RR interval after standing minus the baseline RR interval all divided by the baseline RR interval) and the brake index (the longest RR interval after standing minus the shortest RR interval all divided by the baseline RR interval). They suggested that the acceleration index provides a measure of baroreceptor-mediated vagal withdrawal, whereas the brake index assesses the vagal response to the sympathetic nervous system-mediated increase in peripheral resistance *(88)*. Others have suggested that the RR interval lengthening does not occur after passive tilting *(84,86)*.

**The Heart-Rate Response to Lying Down** A related test measures the heart rate response to assuming the supine position. After lying down, there is a decrease in the RR interval that is maximal around the third or fourth beat that is followed by an increase in the RR interval value (greater than the resting value) at approx the 25th to 30th beat. Autonomic blockade studies with atropine and propranolol have suggested that the initial RR interval shortening is mediated by the vagus nerve, whereas the latter lengthening of the RR interval is predominantly mediated by the sympathetic nervous system. The initial tachycardia is most likely a manifestation of the "exercise" or "muscle-heart" reflex *(89,90)*.

**The Heart-Rate Response to Squatting** The cardiovascular response to squatting has been measured in a group of controls and diabetic subjects *(91,92)*. In their test, protocol subjects stood still for 3 min, squatted for 1 min, and finally stood up during inspiration. Squatting resulted in lengthening of the RR interval that is abolished by atropine, suggesting a vagal-mediated response, and the shortening of the RR interval that occurred after standing from a squatting position was attenuated by propranolol. A vagal ratio based on this test (the ratio between the RR interval mean before squatting and the longest RR interval after squatting) was calculated that was outside the 99% confidence interval in 42% of diabetic patients and 1.3% of the control subjects. The test results showed an inverse correlation with age *(91)*.

**The Heart-Rate Response to Apneic Facial Immersion** The diving reflex, a reflex present in mammals, is provoked by facial cooling and consists of bradycardia, apnea, decreased cardiac output, and vasoconstriction *(93)*. As a clinical test, the diving reflex can be induced by apneic facial immersion. This test assesses trigeminal-vagal-cardiac and trigeminal-sympathetic-vascular smooth muscle pathways and does not directly involve the baroreflex or its primary central connections *(94)*. The test can also be performed on uncooperative or unconscious patients *(95)*. Some, however, have suggested that this test does not add significantly to other measures of autonomic function *(96)*.

**Long-Term Measures of Heart-Rate Variability** Ewing et al. drew attention to the large, irregular, episodic changes in heart rate that occur in normal subjects. They quantified these steps using a threshold value of a 50 ms difference from the preceding RR interval (NN50) and demonstrated a reduced number of these steps in diabetic subjects with autonomic neuropathy, some diabetic patients without autonomic neuropathy, and patients with cardiac transplants. The number of such steps or "RR counts" in normal subjects shows an inverse relationship with age and the steps show a significant increase during sleep *(19,97)*. Twenty-four percent of diabetic subjects with normal cardiovascular reflexes, had 24-h RR count results that were less than the lower 95% confidence limit for healthy controls related to age. Based on these results, the authors suggested that this method of heart-rate variability analysis is more sensitive than the conventional tests of cardiovascular reflexes *(97)*. This measure and the related pNN50 (the proportion of differences in consecutive normal RR intervals that are greater than 50 ms) correlates with the rMSSD and power in the high frequency of the heart-rate power spectrum ($>0.15$ Hz) *(72,98,99)*.

#### Evaluation of Adrenergic Function

The most frequently performed cardiovascular tests of sympathetic nervous system function are the blood-pressure response to postural change (active standing or passive tilting). The assumption of the upright posture results in a reflex increase in sympathetic and decrease in parasympathetic outflow. Measurements of the changes in blood pressure and heart rate induced by active standing or passive tilt are an essential part of the laboratory and bedside evaluation of patients with suspected adrenergic failure. When severe autonomic failure is present, blood pressure and heart rate abnormalities are apparent after 5–10 min of head up tilt or active standing. Early or mild adrenergic failure may require a longer period of standing or duration of tilt *(88,100,101)*.

Sustained muscle contraction causes a rise in blood pressure and heart rate. Stimuli from exercising muscle and the central nervous system ("central command"), generate an increase in efferent sympathetic activity that increases cardiac output, blood pressure, and heart. The blood-pressure and heart-rate changes induced by a sustained handgrip have been used as a clinical test of sympathetic function. The response to this test is subject to marked variability caused in part by difficulty standardizing muscular effort *(102)*.

A direct measure of the hemodynamic response to the Valsalva maneuver can be made with a noninvasive beat-to-beat blood-pressure monitors such as the Finapres. The availability of these noninvasive blood-pressure measurements permits the determination of the role played by the sympathetic nervous system in the physiological

Table 5
Tests Assessing Cardiovascular Adrenergic (Sympathetic Nervous System) Function

| |
|---|
| Blood-pressure response to standing |
| Blood-pressure response to upright tilt |
| Blood-pressure response to the Valsalva maneuver |
| Blood-pressure response to isometric exercise |
| Blood-pressure response to mental stress |
| Cold pressor test |
| Low frequency heart-rate and blood pressure spectral power |

responses to this maneuver. There is a fall in blood pressure during phase 2 and an increase in blood pressure during phase 4 of the Valsalva maneuver. The measurement of these blood pressure changes during phase 2 and phase 4 of the Valsalva maneuver provides a measure of vasomotor adrenergic function. Indices of abnormality include a fall in blood pressure during phase 2 of <20 mmHg, failure of BP in phase 2 to stabilize or return to baseline and the absence of the "overshoot" of blood pressure in phase 4 *(103)* (see Fig. 1).

The blood-pressure response to cold water immersion *(104)* and mental stress tests *(105)* are less frequently performed tests of adrenergic function. These tests have lower sensitivity and specificity (see Table 5).

### Power Spectral Analysis

Power spectral analysis provides a useful noninvasive technique for analyzing the autonomic mechanisms that control heart rate. The increasing availability of microcomputers and the ensuing ease with which digital signals can be processed has been largely responsible for the recent emergence of measures of autonomic function in the frequency domain *(106,107)*. Spectral analysis reduces a signal to the sum of its component sine waves of different amplitudes and frequencies. The power spectrum displays the squared amplitude of these sine waves as a function of frequency, thus expressing the variance as a function of frequency. Heart-rate fluctuations, which reflect modulation of sinus node activity by autonomic and other homeostatic mechanisms, can be quantified and displayed using this technique.

Spectral analysis of the resting heart rate commonly produces several prominent peaks. A number of animal and human experiments with pharmacological blockade of the autonomic nervous system have shown that the sympathetic and parasympathetic nervous systems mediate heart-rate fluctuations in different frequency bands. The peak found at the highest frequency (>0.15 Hz) reflects oscillations of heart rate that occur with respiration—the respiratory sinus arrhythmia. Quantification of these oscillations provides a measure of the response of the sinus node to fluctuations in vagal-nerve activity at the respiratory frequency and is reduced by parasympathetic pharmacological blockade. Oscillations in heart rate at frequencies less than 0.15 Hz are mediated by both the vagus and the cardiac sympathetic nerves. Spectral power within the 0.05–0.15 Hz frequency band may represents baroreceptor feedback activity, whereas the spectral power at less than 0.05 Hz may reflect both cardiac autonomic input as well as the influence of circulating neurohumoral factors. In normal subjects, the move from the supine to upright position produces a shift in the power spectrum from high to low frequencies (see Fig. 2A). This shift in spectral power, induced by a postural change, is reduced by beta-adrenergic-receptor blockade and may provide an index of sympathetic activity. In diabetic patients, quantification of autonomic function using indices derived from the power spectrum also correlates with the results of standard time domain tests of autonomic function *(107)*. Power spectral analysis may thus provide a measure of both sympathetic and parasympathetic nervous system function that requires minimal patient cooperation *(108,109)*. There is a progressive decline in low- and high-frequency power with progression of diabetic autonomic neuropathy *(107,110)* (see Fig. 2A–C). Some authors have suggested that measures derived from the heart-rate power spectrum provide a more sensitive measure of diabetic autonomic neuropathy *(111,112)*.

## URINARY SYSTEM

### *Clinical Features*

Symptoms of bladder dysfunction have been observed in 37–50% of diabetic patients and there is physiologic evidence of bladder dysfunction in 43–87% of insulin-dependent diabetic patients *(113–115)*. Bladder symptoms associated with autonomic neuropathy include hesitancy, poor stream, increased intervals between micturition, and a sense of inadequate bladder emptying. These symptoms may be followed by urinary retention and overflow incontinence *(113,116,117)*.

The bladder wall is comprised of three layers of interdigitating smooth muscle (the detrusor muscle) and serves as a receptacle for the storage and appropriate evacuation of urine. The detrusor muscle forms the internal sphincter at the junction of the bladder neck and urethra. This sphincter is not anatomically discrete and functions as a physiological sphincter. Afferent fibers mediating bladder sensation and reflex bladder contraction are carried by sympathetic, parasympathetic, and somatic nerves to the spinal cord *(118)*. Detrusor-muscle sensory abnormalities are the earliest bladder autonomic abnormality to occur, producing impaired bladder sensation and increasing the threshold for initiating the micturition reflex. This results in an asymptomatic increase in bladder capacity and retention.

The parasympathetic nerves that originate in the intermediolateral column of the 2nd, 3rd, and 4th sacral segments of the spinal cord provide the major excitatory input to the urinary bladder. Activation of these muscarinic, cholinergic, postganglionic pelvic nerves produces detrusor muscle contraction. When the function of these efferent parasympathetic fibers to the detrusor muscle is impaired, symptoms such as incomplete voiding, hesitancy in micturition, weak stream, and dribbling ensue. A decrease in detrusor activity (detrusor areflexia) follows that leads to incomplete bladder emptying, an increased postvoid residual, decreased peak urinary flow rate, bladder overdistension, and urinary retention. Finally, overflow incontinence occurs because of denervation of the external sphincter (innervated by the somatic pudendal nerve) and internal sphincter (innervated by the sympathetic hypogastric nerves) in combination with urinary retention *(114,116)*. These changes predispose to the development of urinary tract infections including pyelonephritis that may accelerate or exacerbate renal failure *(119,120)*.

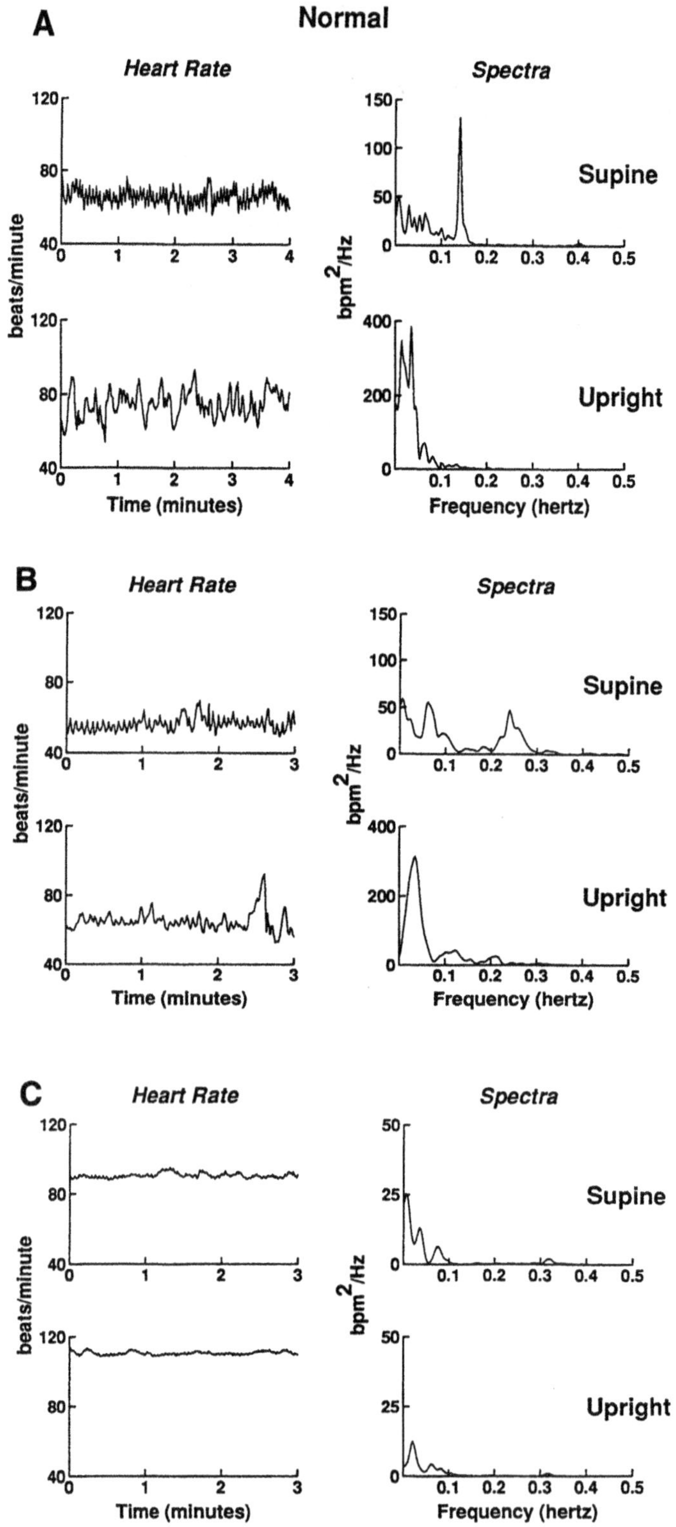


**Fig. 2.** **(A)** The heart-rate tachogram and power spectrum of a control subject. (bpm indicates beats per minute). **(B)** The heart-rate tachogram and power spectrum of a diabetic subject with moderate autonomic neuropathy (bpm indicates beats per minute). **(C)** The heart-rate tachogram and power spectrum of a diabetic subject with severe autonomic neuropathy. Note the lower y-axis scale of the heart rate power spectrum (bpm indicates beats per minute). (Adapted from ref. *107*.)

### *Laboratory Testing*

The urological evaluation of diabetic patients with autonomic dysfunction includes the measurement of residual urinary volume, the excretory urogram (iv pyelogram), the cystometrogram, the voiding cystourethrogram, uroflometry, and electromyography of the periurethral striated muscle. The simplest yet most important of these investigations, the measurement of residual urinary volume, entails only transurethral catheterization immediately after micturition. This provides a measure of bladder evacuation and can also gage the effectiveness of any therapeutic interventions. The cystometrogram documents intravesical compliance, capacity, sensation, and the presence of detrusor contractions as the bladder is progressively distended, usually by a transurethral water or carbon dioxide infusion. The perception of bladder filling occurs at approx 100–200 mL, and patients normally feel a strong desire to void at 400–500 mL. Patients with detrusor hyperreflexia caused by upper motor-neuron disease display uninhibited bladder contractions at volumes considerably lower than this. In contrast, the large-capacity atonic bladder produced by lower motor-neuron disease, as is usually the case in patients with diabetic autonomic neuropathy, show no increase in intravesical pressure despite the introduction of large volumes of fluid. The coordination of bladder contraction and sphincter relaxation can be determined by carrying out simultaneous sphincter electromyography. The voiding cystourethrogram is a radiologic study that provides structural and dynamic measures of bladder function. The patient is requested to void after the introduction of contrast material. Radiography carried out during micturition displays bladder size and shape, sphincter function, and urinary flow *(114,116)*.

### *Treatment*

The goal of treatment is to improve bladder emptying and includes the institution of regular voiding patterns, the Crede maneuver and clean intermittent self-catheterization. Pharmacotherapeutic agents include the cholinergic agonists such as bethanechol and carbachol, which stimulate the muscarinic, postganglionic receptors and result in enhanced bladder contractility *(121)*. Bethanechol chloride is a parasympathomimetic drug with relatively selective action at the urinary bladder. Typical oral doses range from 25–100 mg four times daily. The cholinergic agonist, carbachol chloride, which may have additional ganglion stimulating properties, also enhances bladder motility *(121)*. Under very rare circumstances, bladder neck surgery may be necessary *(113)*.

## THE GENITAL SYSTEM

### *Clinical Features*

Erectile dysfunction is a frequent and disturbing symptom in male diabetic patients. Reported incidence has ranged from 30–75% *(122–125)*. Impotence may be the earliest symptom of diabetic autonomic neuropathy although sensory, vascular, hormonal, and psychogenic etiologies, alone or in combination, may also be implicated. A significant proportion of diabetic patients, presenting with impotence alone, will develop other autonomic symptoms and abnormalities on autonomic testing when studied prospectively *(60)*.

Cholinergic and noncholinergic nonadrenergic neurotransmitters mediate erectile function by relaxing the smooth muscle of the corpus cavernosum *(126–129)*. Nitric oxide is an important mediator of noncholinergic nonadrenergic corpus cavernosum relaxation *(130)*. In vivo studies of isolated corpus cavernosum tissue from diabetic men have demonstrated functional impairment in autonomic and endothelial-dependent relaxation of corpus cavernosum smooth muscle *(128)*. Endothelial-independent relaxation of cavernosal tissue is maintained with administration of the vasodilators such as papaverine and sodium nitroprusside *(128)*. Impotence caused by autonomic neuropathy progresses gradually but is usually permanent 2 yr after onset. Sympathetically mediated ejaculatory failure may precede the appearance of impotence, although impotence can occur with retained ability to ejaculate and experience orgasm. Retrograde ejaculation will occur if the bladder neck fails to close. This function is also controlled by the sympathetic nervous system *(126,127)*. There are few studies of genital autonomic neuropathy in female diabetic patients *(131)*.

### *Laboratory Evaluation*

Erectile function is measured by evaluating nocturnal penile tumescence and rigidity *(132)* or with circumferential penile expansion measures *(133,134)*. Other endocrine causes of erectile dysfunction should be excluded by measuring serum testosterone and prolactin. Vascular function is determined with penile Doppler ultrasonography of the penile circulation *(135)* and penile blood-pressure measures *(136)*. Neurophysiological studies frequently used to evaluate erectile function include nerve conduction studies of the dorsal nerve of the penis *(137)* and bulbocavernosus reflex latency measurement *(138)*. The bulbocavernosus reflex latency, which is predominantly a measure of large fiber function, is not a sensitive or specific test for neurogenic impotence. Pudendal-evoked potentials may be helpful in evaluating erectile function in males with myelopathy.

### *Treatment*

Medications influencing autonomic function such as psychotropic and antihypertensive agents should be discontinued. Therapy for this erectile failure entails the use of mechanical devices such as the vacuum erection device *(139)* or the auto-injection of vasoactive substances (papaverine, phentolamine, and prostaglandin E1) into the corpus cavernosum *(140–144)*. The vasoactive agents simulate the natural erectile process by relaxing the arterial and trabecular smooth muscle, which increases the flow of blood into the sinusoidal spaces of the corpora cavernosum. The resulting corporeal engorgement produces veno-occlusion by compression of the subtunical emissary veins against the tunica albuginea. Prostaglandin E1, its synthetic analog alprostadil, and papaverine are direct smooth-muscle relaxants, whereas phentolamine is an alpha-adrenoreceptor antagonist. Pain, priapism, prolonged erection, penile hematomas, and fibrosis are the most frequent side effects of injection therapy. Severe arterial disease and venous leakage are the most common causes of treatment failure. Penile prosthetic implants may be used if auto-injection or the vacuum erection device fails or is not tolerated by the patient *(145)*. A recent study has demonstrated that the synthetic prostaglandin E1 analog, alprostadil, can be successfully delivered transurethrally, resulting in an erection sufficient for intercourse *(146)*.

## GASTROINTESTINAL SYSTEM

Autonomic dysfunction occurs throughout the gastrointestinal tract, producing several specific clinical syndromes. Gastrointestinal autonomic neuropathy results in disordered gastrointestinal motility, secretion, and absorption. Up to 76% of unselected diabetic patients are reported to acknowledge gastrointestinal symptoms *(147,148)*.

The autonomic control of the gastrointestinal tract is mediated by the extrinsic parasympathetic and sympathetic nervous systems and the intrinsic enteric nervous system. The parasympathetic input to the gut originates from the vagus and pelvic nerves from the second through fourth sacral segments. The postsynaptic cholinergic neurons provide excitatory input to the gastrointestinal tract. The sympathetic nervous system provides inhibitory input to the gastrointestinal tract. Extrinsic sympathetic efferents arising in the intermediolateral gray column synapse in the celiac, superior, and inferior mesenteric ganglia, and ramify throughout the gastrointestinal tract in the distribution of their respective arterial trunks. The upper gastrointestinal tract is innervated by the greater splanchnic nerve, which synapses in the celiac ganglion and travels with the celiac artery; the small intestine (midgut) is innervated by the lesser splanchnic nerve, which synapses in the superior mesenteric ganglion and travels with the superior mesenteric artery; and the large intestine is innervated by the lumbar splanchnic nerve, which synapses in the inferior mesenteric ganglion and travels with the inferior mesenteric ganglion *(149–151)*.

The enteric nervous system is comprised of a myenteric plexus located between the inner-circular and outer-longitudinal smooth-muscle layers (Auerbach's plexus) and a submucosal plexus (Meissner's plexus). At least five types of intrinsic enteric neurons have been identified, and any individual neuron may contain multiple neuropeptides *(150)*. Motor excitation is mediated by the cholinergic substance P neurons and inhibition is mediated by the dynorphin-vasoactive intestinal polypeptide neurons. Even in the absence of extrinsic autonomic nervous system influences, the enteric nervous system governs basic gut functions *(150)*.

## *Gastroparesis*

### Clinical Features

Gastric emptying is delayed in 30–50% of both type I and type II diabetic patients *(152,153)*. The term gastroparesis diabeticorum was first introduced by Kassander to describe the altered gastrointestinal motility in diabetic patients *(154)*. Food residue is retained in the stomach because of absent or decreased gastric peristalsis compounded by lower intestinal dysmotility *(155)*. Diabetic gastroparesis may manifest as nausea, postprandial vomiting, bloating, abdominal distension and pain, belching, loss of appetite, and early satiety. Many patients, however, are asymptomatic despite impaired gastric motility *(153)*. A gastric splash may be elicited on clinical examination. Gastroparesis is also associated with the development of bezoars *(156)* and bacterial overgrowth of stomach and small intestine, esophagitis, gastric ulcers, and gastritis *(157)*. Gastroparesis may impair the establishment of adequate glycemic control by mismatching plasma glucose and insulin levels. The absorption of orally administered drugs may also be affected *(154,158)*.

Impaired gastric emptying is frequently associated with cardiovagal neuropathy and small-fiber dysfunction *(159)*. Morphological changes in the vagus nerve are reported in some *(160,161)*, but not all studies *(162)*. Recent studies have implicated hyperglycemia as a cause of impaired gastric and small intestinal motility during fasting and after food intake. Hyperglycemia delays gastric emptying in healthy and diabetic subjects *(163–166)*.

### Laboratory Evaluation

Scintigraphic studies with radionuclide markers provide the most useful measures of gastric motility. Because a difference between the emptying rates of liquids and solids may be observed, both solid and liquid components of a meal should be evaluated. Other diagnostic investigations to study gastric motility include upper gastrointestinal X-rays, ultrasound, gastroscopy, intraluminal pressure manometry, and recordings of gastric electrical activity using surface electrodes (electrogastrography) *(64,167–170)*.

### Treatment

Frequent small meals and pharmacotherapy are standard treatments for this disorder. Metoclopramide (5–20 mg orally, 30 min before meals and at bedtime) accelerates gastric emptying, and has a central antiemetic action *(171–173)*. This agent is a dopamine antagonist and also may release acetylcholine from intramural cholinergic neurons or directly stimulate antral muscle *(174)*. Bethanechol may be used in combination with metoclopramide or in cases of metoclopramide resistance *(147,175)*. Domperidone (10–20 mg four times a day), a peripheral D2 receptor antidopaminergic agent *(176,177)* and cisapride (10 mg four times a day), a cholinomimetic agent that increases gastrointestinal motility by enhancing release of acetylcholine from neurons of the myenteric plexus may also be of benefit *(178)*. Infusions of motilin in diabetic patients with gastroparesis result in accelerated gastric emptying, but therapeutic use of the agent is limited by its need for iv administration and by its short half life *(179)*. Erythromycin and related macrolide compounds exhibit strong in vitro affinity for motilin receptors, and may have motilin-agonist properties *(180,181)*. Intravenous and oral erythromycin (250 mg three times a day) improve gastric-emptying time in diabetic patients with gastroparesis *(182)*.

## *Diabetic Diarrhea*

### Clinical Features

Diarrhea and other lower gastrointestinal tract symptoms may also occur. Diabetic diarrhea manifests as a profuse, watery, typically nocturnal diarrhea that can last for hours or days and frequently alternates with constipation *(183)*. Abdominal discomfort is commonly associated. The pathogenesis of diabetic diarrhea includes reduced gastrointestinal motility *(184)*, abnormalities in gut transit time *(185,186)*, reduced alpha-2 adrenergic receptor-mediated fluid absorption *(187)*, bacterial overgrowth *(188)*, pancreatic insufficiency, coexistent celiac disease *(189)*, and abnormalities in bile-salt metabolism *(190)*. Fecal incontinence, because of anal-sphincter incompetence or reduced rectal sensation is another manifestation of diabetic intestinal neuropathy *(187,191)*. Incontinence is often exacerbated by diarrhea.

### Treatment

The treatment of diabetic diarrhea includes symptomatic treatment with loperamide, diphenoxylate, or codeine phosphate. Possible bacterial overgrowth is treated with antibiotics such as tetracycline or metronidazole *(192)*. Cholestyramine (4–12 g/d) may be used to treat bile-acid malabsorption and the alpha-2 agonist, clonidine, (0.1–0.5 mg twice daily) improves the reduced alpha-2 adrenoreceptor-mediated intestinal absorption *(187)*. The somatostatin analog, octreotide, (50–75 μg twice daily subcutaneously) reverses diarrhea by decreasing fluid secretion and suppressing prokinetic hormone release *(193)*. Fecal incontinence may be improved by the diarrhea treatment and by biofeedback techniques to improve rectal sensation *(191)*.

### *Constipation*

Constipation is the most frequently reported gastrointestinal autonomic symptom and is found in up to 60% of diabetic patients *(147)*. The pathophysiology of diabetic constipation is poorly understood, but may reflect intestinal denervation and loss of the postprandial gastrocolic reflex *(148)*. Diabetic patients with severe constipation have no postprandial increase in colonic smooth-muscle activity, although the ability to respond to exogenous neostigmine and metoclopramide is retained *(194,195)*. Therapeutic interventions include increasing dietary fiber and stool softeners, in combination with prokinetic agents such as metoclopramide, bethanechol, and cisapride *(147,194,195)*.

### *Esophagus and Gall Bladder*

Esophageal motility abnormalities and reduced lower esophageal-sphincter pressures have also been demonstrated. Although usually asymptomatic, these abnormalities may result in symptoms such as dyspepsia, dysphagia, and an increased predisposition to esophageal ulceration *(196)*. These symptoms may be relieved by metoclopramide, domperidone, and other prokinetic agents *(197)*.

Impaired muscular contraction and enlargement of the gallbladder have been described in patients with diabetic autonomic dysfunction resulting in decreased gallbladder emptying. This may be responsible for the observed increased incidence of cholesterol gallstones in diabetic patients *(198)*.

## THE PUPIL

Pupillary manifestations of diabetic autonomic neuropathy include miosis, impaired light reflexes, and decreased hippus (the fluctuations in pupil diameter that occur during continuing illumination). Some diabetic patients demonstrate corectopia (oval pupils) *(199)*. Quantitative assessment of pupillary function can be obtained with infrared television pupillometry *(63,200)*, Polaroid photography *(201)*, and pharmacological testing *(202,203)*.

The dark-adapted pupil diameter or area, an index of sympathetic innervation of the dilator pupillae, is reduced in diabetic subjects *(63,204)*. The sensitivity of this test may be improved by parasympathetic blockade *(204)*. Because the pupil size decreases with advancing age, age-based norms are required for this measure. The amplitude of the light reflex also is reduced in diabetic patients, particularly those with small pupils (less than 6 mm) *(63)*. Abnormalities have also been demonstrated in the latency, constriction velocity, and dilation velocity of the light reflex *(11,63,204)*. The velocity of redilation in the latter part of the redilation curve of the light reflex also may provide a measure of sympathetic function. This measure, in contrast to the latency and constriction velocity, may be independent of the light-reflex amplitude reduction *(63)*. Abnormalities in the pupillary light-reflex latency, which is predominantly a measure of parasympathetic nervous system pupillomotor function, occur more frequently than abnormalities in the sympathetic nervous system-mediated dark-adapted pupil diameter *(205)*. Abnormalities are present within 2 yr of the diagnosis of diabetes in both insulin- and non-insulin-dependent diabetes mellitus *(11)*.

The oscillations of the pupil, induced by focusing a narrow beam of light from a slit lamp on the pupillary margin, may provide an index of parasympathetic pupillomotor function. The pupil-cycle time, a measure of these oscillations, was prolonged in a large proportion of patients with autonomic neuropathy *(206)*. Diabetic patients may display enhanced mydriasis to direct sympathomimetic agents that is consistent with denervation supersensitivity. The response to hydroxyamphetamine instillation is normal, suggesting that the major pathology is not in the postganglionic neuron *(63)*. Parasympathetic denervation supersensitivity has also been demonstrated. These indices of pupillary function correlate with cardiovascular autonomic dysfunction *(63,207)*, small-nerve fiber function *(195)*, somatic peripheral neuropathy *(199)*, and disease duration *(208)*.

## SUDOMOTOR SYSTEM

### *Clinical Features and Treatment*

Sudomotor dysfunction is a common feature of diabetic autonomic neuropathy. This generally manifests as anhidrosis of the extremities, which may be accompanied by hyperhidrosis in the trunk *(209)*. Rundles et al. demonstrated an 85% prevalence of thermoregulatory sweating abnormalities in diabetic patients *(210)*. Fealey et al. observed a 92% rate of sweat abnormality in patients with diabetic neuropathy and characterized the different thermoregulatory sweat patterns. Most patients (65%) exhibited a distal distribution of hypohidrosis and anhidrosis *(211)*. Initially, patients displayed a loss of thermoregulatory sweating in a glove and stocking distribution *(209–212)*, which, with progression of autonomic neuropathy, extended from the lower to the upper extremities and to the anterior abdomen, conforming to the well-recognized length dependency of diabetic neuropathy. This process ultimately resulted in a global anhidrosis that usually accompanied a profound generalized autonomic neuropathy. Kennedy et al. documented a decrease in the number of active sweat glands and a low sweat rate per unit area of skin *(213)*. Focal areas of anhidrosis may accompany diabetic truncal neuropathy and other mononeuropathies *(211)*. Histological studies suggest that the sudomotor dysfunction is caused by degeneration of postganglionic unmyelinated sudomotor axons *(214)*.

Diabetic anhidrosis is associated with other deficits of autonomic function including orthostatic hypotension, cardiac vagal abnormalities, and absence of sympathetic activation on microneurographic studies *(215–217)*. A decrease in pain perception frequently accompanies loss of distal sweating *(218)*. There is no treatment for diabetic anhidrosis. Hyperhidrosis may also accompany diabetic autonomic neuropathy. Excessive sweating may occur as a compensatory phenomenon involving proximal regions such as the head and trunk that are spared in a dying-back neuropathy. Alternately, distal hyperhidrosis may occur occasionally, particularly early in the course of a distal autonomic neuropathy. This phenomenon is most likely caused by spontaneous firing of injured neurons.

Gustatory sweating, the abnormal production of sweat that appears over the face, head, neck, shoulders, and chest after eating even nonspicy foods, is occasionally observed *(219)*. In contrast to truncal hyperhidrosis, which does not occur in response to eating, gustatory hyperhidrosis is not likely to be a compensatory response to anhidrosis *(220)*. This poorly understood, socially embarrassing phenomenon may be treated with anticholinergic agents such as trihexyphenidyl, probanthine, or scopolamine. High

Table 6
Tests Assessing Sudomotor Function

| |
|---|
| The thermoregulatory sweat test |
| The quantitative sudomotor axon reflex test |
| Skin potentials |
| The sweat imprint |

doses of these agents are usually required and therapy is usually limited by other anticholinergic side effects, such as dry mouth, urinary retention, and constipation.

### *Laboratory Evaluation*

Testing of the eccrine sweat glands has provided a useful means of assessing and localizing sympathetic nervous system function in patients with autonomic failure. Thermoregulatory sweat testing assesses both central and peripheral aspects of the efferent sympathetic nervous system, from the hypothalamus to the sweat glands, but is not able to differentiate between pre- and postganglionic causes of anhidrosis. Postganglionic sudomotor function can be determined by measuring sweat output after iontophoresis or intradermal injection of cholinergic agonists such as pilocarpine, nicotine, or methacholine. These agents either stimulate sweat glands directly *(213)* or effect a neighboring population of sweat glands via an axonal reflex *(216)*. The site of a lesion can be established when the thermoregulatory sweat test is combined with a test measuring postganglionic sudomotor function. For example, an abnormal thermoregulatory sweat test with normal postganglionic function indicates a preganglionic cause of anhidrosis, whereas an abnormal thermoregulatory sweat test with abnormal postganglionic function indicates a postganglionic cause of anhidrosis. Skin potential recordings measuring skin conductance, skin resistance, or the sympathetic skin potential provide an alternate measure of sudomotor function (see Table 6).

### *Thermoregulatory Sweat Test*

Thermoregulatory sweating can be tested by raising the body temperature with an external heating source. An increase in oral temperature of 1°C is sufficient to induce generalized sweating. This test evaluates the distribution of sweating by measuring the change in color of an indicator powder such as iodine with starch, quinizarin *(221,222)*, or alizarin-red *(211)* in response to a rise in core body temperature. Test results may be expressed semiquantitatively as the percentage of body anhidrosis. The test is well-standardized and hypohidrosis and anhidrosis in patients with autonomic failure have been documented using this technique by many investigators.

### *The Quantitative Sudomotor Axon Reflex Test*

The quantitative sudomotor axon reflex test (QSART) provides a quantitative measure of postganglionic sudomotor function. The sudomotor response measured by the QSART is mediated by an "axon-reflex" that is elicited by iontophoresis of a cholinergic agonist. To evaluate the distribution of postganglionic sudomotor deficits, recordings are made from the forearm and lower extremity skin sites *(216)*.

## The Sweat Imprint

A sweat imprint is formed by the secretion of active sweat glands into a plastic or silicone mold in response to iontophoresis of a cholinergic agonist. This test can be used to determine sweat-gland density, sweat-droplet size, and sweat volume per area *(213)*.

## Skin Potentials

Electrodermal activity is generated by the sweat glands and overlying epidermis and mediated by supraspinal sites. This response, which occurs spontaneously and can be evoked by stimuli such as respiration, startle, and mental stress is referred to as the sympathetic skin response or the peripheral autonomic surface potential. The sympathetic skin response can be measured with surface electrodes connected to a standard EMG instrument. The active recording electrode is placed on the palmar or plantar surface and the indifferent electrode on the volar surface. The response habituates with repeated stimuli and is subject to marked variability. Habituation may be minimized by delivering stimuli at irregular intervals. Concordance between the sympathetic skin response and sudomotor function has been shown in some but not all studies *(223,224)*.

# REFERENCES


1. Neil HA, Thompson AV, John S, McCarthy ST, Mann JI. Diabetic autonomic neuropathy: the prevalence of impaired heart rate variability in a geographically defined population. Diabetic Med 1989;6:20–24.
2. Dyck PJ, Kratz KM, Karnes JL, Litchy WJ, Klein R, Pach JM, Wilson DM, O'Brien PC, Melton LJ, Service FJ. The prevalence by staged severity of various types of diabetic neuropathy, retinopathy, and nephropathy in a population-based cohort: the Rochester Diabetic Neuropathy Study. Neurology 1993;43:817–824.
3. Ewing DJ, Martyn CN, Young RJ, Clarke BF. The value of cardiovascular autonomic function tests: 10 years experience in diabetes. Diabetes Care 1985;8:491–498.
4. Masaoka S, Lev-Ran A, Hill LR, Vakil G, Hon EH. Heart rate variability in diabetes: relationship to age and duration of the disease. Diabetes Care 1985;8:64–68.
5. Niakan E, Harati Y, Comstock JP. Diabetic autonomic neuropathy. Metab Clin Exp 1986;35:224–234.
6. O'Brien IA, O'Hare JP, Lewin IG, Corrall RJ. The prevalence of autonomic neuropathy in insulin-dependent diabetes mellitus: a controlled study based on heart rate variability. Q J Med 1986;61:957–967.
7. Ziegler D, Gries FA, Muhlen H, Rathmann W, Spuler M, Lessmann F. Prevalence and clinical correlates of cardiovascular autonomic and peripheral diabetic neuropathy in patients attending diabetes centers. The Diacan Multicenter Study Group. Diabete Metab 1993;19:143–151.
8. Maser RE, Pfeifer MA, Dorman JS, Kuller LH, Becker DJ, Orchard TJ. Diabetic autonomic neuropathy and cardiovascular risk. Pittsburgh Epidemiology of Diabetes Complications Study III. Arch Intern Med 1990;150:1218–1222.
9. Fraser DM, Campbell IW, Ewing DJ, Murray A, Neilson JM, Clarke BF. Peripheral and autonomic nerve function in newly diagnosed diabetes mellitus. Diabetes 1977;26:546–550.
10. Young RJ, Ewing DJ, Clarke BF. Nerve function and metabolic control in teenage diabetics. Diabetes 1983;32:142–147.
11. Pfeifer MA, Weinberg CR, Cook DL, Reenan A, Halter JB, Ensinck JW, et al. Autonomic neural dysfunction in recently diagnosed diabetic subjects. Diabetes Care 1984;7:447–453.
12. Wheeler T, Watkins PJ. Cardiac denervation in diabetes. Br Med J 1973;4:584–586.
13. Sundkvist G, Almer L, Lilja B. Respiratory influence on heart rate in diabetes mellitus. Br Med J 1979;1:924, 925.
14. Lloyd-Mostyn RH, Watkins PJ. Defective innervation of heart in diabetic autonomic neuropathy. Br Med J 1975;3:15–17.
15. Bennett T, Hosking DJ, Hampton JR. Cardiovascular control in diabetes mellitus. Br Med J 1975;2:585–587.

16. Ewing DJ, Campbell IW, Clarke BF. Heart rate changes in diabetes mellitus. Lancet 1981;1:183–186.
17. Furlan R, Guzzetti S, Crivellaro W, Dassi S, Tinelli M, Baselli G, Cerutti S, Lombardi F, Pagani M, Malliani A. Continuous 24-hour assessment of the neural regulation of systemic arterial pressure and RR variabilities in ambulant subjects. Circulation 1990;81:537–547.
18. Bernardi L, Ricordi L, Lazzari P, Solda P, Calciati A, Ferrari MR, Vandea I, Finardi G, Fratino P. Impaired circadian modulation of sympathovagal activity in diabetes. A possible explanation for altered temporal onset of cardiovascular disease. Circulation 1992;86:1443–1452.
19. Ewing DJ, Neilson JM, Travis P. New method for assessing cardiac parasympathetic activity using 24 hour electrocardiograms. Br Heart J 1984;52:396–402.
20. Ewing DJ, Borsey DQ, Travis P, Bellavere F, Neilson JM, Clarke BF. Abnormalities of ambulatory 24-hour heart rate in diabetes mellitus. Diabetes 1983;32:101–105.
21. Malpas SC, Maling TJ. Heart-rate variability and cardiac autonomic function in diabetes. Diabetes 1990;39:1177–1181.
22. Spallone V, Bernardi L, Maiello MR, Cicconetti E, Ricordi L, Fratino P, Menzinger G. Twenty-four-hour pattern of blood pressure and spectral analysis of heart rate variability in diabetic patients with various degrees of autonomic neuropathy. Comparison to standard cardiovascular tests. Clin Sci (Colch) 1996;91(Suppl.):105–107.
23. Liniger C, Favre L, Assal JP. Twenty-four hour blood pressure and heart rate profiles of diabetic patients with abnormal cardiovascular reflexes. Diabetic Med 1991;8:420–427.
24. Nakano S, Uchida K, Kigoshi T, Azukizawa S, Iwasaki R, Kaneko M, Morimoto S. Circadian rhythm of blood pressure in normotensive NIDDM subjects. Its relationship to microvascular complications. Diabetes Care 1991;14:707–711.
25. Zola B, Kahn JK, Juni JE, Vinik AI. Abnormal cardiac function in diabetic patients with autonomic neuropathy in the absence of ischemic heart disease. J Clin Endocrinol Metab 1986;63:208–214.
26. Kahn JK, Zola B, Juni JE, Vinik AI. Radionuclide assessment of left ventricular diastolic filling in diabetes mellitus with and without cardiac autonomic neuropathy. J Am Coll Cardiol 1986;7: 1303–1309.
27. Faerman I, Faccio E, Milei J, Nunez R, Jadzinsky M, Fox D, Rapaport M. Autonomic neuropathy and painless myocardial infarction in diabetic patients. Histologic evidence of their relationship. Diabetes 1977;26:1147–1158.
28. Nesto RW, Phillips RT. Asymptomatic myocardial ischemia in diabetic patients. Am J Med 1986;80:40–47.
29. Ewing DJ, Campbell IW, Clarke BF. Mortality in diabetic autonomic neuropathy. Lancet 1976;1:601–603.
30. Burgos LG, Ebert TJ, Asiddao C, Turner LA, Pattison CZ, Wang-Cheng R, Kampine JP. Increased intraoperative cardiovascular morbidity in diabetics with autonomic neuropathy. Anesthesiology 1989;70:591–597.
31. Soler NG, Eagleton LE. Autonomic neuropathy and the ventilatory responses of diabetics to progressive hypoxemia and hypercarbia. Diabetes 1982;31:609–614.
32. Page MM, Watkins PJ. Cardiorespiratory arrest and diabetic autonomic neuropathy. Lancet 1978;1:14–16.
33. Kahn JK, Sisson JC, Vinik AI. QT interval prolongation and sudden cardiac death in diabetic autonomic neuropathy. J Clin Endocrinol Metab 1987;64:751–754.
34. Bellavere F, Ferri M, Guarini L, Bax G, Piccoli A, Cardone C, Fedele D. Prolonged QT period in diabetic autonomic neuropathy: a possible role in sudden cardiac death? Br Heart J 1988;59:379–383.
35. Chambers JB, Sampson MJ, Sprigings DC, Jackson G. QT prolongation on the electrocardiogram in diabetic autonomic neuropathy. Diabetic Med 1990;7:105–110.
36. Jermendy G, Toth L, Voros P, Koltai MZ, Pogatsa G. Cardiac autonomic neuropathy and QT interval length. A follow-up study in diabetic patients. Acta Cardiologica 1991;46:189–200.
37. Ewing DJ, Neilson JM. QT interval length and diabetic autonomic neuropathy. Diabetic Med 1990;7:23–26.
38. Jermendy G, Koltai MZ, Pogatsa G. QT interval prolongation in type 2 (non-insulin-dependent) diabetic patients with cardiac autonomic neuropathy. Acta Diabetologica Latina 1990;27:295–301.
39. Gonin JM, Kadrofske MM, Schmaltz S, Bastyr EJ, Vinik AI. Corrected Q-T interval prolongation as diagnostic tool for assessment of cardiac autonomic neuropathy in diabetes mellitus. Diabetes Care 1990;13:68–71.

40. Veglio M, Chinaglia A, Borra M, Perin PC. Does abnormal QT interval prolongation reflect autonomic dysfunction in diabetic patients? QTc interval measure versus standardized tests in diabetic autonomic neuropathy. Diabet Med 1995;12:302–306.
41. Oka H, Mochio S, Sato K, Sato H, Katayama K. Prolongation of QTc interval and autonomic nervous dysfunction in diabetic patients. Diabetes Res Clin Pract 1996;31:63–70.
42. Anonymous. Position paper: Orthostatic hypotension, multiple system atrophy (the Shy Drager syndrome) and pure autonomic failure. J Auton Nerv Syst 1996;58:123–124.
43. Low PA, Walsh JC, Huang CY, McLeod JG. The sympathetic nervous system in diabetic neuropathy. A clinical and pathological study. Brain 1975;98:341–356.
44. Hilsted J, Parving HH, Christensen NJ, Benn J, Galbo H. Hemodynamics in diabetic orthostatic hypotension. J Clin Invest 1981;68:1427–1434.
45. Hilsted J, Galbo H, Christensen NJ. Impaired cardiovascular responses to graded exercise in diabetic autonomic neuropathy. Diabetes 1979;28:313–319.
46. Cryer PE, Silverberg AB, Santiago JV, Shah SD. Plasma catecholamines in diabetes. The syndromes of hypoadrenergic and hyperadrenergic postural hypotension. Am J Med 1978;64:407–416.
47. Tohmeh JF, Shah SD, Cryer PE. The pathogenesis of hyperadrenergic postural hypotension in diabetic patients. Am J Med 1979;67:772–778.
48. Page MM, Watkins PJ. Provocation of postural hypotension by insulin in diabetic autonomic neuropathy. Diabetes 1976;25:90–95.
49. Mathias CJ, da Costa DF, Fosbraey P, Christensen NJ, Bannister R. Hypotensive and sedative effects of insulin in autonomic failure. Br Med J Clin Res 1987;295:161–163.
50. Winocour PH, Dhar H, Anderson DC. The relationship between autonomic neuropathy and urinary sodium and albumin excretion in insulin-treated diabetics. Diabetic Med 1986;3:436–440.
51. Freeman R. Treatment of orthostatic hypotension - Midodrine and other pressor drugs. In: Robertson D, Low PA, Polinsky RJ, eds. Primer on the autonomic nervous system. Academic, New York, 1996, pp. 326–332.
52. Fealey RD, Robertson D. Management of orthostatic hypotension. In: Low PA, ed. Clinical autonomic disorders. Little, Brown, Boston, 1993, pp. 731–743.
53. Hoeldtke RD, Streeten DHP, Streeten DH. Treatment of orthostatic hypotension with erythropoietin. N Engl J Med 1993;329:611–615.
54. Perera R, Isola L, Kaufmann H. Effect of recombinant erythropoietin on anemia and orthostatic hypotension in primary autonomic failure. Clin Auton Res 1995;5:211–213.
55. Gasser HS. The classification of nerve fibers. Ohio J Sci 1941;41:145–159.
56. Bennett T, Farquhar IK, Hosking DJ, Hampton JR. Assessment of methods for estimating autonomic nervous control of the heart in patients with diabetes mellitus. Diabetes 1978;27:1167–1174.
57. Ewing DJ, Borsey DQ, Bellavere F, Clarke BF. Cardiac autonomic neuropathy in diabetes: comparison of measures of R-R interval variation. Diabetologia 1981;21:18–24.
58. McLeod JG, Tuck RR. Disorders of the autonomic nervous system: Part 1. Pathophysiology and clinical features. Ann Neurol 1987;21:419–430.
59. Ewing DJ, Clarke BF. Diagnosis and management of diabetic autonomic neuropathy. Br Med J Clin Res 1982;285:916–918.
60. Ewing DJ, Campbell IW, Clarke BF. The natural history of diabetic autonomic neuropathy. Q J Med 1980;49:95–108.
61. Mackay JD, Page MM, Cambridge J, Watkins PJ. Diabetic autonomic neuropathy. The diagnostic value of heart rate monitoring. Diabetologia 1980;18:471–478.
62. Pfeifer MA, Cook D, Brodsky J, Tice D, Reenan A, Swedine S, Halter JB, Porte D. Quantitative evaluation of cardiac parasympathetic activity in normal and diabetic man. Diabetes 1982;31:339–345.
63. Smith SA, Smith SE. Reduced pupillary light reflexes in diabetic autonomic neuropathy. Diabetologia 1983;24:330–332.
64. Campbell IW, Heading RC, Tothill P, Buist TA, Ewing DJ, Clarke BF. Gastric emptying in diabetic autonomic neuropathy. Gut 1977;18:462–467.
65. Ewing DJ, Bellavere F, Espi F, McKibben BM, Buchanan KD, Riemersma RA, et al. Correlation of cardiovascular and neuroendocrine tests of autonomic function in diabetes. Metab Clin Exp 1986;35:349–353.
66. Low PA, Zimmerman BR, Dyck PJ. Comparison of distal sympathetic with vagal function in diabetic neuropathy. Muscle Nerve 1986;9:592–596.
67. Freeman R. Heart rate variability - the time domain. In: Low PA, ed. Clinical Autonomic Disorders, 2nd ed. Little, Brown, Boston, 1997;297–308.

68. Gundersen HJG, Neubauer B. A long-term diabetic autonomic nervous abnormality. Diabetologia 1977;13:137–140.
69. Weinberg CR, Pfeifer MA. An improved method for measuring heart-rate variability: assessment of cardiac autonomic function. Biometrics 1984;40:855–861.
70. Genovely H, Pfeifer MA. RR-variation: the autonomic test of choice in diabetes. Diab/Met Rev 1988;4:255–271.
71. Anonymous. The effect of intensive diabetes therapy on the development and progression of neuropathy. The Diabetes Control and Complications Trial Research Group. Ann Intern Med 1995;122:561–568.
72. Bigger JT Jr, Albrecht P, Steinman RC, Rolnitzky LM, Fleiss JL, Cohen RJ. Comparison of time- and frequency domain-based measures of cardiac parasympathetic activity in Holter recordings after myocardial infarction. Am J Cardiol 1989;64:536–538.
73. Harry JD, Freeman R. Assessing heart rate variability: A computer simulated comparison of methodologies. Muscle Nerve 1993;16:267–277.
74. Ziegler D, Laux G, Dannehl K, Spüler M, Mühlen P, Mayer P, Gries FA. Assessment of cardiovascular autonomic function: age related normal ranges and reproducibility of spectral analysis, vector analysis, and standard tests of heart rate variation and blood pressure responses. Diabetic Med 1992;9:166–175.
75. Smith SA. Diagnostic value of the Valsalva ratio reduction in diabetic autonomic neuropathy: use of an age-related normal range. Diabetic Med 1984;1:295–297.
76. Levin AB. A simple test of cardiac function based upon the heart rate changes induced by a Valsalva maneuver. Am J Cardiol 1966;18:90–99.
77. Baldwa VS, Ewing DJ. Heart rate response to Valsalva manoeuvre. Reproducibility in normals, and relation to variation in resting heart rate in diabetics. Br Heart J 1977;39:641–644.
78. Benarroch EE, Opfer-Gehrking TL, Low PA. Use of the photoplethysmographic technique to analyze the Valsalva maneuver in normal man. Muscle Nerve 1991;14:1165–1172.
79. Ferrer MT, Kennedy WR, Sahinen F. Baroreflexes in patients with diabetes mellitus. Neurology 1991;41:1462–1466.
80. Eckberg DL. Parasympathetic cardiovascular control in human disease: a critical review of methods and results. [Review]. Am J Physiol 1980;239:H581–H593.
81. Ewing DJ, Campbell IW, Burt AA, Clarke BF. Vascular reflexes in diabetic autonomic neuropathy. Lancet 1973;2:1354–1356.
82. Persson A, Solders G. R-R variations, a test of autonomic dysfunction. Acta Neurologica Scandinavica 1983;67:285–293.
83. van Lieshout JJ, Wieling W, Wesseling KH, Karemaker JM. Pitfalls in the assessment of cardiovascular reflexes in patients with sympathetic failure but intact vagal control. Clin Sci 1989;76:523–528.
84. Borst C, Weiling W, van Brederode JFM, Hond A, DeRijk LG, Dunning AJ, Wieling W, Van Brederode JF, de Rijk LG. Mechanisms of initial heart rate response to postural change. Am J Physiol 1982;243:H676–H681.
85. Sprangers RL, Wesseling KH, Imholz AL, Imholz BP, Wieling W. Initial blood pressure fall on stand up and exercise explained by changes in total peripheral resistance. J Appl Physiol 1991;70:523–530.
86. Ewing DJ, Hume L, Campbell IW, Murray A, Neilson JM, Clarke BF. Autonomic mechanisms in the initial heart rate response to standing. J Appl Physiol: Respir Environ Exer Physiol 1980;49:809–814.
87. Ewing DJ, Campbell IW, Murray A, Neilson JM, Clarke BF. Immediate heart-rate response to standing: simple test for autonomic neuropathy in diabetes. Br Med J 1978;1:145–147.
88. Sundkvist G, Lilja B, Almer LO. Abnormal diastolic blood pressure and heart rate reactions to tilting in diabetes mellitus. Diabetologia 1980;19:433–438.
89. Bellavere F, Ewing DJ. Autonomic control of the immediate heart rate response to lying down. Clin Sci 1982;62:57–64.
90. Bellavere F, Cardone C, Ferri M, Guarini L, Piccoli A, Fedele D. Standing to lying heart rate variation. A new simple test in the diagnosis of diabetic autonomic neuropathy. Diabetic Med 1987;4:41–43.
91. Marfella R, Giugliano D, di Maro G, Acampora R, Giunta R, D'Onofrio F. The squatting test. A useful tool to assess both parasympathetic and sympathetic involvement of the cardiovascular autonomic neuropathy in diabetes. Diabetes 1994;43:607–612.
92. Marfella R, Salvatore T, Giugliano D, di Maro G, Giunta R, Torella R, Juchmes J, Scheen A, Lefebure PJ. Detection of early sympathetic cardiovascular neuropathy by squatting test in NIDDM. Diabetes Care 1994;17:149–151.

93. Finley JP, Bonet JF, Waxman MB. Autonomic pathways responsible for bradycardia on facial immersion. J Appl Physiol 1979;47:1218–1222.
94. Eckberg DL, Mohanty SK, Raczkowska M. Trigeminal-baroreceptor reflex interactions modulate human cardiac vagal efferent activity. J Physiol (Lond) 1984;347:75–83.
95. Khurana RK, Watabiki S, Hebel JR, Toro R, Nelson E. Cold face test in the assessment of trigeminal-brainstem-vagal function in humans. Ann Neurol 1980;7:144–149.
96. Bennett T, Hosking DJ, Hampton JR. Cardiovascular reflex responses to apnoeic face immersion and mental stress in diabetic subjects. Cardiovasc Res 1976;10:192–199.
97. Ewing DJ, Neilson JM, Shapiro CM, Stewart JA, Reid W. Twenty four hour heart rate variability: effects of posture, sleep, and time of day in healthy controls and comparison with bedside tests of autonomic function in diabetic patients. Br Heart J 1991;65:239–244.
98. Kleiger RE, Bigger JT, Bosner MS, Chung MK, Cook JR, Rolnitzky LM, Steinman R, Fleiss JL. Stability over time of variables measuring heart rate variability in normal subjects. Am J Cardiol 1991;68:626–630.
99. Bigger JT Jr, Fleiss JL, Steinman RC, Rolnitzky LM, Kleiger RE, Rottman JN. Correlations among time and frequency domain measures of heart period variability two weeks after acute myocardial infarction. Am J Cardiol 1992;69:891–898.
100. Wieling W, ten Harkel AD, van Lieshout JJ. Spectrum of orthostatic disorders: classification based on an analysis of the short-term circulatory response upon standing. Clin Sci 1991;81:241–248.
101. Imholz BP, Settels JJ, van der Meiracker AH, Wesseling KH, Wieling W. Non-invasive continuous finger blood pressure measurement during orthostatic stress compared to intra-arterial pressure. Cardiovasc Res 1990;24:214–221.
102. Ewing DJ, Irving JB, Kerr F, Wildsmith JA, Clarke BF. Cardiovascular responses to sustained handgrip in normal subjects and in patients with diabetes mellitus: a test of autonomic function. Clin Sci Mol Med 1974;46:295–306.
103. Sandroni P, Benarroch EE, Low PA. Pharmacological dissection of components of the Valsalva maneuver in adrenergic failure. J Appl Physiol 1991;71:1563–1567.
104. Hines EA, Brown GE. The cold pressor test for measuring the reactibility of the blood pressure: data concerning 571 normal and hypertensive subjects. Am Heart J 1936;11:1–9.
105. Pagani M, Furlan R, Pizzinelli P, Crivellaro W, Cerutti S, Malliani A. Spectral analysis of R-R and arterial pressure variabilities to assess sympatho-vagal interaction during mental stress in humans. J Hypertens Suppl 1989;7:S14–S15.
106. Pagani M, Malfatto G, Pierini S, Casati R, Masu AM, Poli M, Guzzetti S, Lombardi F, Cerutti S, Malliani A. Spectral analysis of heart rate variability in the assessment of autonomic diabetic neuropathy. J Auton Nerv Syst 1988;23:143–153.
107. Freeman R, Saul JP, Roberts MS, Berger RD, Broadbridge C, Cohen RJ. Spectral analysis of heart rate in diabetic autonomic neuropathy. A comparison with standard tests of autonomic function. Arch Neurol 1991;48:185–190.
108. Akselrod S, Gordon D, Ubel FA, Shannon DC, Berger AC, Cohen RJ. Power spectrum analysis of heart rate fluctuation: a quantitative probe of beat-to-beat cardiovascular control. Science 1981;213:220–222.
109. Pomeranz B, Macaulay RJ, Caudill MA, Kutz I, Adam D, Gordon D, Killborn KM, Barger AC, Shannon DC, Cohen RJ, and Benson H. Assessment of autonomic function in humans by heart rate spectral analysis. Am J Physiol 1985;248:H151–H153.
110. Freeman R, Cohen RJ, Saul JP. Transfer fuction analysis of respiratory sinus arrythmia-a measure of autonomic function in diabetic neuropathy. Muscle Nerve 1995;18:74–84.
111. Comi G, Sora MG, Bianchi A, Bontempi B, Gianoglio P, Cerutti S, Micossi P, Canal N. Spectral analysis of short-term heart rate variability in diabetic patients. J Auton Nerv Syst 1990;30(Suppl):S45–S49.
112. Lishner M, Akselrod S, Avi VM, Oz O, Divon M, Ravid M. Spectral analysis of heart rate fluctuations. A non-invasive, sensitive method for the early diagnosis of autonomic neuropathy in diabetes mellitus. J Auton Nerv Syst 1987;19:119–125.
113. Frimodt-Moller C, Mortensen S. Treatment of diabetic cystopathy. Ann Intern Med 1980;92: 327–328.
114. Ellenberg M. Development of urinary bladder dysfunction in diabetes mellitus. Ann Intern Med 1980; 92:321–323.
115. Ioanid CP, Noica N. Incidence and diagnostic aspects of the bladder disorders in diabetics. Eur Urol 1981;7:211–214.

116. Bradley WE. Diagnosis of urinary bladder dysfunction in diabetes mellitus. Ann Intern Med 1980;92:323–326.
117. Appell RA, Whiteside HV. Diabetes and other peripheral neuropathies affecting lower urinary tract function. In: Krane RJ, Siroky MB, eds. Clinical Neuro-Urology. Little, Brown, Boston, 1992, pp. 365–373.
118. Blaivas JG. The neurophysiology of micturition. a clinical study of 550 patients. J Urol 1982;127:958–963.
119. Beylot M, Marion D, Noel G. Ultrasonographic determination of residual urine in diabetic subjects: relationship to neuropathy and urinary tract infection. Diabetes Care 1982;5:501–505.
120. Norden G, Granerus G, Nyberg G. Diabetic cystopathy—a risk factor in diabetic nephropathy? J Diabet Complications 1988;2:203–206.
121. Wein AJ, Van Arsdalen K, Levin RM. Pharmacologic Therapy. In: Krane RJ, Siroky MB, eds. Clinical Neuro-Urology, 2nd ed. Little, Brown and Company, Boston, 1992, pp. 523–557.
122. McCulloch DK, Campbell IW, Wu FC, Prescott RJ, Clarke BF. The prevalence of diabetic impotence. Diabetologia 1980;18:279–283.
123. Ellenberg M. Impotence in diabetics. Ann Intern Med 1971;75:213–219.
124. Kaiser FE, Korenman SG. Impotence in diabetic men. Am J Med 1988;85(Suppl. 5A):147–152.
125. Hakim LS, Goldstein I. Diabetic sexual dysfunction. Endocrinol Metab Clin North Am 1996;25:379–400.
126. DeGroat WC, Booth AM. Physiology of male sexual function. Ann Intern Med 1980;329:31.
127. Krane RJ, Siroky MB. Neurophysiology of erection. Neurol Clin North Am 1981;8:91–102.
128. de Tejada IS, Goldstein I, Azadzoi K, Krane RJ, Cohen RA. Impaired neurogenic and endothelium-mediated relaxation of penile smooth muscle from diabetic men with impotence. N Engl J Med 1989;320:1025–1030.
129. Lue TF, Tanagho EA. Physiology of erection and pharmacological management of impotence. J Urol 1987;137:829–836.
130. Rajfer J, Aronson WJ, Bush PA, Dorey FJ, Ignarro LJ. Nitric oxide as a mediator of relaxation of the corpus cavernosum in response to nonadrenergic, noncholinergic neurotransmission. N Engl J Med 1992;326:90–94.
131. Ellenberg M. Sexual function in diabetic patients. Ann Intern Med 1980;92:331–333.
132. Karacan I. Diagnosis of erectile impotence in diabetes mellitus. Ann Intern Med 1980;29:334–337.
133. Anders EK, Bradley WE, Krane RJ. Nocturnal penile rigidity measured by the snap-gauge band. J Urol 1983;129:964–966.
134. Barry JM, Blank B, Boileau M. Nocturnal penile tumescence monitoring with stamps. Urology 1980;15:171–172.
135. Lue TF, Hricak H, Marich KW, Tanagho EA. Vasculogenic impotence evaluated by high-resolution ultrasonography and pulsed Doppler spectrum analysis. Radiology 1985;155:777–781.
136. Abelson D. Diagnostic value of the penile pulse and blood pressure: A Doppler study of impotence in diabetics. J Urol 1975;113:636–639.
137. Bradley WE, Lin JTY, Johnson B. Measurement of the conduction velocity of the dorsal nerve of the penis. J Urol 1984;131:1127–1129.
138. Sarica Y, Karacan I. Bulbocavernosus reflex to somatic and visceral nerve stimulation in normal subjects and in diabetics with erectile impotence. J Urol 1987;138:55–58.
139. Witherington R. Suction device therapy in the management of erectile impotence. Urol Clin North Am 1988;15:123–128.
140. Virag R. Intracavernous injection of papaverine for erectile failure. Lancet 1982;2:938.
141. Zorgniotti AW, LeFleur RS. Auto-injection of the corpus cavernosum with a vasoactive drug combination for vasculogenic impotence. J Urol 1985;133:39–41.
142. Stackl W, Hasun R, Marberger M. Intracavernous injection of prostaglandin E1 in impotent men. J Urol 1988;140:66–68.
143. Veves A, Webster L, Chen TF, Payne S, Boulton AJM. Aetiopathogenesis and management of impotence in diabetic males: four years experience from a combined clinic. Diabetic Med 1995;12:77–82.
144. Linet OI, Ogrinc FG. Efficacy and safety of intracavernosal alprostadil in men with erectile dysfunction. The Alprostadil Study Group. N Engl J Med 1996;334:873–877.
145. Beaser RS, Van der Hoek C, Jacobson AM, Flood TM, Desautels RE. Experience with penile prostheses in the treatment of impotence in diabetic men. JAMA 1982;248:943–948.

146. Padma-Nathan H, Hellstrom WJ, Kaiser FE, Labasky RF, Lue TF, Nolten WE, Norwood PC, Peterson CA, Shabsigh R, Tam PY, Place VA, Gesundheit N. Treatment of men with erectile dysfunction with transurethral alprostadil. Medicated Urethral System for Erection (MUSE) Study Group. N Engl J Med 1997;336:1–7.
147. Feldman M, Schiller LR. Disorders of gastrointestinal motility associated with diabetes mellitus. Ann Intern Med 1983;98:378–384.
148. Feldman M, Corbelt DB, Ramsey EJ. Abnormal gastric function in longstanding insulin-dependent diabetic patients. Gastroenterology 1979;77:12–17.
149. Wingate DL. Autonomic dysfunction and the gut. In: Bannister R, Mathias CJ, eds. Autonomic failure, 3rd ed. Oxford University Press, Oxford, 1992, pp. 510–528.
150. Wood JD. Physiology of the Enteric Nervous System. In: Johnson LR, Christensen J, Jackson MJ, Jacobson ED, Walsh JH, eds. Physiology of the Gastrointestinal Tract. Raven Press, New York, 1987, pp. 67–109.
151. Camilleri M. Disorders of gastrointestinal motility in neurologic diseases. Mayo Clin Proc 1990;65:825–846.
152. Wegener M, Borsch G, Schaffstein J, Luerweg C, Leverkus F. Gastrointestinal transit disorders in patients with insulin-treated diabetes mellitus. Dig Dis 1990;8:23–36.
153. Horowitz M, Harding PE, Maddox AF, Wishart JM, Akkermans LMA, Chatterton BE, Shearman DJC. Gastric and oesophageal emptying in patients with Type 2 (non-insulin-dependent) diabetes mellitus. Diabetologia 1989;32:151–159.
154. Kassander P. Asymptomatic gastric retention in diabetics (gastroparesis diabeticorum). Ann Intern Med 1958;48:797–812.
155. Vogelberg KH, Rathmann W, Helbig G. Sonographic examination of gastric motility in diabetics with autonomic neuropathy. Diabetes Res 1987;5:175–179.
156. Brady PG, Richardson R. Gastric bezoar formation secondary to gastroparesis diabeticorum. Arch Intern Med 1977;137:1729.
157. Parkman HP, Schwartz SS. Esophagitis and gastroduodenal disorders associated with diabetic gastroparesis. Arch Intern Med 1987;147:1477–1480.
158. Loo FD, Palmer DW, Soergel KH, Kalbfleisch JH, Wood CM. Gastric emptying in patients with diabetes mellitus. Gastroenterology 1984;86:485–495.
159. Westerman RA, Delaney C, Ivamy-Phillips A, Horowitz M, Roberts A. Concordance between different measures of small sensory and autonomic fibre neuropathy in diabetes mellitus. Clin Exp Neurol 1989;26:51–63.
160. Guy RJ, Dawson JL, Garrett JR, Laws JW, Thomas PK, Sharma AK, Watkins PJ. Diabetic gastroparesis from autonomic neuropathy: surgical considerations and changes in vagus nerve morphology. J Neurol Neurosurg Psychiatry 1984;47:686–691.
161. Britland ST, Young RJ, Sharma AK, Lee D, Ah-See AK, Clarke BF. Vagus nerve morphology in diabetic gastropathy. Diabetic Med 1990;7:780–787.
162. Yoshida MM, Schuffler MD, Sumi SM. There are no morphologic abnormalities of the gastric wall or abdominal vagus in patients with diabetic gastroparesis. Gastroenterology 1988;94:907–914.
163. Fraser R, Horowitz M, Dent J. Hyperglycaemia stimulates pyloric motility in normal subjects. Gut 1991;32:475–478.
164. Bjornsson ES, Urbanavicius V, Eliasson B, Attvall S, Smith U, Abrahamsson H. Effects of hyperglycemia on interdigestive gastrointestinal motility in humans. Scand J Gastroenterol 1994;29:1096–1104.
165. Horowitz M, Fraser R. Disordered gastric motor function in diabetes mellitus. Diabetologia 1994;37:543–551.
166. Jones KL, Horowitz M, Wishart MJ, Maddox AF, Harding PE, Chatterton BE. Relationships between gastric emptying, intragastric meal distribution and blood glucose concentrations in diabetes mellitus. J Nucl Med 1995;36:2220–2228.
167. DePonti F, Fealey RD, Malagelada JR. Gastrointestinal syndromes due to diabetes mellitus. In: Dyck PJ, Thomas PK, Asbury AK, Winegard AL, Porte D, eds. Diabetic Neuropathy. Saunders, Philadelphia, 1987, pp. 155–161.
168. Wright RA, Clemente R, Wathen R. Diabetic gastroparesis: an abnormality of gastric emptying of solids. Am J Med Sci 1985;289:240–242.
169. Keshavarzian A, Iber FL, Vaeth J. Gastric emptying in patients with insulin-requiring diabetes mellitus. Am J Gastroenterol 1987;82:29–35.

170. Smout A, Horowitz M, Armstrong D. Methods to study gastric emptying. Frontiers in gastric emptying. Dig Dis Sci 1994;39(Suppl.):130S–132S.
171. Snape WJ Jr, Battle WM, Schwartz SS, Braunstein S, Goldstein HH, Alavi A. Metoclopramide to treat gastoparesis due to diabetes mellitus: a double-blind, controlled trial. Ann Intern Med 1982;96:444–446.
172. Longstreth GF, Malagelada J, Kelly KA. Metoclopramide stimulation of gastric motility and emptying in diabetic gastroparesis. Ann Intern Med 1977;86:195–196.
173. Perkel MS, Moore C, Hersh T, Davidson ED. Metoclopramide therapy in patients with delayed gastric emptying A randomized, double-blind study. Dig Dis Sci 1979;24:662–666.
174. Fox S, Behar J. Pathogenesis of diabetic gastroparesis: a pharmacologic study. Gastroenterology 1980;78:57–63.
175. Malagelada JR, Rees WDW, Mazzotta LJ, Go VLW. Gastric motor abnormalities in diabetic and postvagotomy gastroparesis: effect of metoclopramide and bethanechol. Gastroenterology 1980;78:286–293.
176. Horowitz M, Harding PE, Chatterton BE, Collins PJ, Shearman DJ. Acute and chronic effects of domperidone on gastric emptying in diabetic autonomic neuropathy. Dig Dis Sci 1985;30:1–9.
177. Watts GF, Armitage M, Sinclair J, Hill RD. Treatment of diabetic gastroparesis with oral domperidone. Diabetic Med 1985;2:491–492.
178. Feldman M, Smith HJ. Effect of cisapride on gastric emptying of indigestible solids in patients with gastroparesis diabeticorum. Gastroenterology 1987;92:171–174.
179. Schmid R, Schusdziarra V, Allescher HD, Bofilias J, Buttermann G, Classen M. Effect of motilin on gastric emptying in patients with diabetic gastroparesis. Diabetes Care 1991;14:65–67.
180. Kondo Y, Torii K, Omura S, Itoh Z. Erythromycin and its derivatives with motilin-like biological activities inhibit the specific binding of 125I-motilin to duodenal muscle. Biochem Biophy Res Comm 1988;150:877–882.
181. Depootere I, Peeters TL, Matthijs G, Vantrappen G. Macrolide antibiotics are motilin receptor agonists. Hepato-Gastroenterol 1988;35:198.
182. Janssens J, Peeters TL, Vantrappen G, et al. Improvement of gastric emptying in diabetic gastroparesis by erythromycin: preliminary studies. N Engl J Med 1990;322:1028–1031.
183. Ogbonnaya KI, Arem R. Diabetic diarrhea. Pathophysiology, diagnosis, and management. Arch Intern Med 1990;150:262–267.
184. Whalen GE, Soergel KH, Geenen JE. Diabetic diarrhea: a clinical and pathophysiological study. Gastroenterology 1969;56:1021–1032.
185. Keshavarzian A, Iber FL. Intestinal transit in insulin-requiring diabetics. Am J Gastroenterol 1986;81:257–260.
186. Scarpello JHB, Greaves M, Sladen JE. Small intestinal transit in diabetics. Br Med J 1976;ii:1225–1226.
187. Fedorak RN, Field M, Chang EB. Treatment of diabetic diarrhea with clonidine. Ann Intern Med 1985;102:197–199.
188. Scarpello JHB, Hague RV, Cullen DR, Sladen GE. The 14C-glycocholate test in diabetic diarrhea. Br Med J 1976;ii:673–675.
189. Walsh CP, Cooper BT, Right AD, Malin JM, Cooke WT. Diabetes mellitus in coeliac disease: a clinical study. Q J Med 1978;47:89–92.
190. Molloy AM, Tomkin GH. Altered bile in diabetic diarrhea. Br Med J 1978;ii:1462–1463.
191. Schiller LR, Santa Ana CA, Schmulen AC, Hendler RS, Harford WV, Fordtran JS. Pathogenesis of fecal incontinence in diabetes mellitus: evidence for internal-anal-sphincter dysfunction. N Engl J Med 1982;307:1666–1671.
192. Green PA, Berge KG, Sprague RG. Control of diabetic diarrhea with antibiotic therapy. Diabetes 1968;17:385–387.
193. Valensi P, Smagghue O, Paries J, Velayoudon P, Nguyen TN, Attali JR. Peripheral vasoconstrictor responses to sympathetic activation in diabetic patients: relationship with rheological disorders. Metabol 1997;46:235–241.
194. Battle WM, Cohen JD, Snape WJ Jr. Disorders of colonic motility in patients with diabetes mellitus. Yale J Biol Med 1983;56:277–283.
195. Battle WM, Snape WJ Jr, Alavi A, Cohen S, Braunstein S. Colonic dysfunction in diabetes mellitus. Gastroenterology 1980;79:1217–1221.
196. Keshavarzian A, Iber FL, Nasrallah S. Radionuclide esophageal emptying and manometric studies in diabetes mellitus. Am J Gastroenterol 1987;82:625–631.

197. Maddern GJ, Horowitz M, Jamieson GG. The effect of domperidone on oesophageal emptying in diabetic autonomic neuropathy. Br J Clin Pharmacol 1985;19:441–444.
198. Stone BG, Gavaler JS, Belle SH, Shreiner DP, Peleman RR, Sarva RP, Yingvorapant N, Van Thief DH. Impairment of gallbladder emptying in diabetes mellitus. Gastroenterology 1988;95:170–176.
199. Smith SE, Smith SA, Brown PM, Fox C, Sonksen PH. Pupillary signs in diabetic autonomic neuropathy. Br Med J 1978;2:924–927.
200. Weinberg CR, Pfeifer MA. Development of a predictive model for symptomatic neuropathy in diabetes. Diabetes 1986;35:873–880.
201. Smith SA, Dewhirst RR. A simple diagnostic test for pupillary abnormality in diabetic autonomic neuropathy. Diabetic Med 1986;3:38–41.
202. Lepore FE. Diagnostic pharmacology of the pupil. Clin Neuropharmacol 1985;8:27–37.
203. Smith SA, Smith SE. Evidence for a neuropathic aetiology in the small pupil of diabetes mellitus. Br J Opthalmol 1983;2:924–927.
204. Pfeifer MA, Cook D, Brodsky J, Tice D, Parrish D, Reenan A, Halter JB, Ensinck JW, Porte D Jr. Quantitative evaluation of sympathetic and parasympathetic control of iris function. Diabetes Care 1982;5:518–528.
205. Lanting P, Bos JE, Aartsen J, Schuman L, Reichert-Thoen J, Heimans JJ. Assessment of pupillary light reflex latency and darkness adapted pupil size in control subjects and in diabetic patients with and without cardiovascular autonomic neuropathy. J Neurol Neurosurg Psychiatry 1990;53:912–914.
206. Martyn CN, Ewing DJ. Pupil cycle time: a simple way of measuring an autonomic reflex. J Neurol Neurosurg Psychiatry 1986;49:771–774.
207. Lanting P, Strijers RL, Bos JE, Faes TJ, Heimans JJ. The cause of increased pupillary light reflex latencies in diabetic patients: the relationship between pupillary light reflex and visual evoked potential latencies. Electroencephalogr Clin Neurophysiol 1991;78:111–115.
208. Straub RH, Zietz B, Palitzsch KD, Scholmerich J. Impact of disease duration on cardiovascular and pupillary autonomic nervous function in IDDM and NIDDM patients. Diabetes Care 1996;19:960–967.
209. Barany FR, Cooper EH. Pilomotor and sudomotor innervation in diabetes. Clin Sci 1956;15:533–540.
210. Rundles RW. Diabetic neuropathy: general review with report of 125 cases. Medicine 1945;24:111–160.
211. Fealey RD, Low PA, Thomas JE. Thermoregulatory sweating abnormalities in diabetes mellitus. Mayo Clin Proc 1989;64:617–628.
212. Odel HM, Roth GM, Keating FR. Autonomic neuropathy simulating the effects of sympathectomy as a complication of diabetes mellitus. Diabetes 1955;4:92–97.
213. Kennedy WR, Sakuta M, Sutherland D, Goetz FC. Quantitation of the sweating deficiency in diabetes mellitus. Ann Neurol 1984;15:482–488.
214. Faerman I, Faccio E, Calb I, Razumny J, Franco N, Dominguez A, et al. Autonomic neuropathy in the skin: a histological study of the sympathetic nerve fibres in diabetic anhidrosis. Diabetologia 1982;22:96–99.
215. Goodman JI. Diabetic anhidrosis. Am J Med 1966;41:831–835.
216. Low PA, Caskey PE, Tuck RR, Fealey RD, Dyck PJ. Quantitative sudomotor axon reflex test in normal and neuropathic subjects. Ann Neurol 1983;14:573–580.
217. Fagius J. Microneurographic findings in diabetic polyneuropathy with special references to sympathetic nerve activity. Diabetologia 1982;23:415–420.
218. Kennedy WR, Sakuta M, Sutherland D, Goetz FC. The sweating deficiency in diabetes mellitus: Methods of quantitative and clinical correlation. Neurology 1984;34:758–763.
219. Watkins PJ. Facial sweating after food: a new sign of diabetic autonomic neuropathy. Br Med J 1973;1:583–587.
220. Stuart DD. Diabetic gustatory sweating. Ann Intern Med 1978;89:223, 224.
221. List CF, Peet M. Sweat secretion in man. I. Sweating responses in normal persons. Arch Neurol Psychiatry 1938;39:1228–1237.
222. Guttman L. Management of the quinizarin sweat test. Postgrad Med J 1947;23:353–355.
223. Low PA. Quantitation of autonomic function. In: Dyck PJ, Thomas PK, Griffin JW, Low PA, Podulso JF, eds. Peripheral Neuropathy, vol. I, 3rd ed. W.B. Saunders, Philadelphia, 1993, pp. 729–745.
224. Shahani BT, Halperin JJ, Boulu P, Cohen J. Sympathetic skin response - a method of assessing unmyelinated axon dysfunction in peripheral neuropathies. J Neurol Neurosurg Psychiatry 1984;47:536–542.

# 13 Autonomic Neuropathy and Heart Disease

*Efthymios N. Deliargyris,* MD
*and Richard W. Nesto,* MD, FACC

*CONTENTS*



## INTRODUCTION

Diabetes mellitus is associated with a high incidence of cardiovascular complications and has been identified as an independent risk factor for the development of coronary artery disease *(1,2)*. Once the diagnosis of coronary disease is established, patients with diabetes have higher complication rates and higher mortality than their nondiabetic counterparts *(3,4)*. Overall, diabetes increases the relative risk of cardiovascular death threefold in males regardless of the presence of other traditional risk factors, with an even more pronounced effect in diabetic females *(5,6)*.

There are many proposed mechanisms responsible for the poor cardiovascular outcome of patients with diabetes including an altered lipid profile leading to more aggressive and extensive atherosclerosis, as well as changes in coagulation and fibrinolysis parameters resulting in accentuated thrombosis. Recently, the potential contribution of autonomic dysfunction to the poor outcome of diabetic patients has generated interest, since autonomic neuropathy is a frequent complication of diabetes. An intact autonomic nervous system is necessary for the maintenance of numerous organ systems and abnor-

From: *Contemporary Endocrinology: Clinical Management of Diabetic Neuropathy*
Edited by: A. Veves © Humana Press Inc., Totowa, NJ

Table 1
Disorders of Autonomic Function

| | |
|---|---|
| **Primary** | |
| | Shy-Drager syndrome (multiple-system atrophy or MSA) |
| | Primary autonomic failure (PAF) (idiopathic) |
| | Progressive autonomic failure associated with Parkinson's disease |
| | Sympathotonic orthostatic hypotension |
| **Secondary** | |
| | Spinal cord lesions |
| | Polyneuropathy: diabetes, amyloidosis, chronic renal and hepatic failure |
| | Autoimmune disorders: Guillain-Barre syndrome, myasthenia gravis, dysautonomia (acute and subacute), rheumatoid arthritis, multiple sclerosis, systemic lupus erythematosus |
| | Metabolic disorders: porphyria, Tangier disease, Fabry disease, vitamin B12 deficiency |
| | Neoplasms: carcinomatous autonomic neuropathy, tumors involving the hypothalamus or midbrain |
| | Infections of the nervous system: neurosyphilis, Chagas disease |
| | Familial disorders: dysautonomia, hyperbradykinism |
| | Drugs: neuroleptics (tranquilizers, antidepressants), cardiovascular agents (prazosin, hydralazine, α-methyldopa, clonidine, phenoxybenzamine, hexamethonium) |
| | Neurotoxins: alcohol, botulism, heavy metals, vincristine |

malities of the parasympathetic and sympathetic systems may lead to significant cardiovascular morbidity and mortality.

## DEFINITION AND PREVALENCE OF CARDIOVASCULAR AUTONOMIC NEUROPATHY

Cardiovascular autonomic neuropathy (CAN) may be a feature of any syndrome that affects the autonomic nervous system. Table 1 lists the syndromes associated with autonomic dysfunction and separates them into primary or secondary causes. Diabetes is by far the leading cause of secondary autonomic neuropathy, which can affect a variety of organ systems and cause a wide array of symptoms (Table 2). Cardiovascular manifestations include resting tachycardia, impaired exercise capacity, and orthostatic hypotension. Either clinical symptoms or abnormal cardiovascular reflex testing such as inadequate heart rate and blood pressure responses to various stimuli are sufficient for the diagnosis of autonomic neuropathy.

Autonomic function declines with age in healthy subjects, as is evident by a decrease in heart-rate variability and a higher incidence of postural hypotension in the elderly (Fig. 1). The presence of diabetes greatly accelerates this process *(8)*. It is estimated that one fourth of patients with type I diabetes and one third of the patients with type II diabetes have abnormal autonomic function *(9,10,12,21)*. In some of these patients, autonomic dysfunction is present as early as at the time of initial diagnosis of diabetes. Furthermore, in a prospective study of newly diagnosed non-insulin dependent diabetic patients and healthy controls, diabetic patients had a threefold increase in their chance of developing autonomic neuropathy at 10-yr follow-up *(11)*. It is not clear which diabetic patients will develop autonomic neuropathy, as reports examining the relation of the duration and/or severity of diabetes to ANS dysfunction have yielded conflicting

Table 2
Clinical Manifestations of Autonomic Neuropathy

| *Systems Involved* | *Manifestations* |
|---|---|
| Cardiovascular | Resting tachycardia, impaired exercise-induced cardiovascular responses, cardiac denervation, orthostatic hypotension, heat intolerance, impaired vasodilation, impaired venarteriolar reflex dependent edema) |
| Eye | Decreased diameter of dark-adapted pupil (dark-adapted miosis) |
| Gastrointestinal | Esophageal enteropathy, gallbladder atony, impaired gastric and colonic motility (gastroparesis, diarrhea, constipation), anorectal sphincter dysfunction (incontinence) |
| Genitourinary | Neurogenic vesical dysfunction (decreased bladder sensitivity/incontinence/retention), sexual dysfunction (male, penile erectile failure and retrograde ejaculation; female, defective lubrication) |
| Sudomotor | Anhidrosis/hyperhidrosis (heat intolerance), gustatory sweating |
| Endocrine | Hypoglycemia-associated autonomic failure |

results. One interesting report however by Barzilay et al. has shown a strong association between the HLA-DR3/4 phenotype and the development of cardiovascular autonomic neuropathy in patients with type I diabetes, raising the possibility of genetic predisposition *(14)*.

## PATHOPHYSIOLOGY AND NATURAL HISTORY OF CARDIOVASCULAR AUTONOMIC NEUROPATHY

Autonomic neuropathy is caused by the same mechanisms that are responsible for the development of peripheral somatic neuropathy *(13)*. The progressive neuronal degeneration and dysfunction is a global process and affects all limbs of the nervous system. Such diffuse involvement has been demonstrated in studies showing that peripheral somatic neuropathy and autonomic neuropathy coexist in 90% of cases of diabetic neuropathy *(23)*.

In regard to cardiovascular autonomic neuropathy, this progressive neuronal degeneration can lead to marked autonomic denervation of the heart and the arterial system. The initial observation of the association between diabetes and cardiac autonomic denervation was based on autopsy reports of patients who died as a result of clinically silent myocardial infarctions. The myocardium of these long-standing diabetic patients was found to be greatly depleted of catecholamine stores. This adrenergic depletion was thought to be at least in part responsible for the inability of these patients to sense myocardial ischemia *(24)*. Modern imaging techniques that can assess myocardial catecholamine stores in live patients have also demonstrated a close correlation between abnormal autonomic innervation and inability to sense myocardial ischemia.

Evidence of deficient parasympathetic innervation is usually the initial finding during autonomic testing. An increase in resting heart rates suggests decreased vagal input to the sinus node. Gradual decline in resting heart rates and finally the appearance of a fixed heart rate indicate progressively decreasing adrenergic input and sympathetic

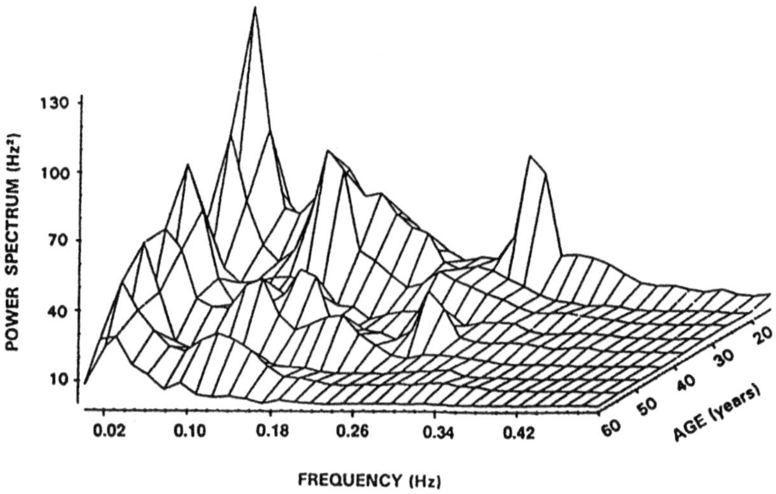


**Fig. 1.** Age-related decline in the Valsalva ratio in normal subjects and 90 and 95% confindence limits. (From O'Brien et al., with permission, ref. *8*).

involvement *(15)*. The "indifference" of heart rate in response to physiologic stimuli seen in many long-term diabetic patients closely resembles the effect of autonomic denervation in cardiac transplant recipients. Postural hypotension, a marker of significant sympathetic dysfunction, usually appears later than heart-rate abnormalities. Although the exact time course is not clear, evidence of sympathetic involvement is usually present within 5 yr of the development of parasympathetic dysfunction.

An intact autonomic nervous system is responsible for maintenance of cardiovascular homeostasis during changing conditions, and subclinical CAN can run a long, indolent course and become apparent only during periods of cardiovascular stress. Burgos et al. showed that 35% of diabetic patients required inotropic support during induction of general anesthesia vs only 5% of nondiabetic controls. Although none of the patients had any clinical symptoms suggesting autonomic neuropathy, those that required vasopressor support all had abnormal autonomic testing during preoperative evaluation *(17)*. From the results of this study, it is apparent that even in the absence of any symptoms, significant autonomic dysfunction may be present that can lead to complications during periods of cardiovascular stress.

The appearance of symptoms, namely orthostatic hypotension, implies severe autonomic dysfunction and is associated with a very grim prognosis. In a landmark study, Ewing and colleagues showed that in type I diabetic patients, the development of symptomatic autonomic neuropathy was associated with mortality rates in excess of 50% at 5-yr follow-up (Fig. 2) *(7)*. Such disturbing statistics underline the importance of detection of autonomic dysfunction in its subclinical phase, since it may help select the patients at risk for progressing to symptomatic neuropathy with its associated poor prognosis.

## METHODS OF ASSESSING CARDIOVASCULAR AUTONOMIC NEUROPATHY

Over the years, numerous tests with varying complexity have been devised to test autonomic integrity of various organ systems. Tests of cardiovascular reflexes however

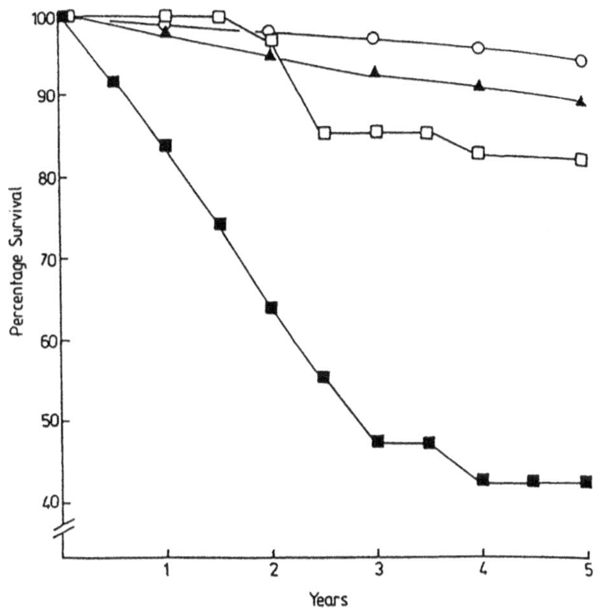


**Fig. 2.** Five-year survival curves for age- and sex-matched general population (open circles), age- and sex-matched diabetic population (black triangles), 33 normal diabetic subjects (open squares) and 40 diabetic subjects with symptoms and abnormal autonomic function tests (black squares). (From Ewing et al., with permission, ref. *7*).

remain the mainstay of making a diagnosis of cardiovascular autonomic neuropathy since they are sensitive, relatively easy to perform, and accurately represent global autonomic function *(22)*. Such tests assess the changes in heart rate and blood pressure in response to various stimuli such as deep respiration, the Valsalva maneuver, changes in bodily position, exercise, carotid massage, mental stress, and others.

### *Heart-Rate Variability*

Heart-rate variability (HRV), which measures beat-to-beat oscillations as well as changes in instantaneous heart rates, is a promising and popular marker of autonomic integrity. HRV can be measured by a variety of tests ranging from bed-side evaluations to 24-hr ambulatory ECG monitoring. It is important to emphasize that HRV measures fluctuations of autonomic input rather than mean autonomic input to the heart. A diminished HRV may therefore represent either autonomic withdrawal or a constantly high autonomic tone *(20)*. Since both conditions have been associated with deleterious effects on the cardiovascular system, an abnormal result during HRV testing maintains its value in either scenario. When possible, 24-hr recordings should be used, since they are superior to shorter measurements of HRV. An example of abnormal HRV is the absence of the physiological "sinus arrhythmia" which is consistently encountered in diabetic patients with autonomic neuropathy (Fig. 3).

The advent of power spectral analysis (PSA) has allowed for translation of conventional heart-rate recordings to frequency amplitude graphs using various mathematical approaches. Using PSA, three distinct frequency peaks have been identified within the spectrum of HRV allowing for selective assessment of the parasympathetic and sympathetic system. The very-low- and low-frequency peaks are mostly under sympathetic

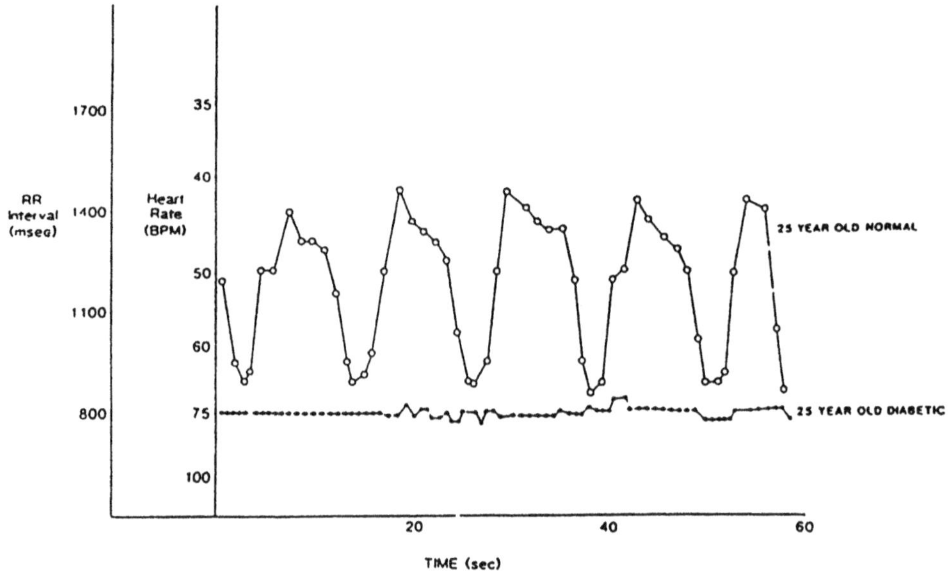


**Fig. 3.** Changes in heart rate during deep breathing in a normal and a diabetic subject. The variation in heart rate (sinus arrhythmia) during breathing is termed RR variation. Its magnitude is clearly less in this 25-yr-old diabetic patient with autonomic neuropathy than in the normal subject. Both patients were breathing at a fixed rate of five breaths per minute. (From Pfeifer et al., Current Concepts. The Upjohn Company, 1985 with permission).

control, whereas high frequencies represent parasympathetic input. During tilt-table testing of patients with postural hypotension, there is an absence of the expected rise of the sympathetic components, suggesting adrenergic dysfunction as the underlying mechanism (Fig. 4). However, since autonomic regulation is such a dynamic process, there can be overlap between sympathetic and parasympathetic input beyond these frequency peaks and interpretations of PSA results must be cautiously made *(21)*.

The clinical relevance of abnormal HRV has been investigated in numerous clinical conditions including coronary artery disease, congestive heart failure, hypertension, sudden death, and cardiac arrest among others with very interesting results. The predictive value of HRV has been demonstrated in acute myocardial infarction survivors and in diabetic patients prone to the development of symptomatic autonomic neuropathy *(18,19)*.

### *Blood-Pressure Testing*

Orthostatic hypotension is the cardinal clinical feature of symptomatic cardiovascular autonomic neuropathy. The presence of lightheadedness, weakness, visual changes, and palpitations can present a clinical dilemma in diabetic patients since it can be mistaken as hypoglycemia. However, since severe autonomic dysfunction can be present long before clinical orthostasis develops, testing in the suclinical phase is justified, particularly in the diabetic population.

The demonstration of a drop in systolic blood pressure of 30 mmHg or a drop in diastolic pressure of 10 mmHg is sufficient for the diagnosis of postural hypotension *(23)*. The most commonly used tests include response of blood pressure to standing, tilting,

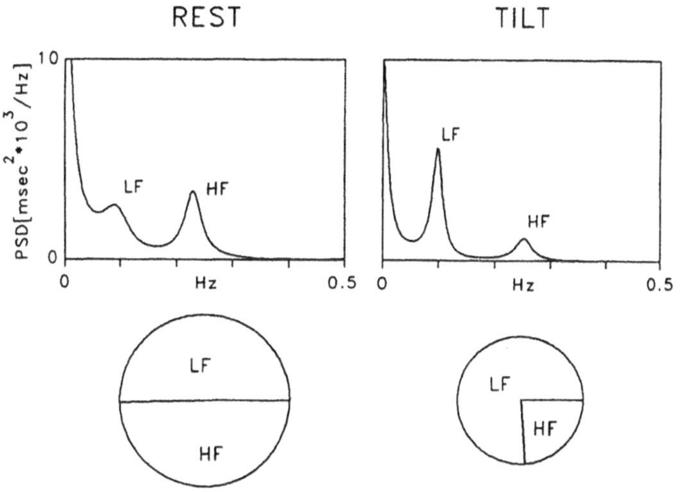


**Fig. 4.** Spectral analysis of RR interval variability in a healthy subject at rest and during 90% head-up tilt. At rest, two major components of similar power are detectable at low and high frequencies. During tilt, there is clear dominance of the LF component, which reflects mostly sympathetic input *(61)*.

during handgrip exercise, and continuous ambulatory 24-hr blood-pressure monitoring. It is important that patients undergoing testing abstain from caffeine, nicotine, and ethanol, and that drugs able to cause postural hypotension, such as tricyclic antidepressants, vasodilators, diuretics, and even insulin are excluded. Unlike HRV, which is determined by both parasympathetic and sympathetic input, abnormal blood pressure responses are thought to represent sympathetic dysfunction, since central and peripheral adrenergic mechanisms are responsible for blood-pressure homeostasis.

### *Radionuclide Imaging*

The use of radioisotope-tagged analogs of naturally occurring neurotransmitters allows for quantitative scintigraphic assessment of autonomic innervation of the heart. Methods for detection of adrenergic defects are currently available, and similar methods should be available in the future for assessment of parasympathetic fibers. Measurement of iodine-123-tagged metaiodobenzylguanidine (I-123 MIBG), a nonmetabolized norepinephrine analog, showed marked uptake deficits in diabetic hearts *(16)*. Single-photon emission computed tomography (SPECT) images have also been used to demonstrate abnormal cardiac sympathetic innervation. These findings suggest that the number of adrenergic fibers in the myocardium of diabetic patients is greatly decreased. There is evidence to support that scintigraphic assessment may be more sensitive than conventional autonomic testing in detecting CAN, since abnormal adrenergic uptake patterns are present even when conventional tests are still normal *(25,26)*.

## CLINICAL IMPLICATIONS OF CARDIOVASCULAR AUTONOMIC NEUROPATHY

Coronary artery disease is the leading cause of mortality in the diabetic population, and patients with diabetes have a worse prognosis than nondiabetic patients with angiographically similar CAD. Diabetic patients also have higher incidence of congestive heart failure and higher mortality following myocardial infarction than nondiabetic patients with similar infarct size *(27,28)*. The exact mechanisms responsible for the worst outcome associated with diabetes are not clear. Proposed theories include an altered lipid profile, accelerated atherosclerosis, endothelial dysfunction, increased platelet aggregability, raised fibrinogen levels, and increased plasminogen-activator inhibitor (PAI-1) activity. Furthermore, the presence of autonomic neuropathy, a common complication of diabetes, has been proven to be an independent predictor of mortality in myocardial infarction survivors. Putative mechanisms by which autonomic neuropathy can adversely affect outcome in these patients include an altered or absent perception of myocardial ischemia, abnormal hemodynamic responses to cardiovascular stress (i.e., myocardial infarction, exercise capacity, general anesthesia), abnormal left ventricular filling patterns, and a predisposition to lethal arrhythmias *(29)*.

## *Silent Ischemia*

Abnormal autonomic function testing reflects damage of efferent autonomic fibers responsible for transmission of central autonomic impulses to the periphery, and probably also indicates concomitant damage of the afferent fibers that are responsible for the sensory innervation of the heart. Damage to these fibers is thought to be the underlying pathogenetic mechanism responsible for the blunted or absent perception of ischemic pain in diabetic patients. There are numerous histopathologic studies supporting the link between diabetes, autonomic neuropathy, and clinically silent coronary disease. Histologic examination of the myocardium in diabetic patients with painless myocardial infarction demonstrated extensive damage of the afferent autonomic fibers *(30)*. In another study, patients with long-term diabetes had markedly reduced norepinephrine stores in their myocardium and arterial system during postmortem examination when compared to nondiabetic controls, again suggesting autonomic-nerve degeneration *(24)*. Finally, newer radioisotope-imaging techniques have demonstrated decreased norepinephrine analog uptake in the hearts of diabetic patients with evidence of silent ischemia *(16)*. All of the above data suggest that the neuronal degeneration associated with diabetes results in autonomic denervation of the heart and is responsible for the diminished perception of ischemic pain and silent ischemia.

Conventional noninvasive testing is adequate for detection of silent ischemia in the diabetic population. Nesto and coworkers showed that 91% of ischemic episodes in this population are clinically silent during 24-hr ECG monitoring, a percentage much higher than that observed in non-diabetic patients with CAD *(31)*. In another report, again using 24-hr Holter monitoring, the prevalence of silent ischemia was markedly higher in diabetic patients with autonomic neuropathy than diabetic patients without autonomic dysfunction *(34)*. Similar results were seen using dypiridamole-thallium scanning, in which 60% of diabetic patients with severe peripheral vascular disease but no clinical evidence of coronary disease had silent ischemia or previous infarctions *(33)*. Even though the above data are very suggestive of the association between diabetes and autonomic neuropathy with silent ischemia, there has been some criticism regarding the lack of similar data using coronary arteriography. A recent study by Marchant et al. however, showed that in patients with angiographically similar coronary disease, silent ischemia was more frequent in patients with diabetes and abnormal autonomic function *(35)*.

Even when diabetic patients do experience symptoms, their anginal perceptual threshold is higher when compared to nondiabetic patients. Ambepityia et al. showed that the onset of angina during treadmill testing in diabetic patients was delayed compared to nondiabetic patients once electrocardiographic evidence of ischemia was present. This delay in the onset of angina allowed diabetic patients to continue exercising with resultant worsening of myocardial ischemia. Further analysis of this study population revealed that patients with abnormal autonomic function testing were especially prone to a prolonged anginal threshold *(32)*.

As a result of their defective perception of warning symptoms, diabetic patients may escape detection or suffer delays in diagnostic and therapeutic interventions. Furthermore, progression of unrecognized atherosclerotic disease can lead to silent myocardial infarctions and serious arrhythmias with congestive heart failure or sudden cardiac death being the initial manifestation of CAD in such patients.

### *Myocardial Infarction*

Diabetes mellitus is associated with high morbidity and mortality rates from coronary disease. In fact, myocardial infarction is the cause of death in approx 30% of diabetic patients *(36)*. Following myocardial infarction the inhospital mortality rate is 28% for all diabetic patients, with an even worse prognosis for diabetic women and patients with a prior infarction, rates that are markedly higher than those of nondiabetic subjects *(37)*. Congestive heart failure, recurrent infarction, atrioventricular and intraventricular conduction abnormalities, and myocardial rupture are also encountered more frequently in diabetic than in nondiabetic patients during the course of acute myocardial infarction *(38–41)*.

So, why do diabetic patients have higher rates of myocardial infarction, more frequent complications, and such an unfavorable outcome? As mentioned earlier in this chapter, the metabolic derangements associated with diabetes create an environment that favors the development and progression of coronary disease. Higher levels of very-low-density lipoprotein (VLDL), decreased levels of high-density lipoprotein (HDL), and a higher fraction of apolipoprotein E (apoE), all contribute to increased cholesterol ester uptake and deposition within the arterial wall with subsequent atherogenesis *(42)*. Diabetes also influences various steps of the coagulation cascade. Platelets from diabetic patients have increased numbers of GpIIb-IIIa receptors on their surface (the integrin that mediates the final common pathway of platelet aggregation) and also demonstrate a hypersensitivity to thrombin, therefore making these platelets more aggregable ("sticky"). Diabetic patients also have decreased antithrombin III activity and lower concentrations of protein C, changes that further predispose to thrombosis. Finally, the fibrinolytic system is impaired in diabetic patients as a result of increased activity of plasminogen activator inhibitor-1 (PAI-1) even though levels of tissue-plasminogen activator (tPA) are normal or increased *(43)*. The alterations in the lipid profile in conjunction with the effects of diabetes on platelet function, coagulation, and fibrinolysis, create an intravascular milieu that favors atherosclerotic plaque formation, fissuring, thrombosis and myocardial infarction.

Coronary disease in diabetic patients can be further complicated by the frequent coexistence of autonomic neuropathy. Silent infarctions are more common in diabetic than in nondiabetic patients; 39 vs 22% of all infarctions *(44)*. This observation is supported by autopsy data demonstrating the presence of myocardial scar in the absence of an antemortem history of infarction three times more frequently in diabetic than nondiabetic patients *(45)*. In other instances, myocardial infarction may not be silent in diabetic patients but may present with atypical symptoms. Nausea and vomiting, dyspnea, or even confusion are the presenting complains in approx 40% of diabetic patients suffering an acute myocardial infarction *(46)*. This atypical symptomatology may result in delayed triage and inappropriate disposition of such patients to the general medical wards rather than the coronary-care unit. Furthermore, diabetic patients may underestimate the importance of such symptoms and not seek medical attention for several hours, therefore depriving themselves of the benefits associated with early pharmacologic or mechanical thrombolysis. Such delays are thought to account in part for the increased morbidity and mortality of diabetic patients with acute myocardial infarction, since early administration of thrombolytic agents has been associated with at least equal if not greater benefit in the diabetic population *(3,60)*.

Besides blunting the perception of ischemic pain, the presence of autonomic neuropathy can precipitate or complicate the course of an acute infarction by several mechanisms. Higher resting heart rates associated with autonomic dysfunction increase myocardial oxygen demand and can therefore precipitate ischemia. This high sympathetic input also results in increased vascular tone and subsequent vasoconstriction at the sites of coronary stenosis, further reducing myocardial perfusion. Furthermore, orthostatic hypotension may itself precipitate myocardial ischemia by decreasing coronary perfusion pressure. The constellation of these mechanisms that can initiate an ischemic episode coupled with the prolonged anginal perceptual threshold that frequently coexists in such patients may lead to prolonged ischemia and infarction.

Finally, the presence of autonomic dysfunction may impair reflex adaptation to hemodynamic stress associated with acute myocardial infarction. Indirect evidence to support this hypothesis comes from the anesthesiology literature. As mentioned earlier in this chapter, diabetic patients with autonomic neuropathy were much more likely to require vasopressor support to counteract the hemodynamic effects of induction of general anesthesia than were nondiabetic patients or diabetic patients without evidence of autonomic dysfunction *(17)*. This impaired reflex adaptation may at least in part explain the higher incidence of congestive heart failure and cardiogenic shock in diabetic patients when compared to nondiabetic patients with similar infarct size *(47)*.

### *Diabetic Cardiomyopathy*

Rubler et al. in 1972 were the first to suggest the existence of a distinct cardiomyopathy associated with diabetes. During autopsy studies of four diabetic patients with an antemortem history of congestive heart failure, they demonstrated the absence of atherosclerotic, valvular, congenital, hypertensive, or alcoholic heart disease and concluded that diabetes itself may play a causative role in the development of cardiomyopathy *(48)*. Since then, numerous epidemiologic studies have supported that hypothesis. For example, in the Framingham Heart Study, diabetic men had more than twice the frequency of congestive heart failure than their nondiabetic counterparts and, in the case of diabetic women, that risk increased to fivefold. This increased risk persisted after controlling for age, hypertension, coronary disease, hypercholesterolemia, and obesity, again implying that diabetes may be the primary cause of cardiomyopathy *(49)*.

Histopathologic studies in both animals and humans have failed to elucidate a single pathogenetic mechanism responsible for the development of diabetic cardiomyopathy. In these studies, interstitial deposition of periodic acid-Schiff (PAS)-positive material, along with myocardial hypertrophy and fibrosis have been the consistent findings during postmortem examination. It is probably a constellation of pathogenic mechanisms that leads to myocardial dysfunction, including small-vessel disease, interstitial changes, metabolic abnormalities, and autonomic dysfunction *(50)*. Using noninvasive testing, diastolic dysfunction as evidenced by a prolonged peak diastolic filling rate along with an augmented atrial contribution to diastolic filling was encountered in diabetic patients with autonomic neuropathy and the severity of diastolic dysfunction correlated with the degree of autonomic neuropathy *(51,52)*. Similarly, systolic function may also be affected, especially during exercise. Vered et al. demonstrated that in young diabetic patients with normal resting ejection fraction and without evidence of coronary disease or hypertension, ejection fraction failed to increase and in some cases decreased during exercise *(53)*. These findings suggest that the development of cardiomyopathy starts early in the course of diabetes and that diabetic patients without any clinical findings suggestive of heart failure may have significant abnormalities of both systolic and diastolic function.

Normal contraction and relaxation of the myocardium relies greatly on an intact autonomic nervous system. Sympathetic stimulation results both in increased left ventricular contractility and also in more rapid left ventricular relaxation, an effect of catecholamine-facilitated calcium uptake by the sarcoplasmic reticulum *(50)*. Myocardium of patients with autonomic neuropathy has greatly depleted catecholamine stores detected both during postmortem pathologic studies, but also using radionuclide studies in live patients *(16,24)*. This autonomic denervation is considered to be the underlying mechanism for the decreased exercise capacity often encountered in this patient population. This inability for adrenergic recruitment is also responsible for the frequent cardiovascular decompensation of these patients during periods of acute hemodynamic stress, such as during induction of general anesthesia and in the course of an acute myocardial infarction.

Autonomic neuropathy is frequently present even in the very early stages of diabetes. Asymptomatic systolic or diastolic dysfunction may also be present early in the course of diabetes and is usually associated with the coexistence of autonomic neuropathy. Decreased heart-rate variability (HRV) is a consistent finding in congestive heart failure, and there is data to support a correlation between the degree of autonomic impairment and the severity of heart failure *(54)*. The presence of subclinical abnormalities in systolic or diastolic function may therefore be helpful in identifying patients at risk of developing overt heart failure and may also help select patients warranting closer monitoring during exercise or while undergoing surgical procedures.

### *Sudden Death*

Symptomatic cardiovascular autonomic neuropathy is associated with a 50% mortality over 5 yr after its onset *(7)*. Sudden death, presumably of cardiac etiology, is responsible for about one-third of these deaths *(55)*. The exact etiology of the high incidence of sudden cardiac death in these patients is not clear but may be related to a combination of silent ischemia, infarction, and/or primary arrhythmia.

Autonomic dysfunction may contribute to life-threatening arrhythmia by two different mechanisms. First, chronically depleted catecholamine stores lead to upregulation of myocardial adrenergic receptors. Such patients demonstrate exaggerated responses to infusions of $\alpha$ and $\beta$ adrenergic agonists, a condition termed "adrenergic denervation hypersensitivity." During conditions that are associated with catecholamine release,

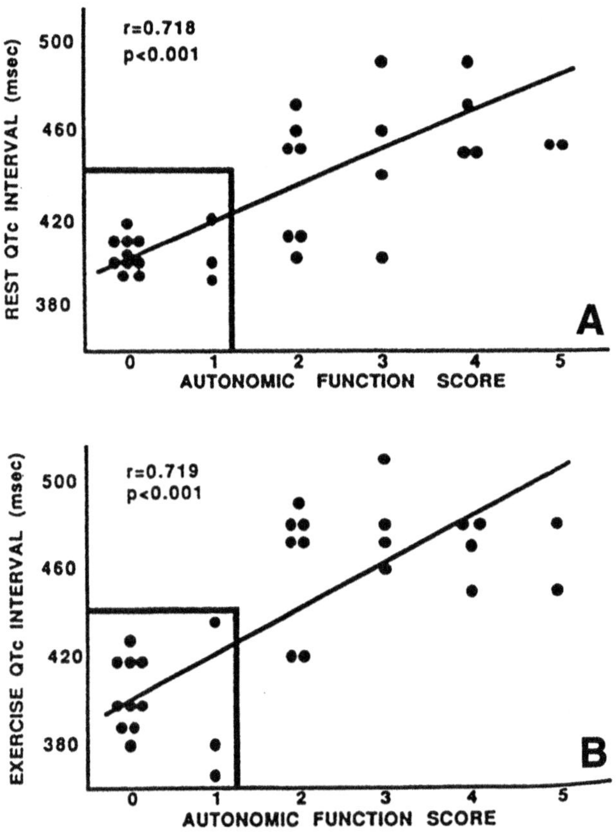


**Fig. 5.** Direct linear relationship between the extent of cardiac autonomic neuropathy and the QT interval at rest (**A**) and with maximal exercise (**B**) in 30 patients with diabetes mellitus. The enclosed box indicates patients who had no cardiac autonomic neuropathy, all of whom had normal (<440 ms) QT intervals. Autonomic scores were assigned based on results of five tests: resting pulse, beat-to-beat heart-rate variability, Valsalva maneuver, heart response to standing and blood pressure response to standing. (From Kahn et al., with permission, ref. *57*).

these patients might have excessive increases in heart rate and myocardial oxygen demand, changes that may, in turn, precipitate a malignant arrhythmia *(56)*. The second mechanism by which autonomic neuropathy may contribute to sudden death is through prolongation of the QT interval. The long QT syndrome has been historically linked with malignant ventricular arrhythmias, namely *torsade de pointes*, and a high incidence of sudden death. Numerous reports exist that correlate the degree of autonomic neuropathy and the extent of QT prolongation, an effect that was further exacerbated by exercise (Fig. 5) *(57)*. These findings suggest an attractive explanation for the high incidence of sudden death in the presence of autonomic dysfunction, however a clear cause-and-effect relationship has not yet been established *(58,59)*.

## CARDIOVASCULAR AUTONOMIC NEUROPATHY AS AN INDEPENDENT RISK FACTOR

The abundance of studies proposing various mechanisms of contribution of autonomic neuropathy to the poor cardiovascular outcome of diabetic patients has resulted in some controversy regarding the exact significance of abnormal testing and the clinical situations were it may be applied. This prompted the European Society of Cardiology and the North American Society of Pacing and Electrophysiology to form a task force that in March of 1996 provided a consensus statement on the measurement, physiological interpretation, and clinical use of heart-rate variability *(61)*. After reviewing the literature on the prognostic value of HRV in numerous cardiac and non-cardiac diseases it was concluded that HRV assessment can be used as an independent prognostic factor in only two clinical scenarios, namely risk stratification after acute myocardial infarction and prediction of development of symptomatic diabetic autonomic neuropathy.

In regard to risk stratification following myocardial infarction, HRV is a powerful and independent predictor of mortality and arrhythmic complications. They suggested that HRV assessment take place soon after the infarction and prior to hospital discharge and also emphasize the need of 24-hr recordings since they are superior to shorter measurements. These recommendations were based on studies that demonstrated that HRV has at least equal predictive power with post-MI left ventricular ejection fraction (LVEF) for overall mortality, and is a more powerful predictor of sudden death and serious arrhythmic events *(18,62)* (Fig. 6).

The second clinical setting in which HRV testing is indicated is in the detection of diabetic patients at risk for development of symptomatic autonomic neuropathy. Diabetic autonomic neuropathy can run a long, indolent course, however once symptoms develop the estimated 5-yr mortality is approx 50% *(7)*. Early subclinical detection of autonomic dysfunction can therefore be very important in risk stratification and potential management of this subgroup of the diabetic population that may be at risk for silent coronary disease, congestive heart failure, or sudden death. Short-and/or long-term HRV measurements have been proven useful for the detection of subclinical autonomic dysfunction *(19,63)*.

## TREATMENT OPTIONS AND RECOMMENDATIONS FOR PATIENTS WITH CARDIOVASCULAR AUTONOMIC NEUROPATHY

Unfortunately, most currently available treatments for cardiovascular autonomic neuropathy are aimed only at the symptomatic relief of orthostatic hypotension. Avoidance of precipitating medications should always be attempted along with measures to maintain optimal intravascular volume and increase venous return, such as elasticized stockings, increased salt intake if not contraindicated, and fludrocortisone (Florinef). Newer therapies include erythropoietin injections for optimization of red-cell mass, and administration of octreotide, a somastatin analog, which increases splanchnic vascular resistance and cardiac output *(64,65)*.

In regard to etiologic treatment of autonomic neuropathy, strict glycemic control should be the primary goal of therapy. The Diabetes Control and Complications Trial (DCCT) demonstrated that in patients with type I diabetes receiving intensive insulin therapy, the development of abnormal autonomic testing was reduced by approx 50% after 5 yr of follow-up when compared with the conventional treatment group *(66)*. Similar beneficial effect on autonomic testing was also seen in patients with type II diabetes who followed intense metabolic and exercise programs, further underlining the need for strict glucose control in all patients with diabetes *(67)*. Novel treatment strategies aimed at the pathogenetic mechanisms responsible for the neuronal degeneration associated with diabetes have yielded promising results in experimental studies. Such

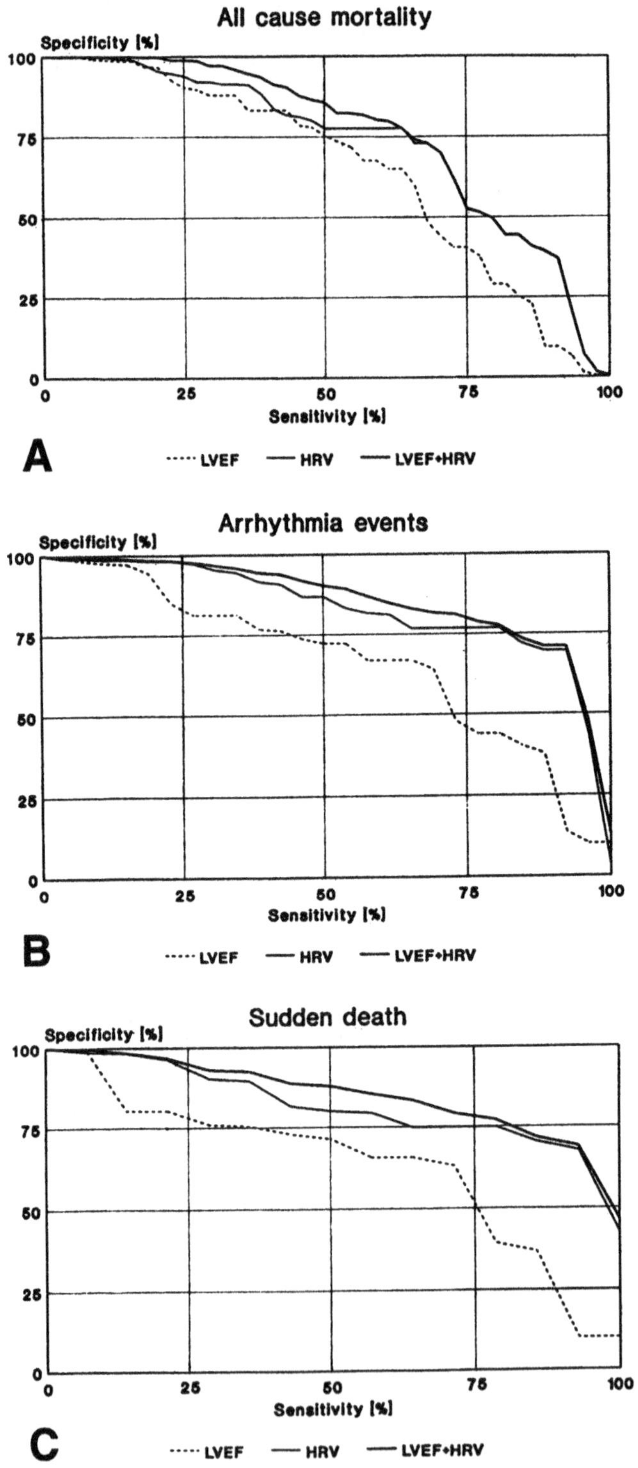


**Fig. 6.** The sensitivity and specificity of left ventricular ejection fraction (LVEF), heart-rate variability (HRV) index, and the combination, for the prediction of all-cause mortality **(A)**, arrhythmic events **(B)**, and sudden deaths **(C)**. (From Odemuyiwa et al., with permission, ref.18.)

agents include aldose reductase inhibitors, antioxidants, gamma-linolenic acid, neurotrophic factors, and inhibitors of advanced glycosylation end-products (AGEs). Numerous clinical trials are currently in progress that in the near future should elucidate the potential of these agents in treating diabetic neuropathy.

Medications commonly used for the treatment of heart disease including α and β blockers, calcium channel blockers, ACE inhibitors, and digoxin have been shown to have complex effects on the autonomic nervous system *(68)*. β blockers have been consistently shown to improve HRV indexes, however their effect is usually modest and there are no available data to suggest actual clinical benefit. On the other hand type IC antiarrhytmic agents decrease heart-rate variability scores, an effect that might provide an insight to the increased mortality associated with these drugs in myocardial-infarction survivors *(69)*. These findings suggest that medications should be continued as indicated by the underlying cardiac condition regardless of autonomic function testing results.

Exercise training has been shown to decrease overall mortality and incidence of sudden cardiac death in myocardial-infarction survivors *(70)*. Regular exercise can also favorably affect autonomic function and accelerate recovery of sympathovagal balance following myocardial infarction *(71)*. Based on these observations, exercise training should be included in the rehabilitation program of all eligible patients surviving myocardial infarction, however special caution should be taken in those patients with coexistent autonomic neuropathy. Such patients may have impaired exercise capacity that can limit their rehabilitation potential, but even more importantly, these same patients may be unable to sense myocardial ischemia during exercise that can lead to serious complications such as myocardial infarction and lethal arrhythmias. It therefore appears prudent that in patients with autonomic dysfunction, noninvasive testing to assess the presence or extent of coronary disease should be undertaken prior to exercise program recommendations.

## REFERENCES


1. Kannel WB, McGee DL. Diabetes and cardiovascular disease: the Framingham study. JAMA 1979;241:2035–2038.
2. Kannel WB, McGee D. Diabetes and cardiovascular risk factors: the Framingham study. Circulation 1979;59:8–13.
3. Granger C, Califf R, Young S, et al. Outcome of patients with diabetes mellitus and acute myocardial infarction treated with thrombolytic agents. J Am Coll Cardiol 1993;21:920.
4. Mueller H, Cohen L, Braunwald E, and the TIMI investigators. Predictors of early morbidity and mortality after thrombolytic therapy for acute myocardial infarction. Circulation 1992;85:1254.
5. Stamler J, Vaccaro O, Neaton J, Wentworth D. Diabetes, other risk factors, and 12-yr cardiovascular mortality for men screened in the Multiple Risk Factor Intervention Trial. Diabetes Care 1993;16:434–444.
6. Pan W-H, Cedres LB, Liu K, et al. Relationship of clinical diabetes and asymptomatic hyperglycemia to risk of coronary heart disease mortality in men and women. Am J Epidemiol 1986;123:504–516.
7. Ewing DJ, Campbell IW, Clarke BF. The natural history of diabetic autonomic neuropathy. Q J Med 1980;49:95–108.
8. O'Brien IA, O'Hare P, Corrall RJ. Heart rate variability in healthy subjects: effect of age and the derivation of normal ranges for tests of autonomic function. Br Heart J 1986;55:348–354.
9. Ewing DJ, Clarke BF. Diagnosis and management of diabetic autonomic neuropathy. Br Med J 1982;295:916–918.
10. Ewing DJ. Cardiac autonomic neuropathy. In Jarrett RJ, ed. Diabetes and Heart Disease. Elsevier, Amsterdam, 1984, pp. 99–132.

11. Toyry JP, Niskannen LK, Uusitupa MI, et al. Occurence, predictors and clinical significance of autonomic neuropathy in NIDDM. Diabetes 1996;45:308–315.
12. O'Brien IA, O'Hare JP, Lewin IG, Corrall RJ. The prevalence of autonomic neuropathy in insulin-dependent diabetes mellitus: a controlled study based on heart rate variability. Q J Med 1986;61:957–967.
13. Pfeifer MA, Schumer MP. Clinical trials of diabetic neuropathy: past, present and future. Diabetes 1995;44:1355–1361.
14. Barzilay J, Warram JH, Krolewski AS, et al. Risk of cardiovascular autonomic neuropathy is associated with the HLA-DR3/4 phenotype in type I diabetes mellitus. Ann Int Med 1992;116:544–549.
15. Ewing DJ, Campbell IW, Clarke BF. Heart range changes in diabetes mellitus. Lancet 1981;1:183–186.
16. Langer A, Freeman MR, Josse RG, et al. Metaiodobenzylguanidine imaging in diabetes mellitus: assessment of cardiac sympathetic denervation and its relation to autonomic dysfunction and silent myocardial ischemia. J Am Coll Cardiol 1995;25:610–618.
17. Burgos LG, Ebert TJ, Assiddao C, et al. Increased intraoperative cardiovascular morbidity in diabetics with autonomic neuropathy. Anesthesiology 1989;70:591–597.
18. Odemuyiwa O, Malik M, Farrell T, et al. Comparison of the predictive characteristics of heart rate variability index and left ventricular ejection fraction for all-cause mortality, arrhythmic events and sudden death after acute myocardial infarction. Am J Cardiol 1991;68:434–439.
19. Bellavere F, Balzani I, De Masi G, et al. Power spectral analysis of heart variation improves assessment of diabetic cardiac autonomic neuropathy. Diabetes 1992;41:633–640.
20. Malik M, Camm AJ. Components of heart rate variability: what they really mean and what we really measure. Am J Cardiol 1993;72:821,822.
21. Ziegler D. Diabetic cardiovascular autonomic neuropathy: prognosis, diagnosis and treatment. Diabetes/Metab Rev 1994;10:4339–4383.
22. Ewing DJ, Clarke BF. Diabetic autonomic neuropathy: present insights and future perspectives. Diabetes Care 1986;9:648–665.
23. Pfeifer MA, Peterson H. Cardiovascular autonomic neuropathy. In: Dyck P, et al. ed. Diabetic Neuropathy. Saunders, Philadelphia, 1987, pp. 122–133.
24. Neubauer B, Christensen NJ. Norepinephrine, epinephrine, and dopamine contents of the cardiovascular system in long-term diabetics. Diabetes 1976;25:6–10.
25. Mantysaari M, Kuikka J, Mustonen J, et al. Noninvasive detection of cardiac sympathetic nervous dysfunction in diabetic patients using [I-123] metaiodobenzylguanidine. Diabetes 1992;41:1069–1075.
26. Allman KC, Stevens MJ, Wieland DM, et al. Noninvasive assessment of cardiac autonomic neuropathy by carbon-11 hydroxyephedrine and positron emission tomography. J Am Coll Cardiol 1993;22:1425–1432.
27. Savage MP, Krolewski AS, Kenien GG, Nunez R, Jadzinky M, Fox D, Rapaport M. Acute myocardial infarction in diabetes mellitus and significance of congestive heart failure as a prognostic factor. Am J Cardiol 1988;62:665–669.
28. Smith JW, Marcus FI, Serokman R. Prognosis of patients with diabetes mellitus after acute myocardial infarction. Am J Cardiol 1984;54:718–721.
29. Leor J, Nesto RW, Kloner RA. Acute myocardial infarction and diabetes mellitus [Commentary]. Cardiovasc Res 1993;27:1913–1915.
30. Faerman I, Faccio E, Milei J, et al. Autonomic neuropathy and painless myocardial infarction in diabetic patients: histologic evidence of their relationship. Diabetes 1977;6:1147–1158.
31. Zarich S, Waxman S, Nesto RW, et al. Effect of autonomic nervous system dysfunction on the circadian pattern of myocardial ischemia in diabetes mellitus. J Am Coll Cardiol 1994;24:956–962.
32. Ambepityia G, Kopelman PG, Ingram D, et al. Exertional myocardial ischemia in diabetes: a quantitative analysis of anginal perceptual threshold and the influence of autonomic function. J Am Coll Cardiol 1990;15:72–77.
33. Nesto RW, Watson FS, Kowalchuk GJ, et al. Silent myocardial ischemia and infarction in diabetics with peripheral vascular disease: assessment by dypiridamole thallium scintigraphy. Am Heart J 1990;120:1073–1077.
34. O'Sullivan JJ, Conroy RM, MacDonald K, et al. Silent ischaemia in diabetic men with autonomic neuropathy. Br Heart J 1991;66:313–315.
35. Marchant B, Umachandran V, Stevenson R, et al. Silent myocardial ischemia: role of subclinical neuropathy in patients with and without diabetes. J Am Coll Cardiol 1993;22:1433–1437.

36. Barrett-Connor E, Orchard T. Insulin dependent diabetes mellitus and ischemic heart disease. Diabetes Care 1985;8:65–70.
37. Savage MP, Krolewski A, Kemien G, et al. Acute myocardial infarction in diabetes mellitus and significance of congestive heart failure as a prognostic factor. Am J Cardiol 1988;62:665–669.
38. Jacoby RM, Nesto RW. Acute myocardial infarction in the diabetic patient: pathophysiology, clinical course and prognosis. J Am Coll Cardiol 1992;20:736–744.
39. Rytter L, Troelsen S, Beck-Nielsen H. Prevalence and mortality of acute myocardial infarction in patients with diabetes. Diabetes Care 1985;8:230–234.
40. Hands M, Rutherford J, Muller J. The in-hospital development of cardiogenic shock after myocardial infarction: incidence, predictors of occurence, outcome and prognostic factors. J Am Coll Cardiol 1989;14:40–46.
41. Partamian JO, Bradley RF. Acute myocardial infarction in 258 cases of diabetes: immediate mortality and five year survival. N Engl J Med 1965;273:455–461.
42. Bierman E. Atherogenesis in diabetes. Atherosclerosis Thrombosis 1992;12:647.
43. Kwaan H. Changes in blood coagulation, platelet function, and plasminogen-plasmin system in diabetes. Diabetes 1992;41(S2):31.
44. Margolis JR, Kannel WB, Feinleib M, Dawber TR, McNamara PM. Clinical features of unrecognized myocardial infarction - silent and symptomatic: eighteen year follow-up: the Framingham study. Am J Cardiol 1973;32:1–7.
45. Cabin HS, Roberts WC. Quantitative comparison of extent of coronary narrowing and size of healed myocardial infarct in 33 necropsy patients with clinically recognized and in 28 with clinically unrecognized ("silent") previous acute myocardial infarction. Am J Cardiol 1982;50:677–681.
46. Nesto RW, Phillips RT. Asymptomatic myocardial ischemia in diabetic patients. Am J Med 1986;80(S4C):40–47.
47. Jaffe AS, Spadaro J, Schectman K, et al. Increased congestive heart failure after myocardial infarction of modest extent in patients with diabetes mellitus. Am Heart J 1984;108:1–7.
48. Rubler S, Dlugash J, Yuceoglu YZ, Kumral T, Branwood AW, Grishman A. New type of cardiomyopathy associated with diabetic glomerulosclerosis. Am J Cardiol 1972;30:595–602.
49. Kannel WB, Hjortland M, Castelli WP. Role of diabetes in congestive heart failure: the Framingham Study. Am J Cardiol 1974;34:29–34.
50. Zarich SW, Nesto RW. Diabetic cardiomyopathy. Am Heart J 1989;118:1000–1012.
51. Kahn JK, Zola B, Juni JE, Vini AI. Radionuclide assessment of left ventricular diastolic filling in diabetes mellitus with and without cardiac autonomic neuropathy. J Am Coll Cardiol 1986;7:1303–1309.
52. Airaksinen KEJ, Koistinen MJ, Ikaheimo MJ, et al. Augmentation of atrial contribution to left ventricular filling in IDDM subjects as assessed by Doppler echocardiography. Diabetes Care 1989;12:159–161.
53. Vered Z, Battler A, Segal P, et al. Exercise-induced left ventricular dysfunction in young men with asymptomatic diabetes mellitus. Am J Cardiol 1984;54:633–637.
54. Kienzle MG, Ferguson DW, Birkett CL, et al. Clinical hemodynamic and sympathetic neural correlates of heart rate variability in congestive heart failure. Am J Cardiol 1992;69:482–485.
55. Nesto RW, Zarich SW, Jacoby RM, Kamalesh M. Heart disease in diabetes, In: Kahn RC, Weir GC, eds. Joslin's Diabetes. Lea & Febiger, Malvern, PA, 1994, pp. 836–851.
56. Hilsted J, Richter E, Madsbad S, et al. Metabolic and cardiovascular responses to epinephrine in diabetic autonomic neuropathy. N Engl J Med 1987;317:421–426.
57. Kahn JK, Sisson JC, Vinik AI. QT interval prolongation and sudden cardiac death in diabetic autonomic neuropathy. J Clin Endocrinol Metab 1987;64:751–754.
58. Ong JJ, Sarma JS, Venkataraman K, Levin SR. Circadian rhythmicity of heart rate and QTc interval in diabetic autonomic neuropathy: implications for the mechanism of sudden death. Am Heart J 1993;125:744–752.
59. Bravenboer B, Hendricksen P-H, Oey LP, et al. Is the corrected QT interval a reliable indicator of the severity of diabetic autonomic neuropathy? Diabetes Care 1993;16:1249–1253.
60. ISIS-2 Collaborative Group. Randomized trial of intravenous streptokinase, oral aspirin, both or neither among 17,817 cases of suspected acute myocardial infarction. Lancet 1988;2:349–360.
61. Task Force of the European Society of Cardiology and the North American Society of Pacing and Electrophysiology. Heart rate variability: standards of measurement, physiological interpretation, and clinical use. Circulation 1996;93:1043–1065.

62. Kleiger RE, Miller JP, Bigger JT, Multicenter Post-Infarction Research Group. Decreased heart rate variability and its association with increased mortality after acute myocardial infarction. Am J Cardiol 1987;59:256–262.
63. Pagani M, Malfatto G, Pierini S, et al. Spectral analysis of heart rate variability in the assessment of autonomic diabetic neuropathy. J Auton Nerv Syst 1988;23:143–153.
64. Hoeldtke RD, Streeten DH. Treatment of orthostatic hypotension with erythropoetin. N Engl J Med 1993;329:611–615.
65. Hoeltdke RD, Davis KM, Joseph J, et al. Hemodynamic effects of octreotide in patients with autonomic neuropathy. Circulation 1991;84:168–176.
66. The Diabetes Control and Complications Trial Research Group. The effects of intensive treatment of diabetes on the development and progression of long-term complications in insulin-dependent diabetes mellitus. N Engl J Med 1993;329:977–986.
67. Vanninen E, Uusitupa M, Lansimie E, et al. Effect of metabolic control on autonomic function in obese patients with newly diagnosed type 2 diabetes. Diabetic Med 1996;10:66–73.
68. van Ravenswaaij-Arts CM, Kolee LA, Hopman JC, et al. Heart rate variability. Ann Intern Med 1993;118:436–447.
69. Zuanetti G, Latini R, Neilson JM, Antiarrhythmic Drug Evaluation Group (ADEG). Heart rate variability in patients with ventricular arrhythmias: effect of antiarrhythmic drugs. J Am Coll Cardiol 1991;17:604–612.
70. O'Connor GT, Buring JE, Yusuf S, et al. An overview of randomized trials of rehabilitation with exercise after myocardial infarction. Circulation 1989;80:234–44.
71. Hull SS, Vanoli E, Adamson PB, et al. Exercise training confers anticipatory protection from sudden death during acute myocardial ischemia. Circulation 1994;89:548–552.

# 14 Diabetic Impotence

*Pathogenesis and Treatment*

*Lynne Webster,* MB, ChB, MSc, FRCPsych

**Contents**



## SEXUAL DYSFUNCTION IN DIABETES

### *Prevalence*

It is not easy to get accurate data about sexual dysfunction because of the personal and sensitive nature of the information. Many factors discourage survey respondents from being entirely truthful, so it has proved difficult to obtain an assessment of the incidence of erectile problems in a representative sample of the general population. Despite this, the male diabetic clinic population has been well researched in this respect. Fairburn et al. *(1)* reviewed seven prevalence studies and found that the rates were between 35 and 59%. Bancroft *(2)* observes that the rate of erectile dysfunction rises with age, so when the prevalence in a diabetic clinic population studied by McCulloch et al. *(3)* is compared with the large general population survey by Kinsey et al. *(4)*, we see an amplification of the age-related pattern (*see* Fig. 1.), a finding that also emerges in the Massachusetts Male Aging Study *(5)*. Throughout these studies it has been consistently found that the prevalence of erectile failure increases with the duration of the diabetes. Not surprisingly, the rate is highest in those who also have evidence of other complications such as proliferative retinopathy, peripheral neuropathy, and autonomic neuropathy. There seems to be little difference between patients needing insulin and those controlled by oral hypoglycaemic agents, though patients using diet alone may be less at risk. In a 5-yr follow-up of 275 men with diabetes who were free from sexual dysfunction at the beginning of the study, McCulloch *(6)* found that 28% developed erectile problems. This was predicted by age, poor glycemic control, alcohol intake, the development of neuropathic symptoms, and vascular disease.

From: *Contemporary Endocrinology: Clinical Management of Diabetic Neuropathy*
Edited by: A. Veves © Humana Press Inc., Totowa, NJ

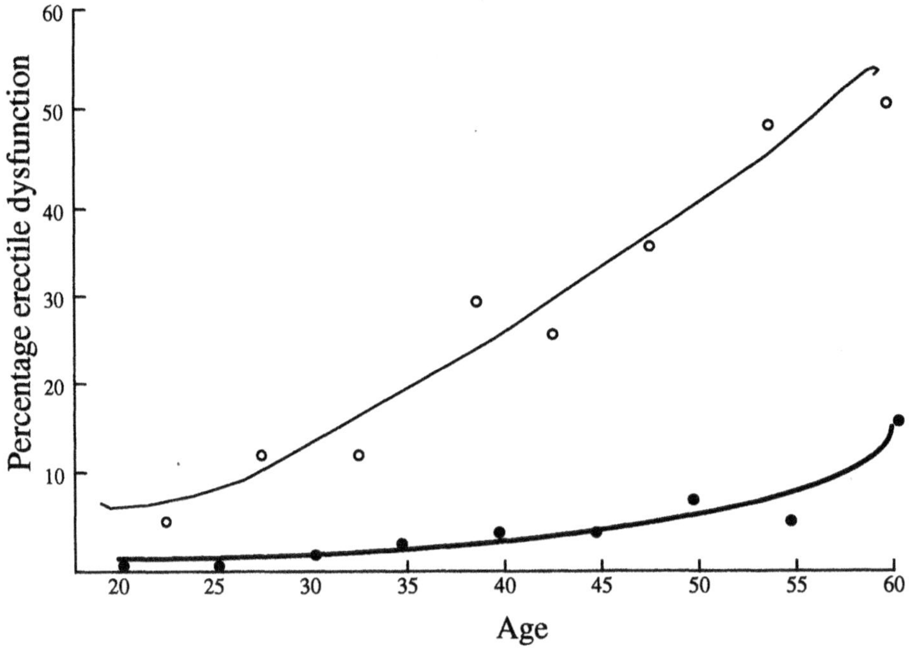


**Fig.1.** Comparing the data from Kinsey *(4)* and McCulloch *(3)*. The age incidence of erectile dysfunction in diabetic and non-diabetic men. (○), diabetic men; (●), non-diabetic men.

### *Neuropathy and Erectile Failure*

Erectile dysfunction in diabetes is a classical example of a multifactorial condition. The difficulty that a patient experiences in achieving and sustaining an erection may be caused by a combination of neuropathy, vascular disease, psychological and interpersonal factors, hormonal imbalance, renal failure, drug side effects, and local genital problems. It can present a considerable diagnostic challenge to unravel which factors are important in any particular case so that a rational treatment plan can be offered. Estimates have been made of the relative contribution of neuropathy to the overall picture of erectile failure in diabetes *(7)*, but the resulting figures vary widely depending on the populations studied and the sophistication of the methods used to detect and quantify neuropathy and vascular disease. Veves et al. *(8)* used clinical examination combined with quantitative sensory testing and electrophysiological measurement to produce a Neuropathy Disability Score in 110 diabetic men complaining of erectile failure. In this group, neuropathy was found to be the main or only cause of the erectile problems in 47% and a contributing factor in another 18%, though other factors were also important (*see* Table 1). Other studies that have used more sensitive tests of vascular function *(9)* have found significant vascular abnormalities in up to 68% of diabetic men with erectile failure. Despite these differences, it is clear that neuropathy is a major etiological factor in diabetic sexual dysfunction.

## PATHOPHYSIOLOGY

### *The Erectile Response*

The peripheral nerves supplying the penis include the pelvic nerves (mainly parasympathetic), the hypogastric nerves (mainly sympathetic), and the pudendal nerve (mainly somatic). The pelvic and hypogastric nerves combine to form the pelvic plexus,

Table 1
Etiopathegenic Factors of Erectile Dysfunction in Diabetic Men

| | *Only factor* | *Main factor* | *Contributing factor* |
|---|---|---|---|
| Neuropathy | 27 | 20 | 18 |
| Psychogenic factors | 11 | 24 | 17 |
| Marital disharmony | 1 | 4 | 17 |
| Medications | 2 | 4 | 19 |
| Peripheral vascular disease | 2 | 6 | 7 |
| Venous leakage | 2 | — | — |
| Endocrine disorders | 1 | — | — |

Results as % of 110 patients, Veves et al. *(8)*.

giving rise to the cavernous nerves that supply the erectile tissue. The pudendal nerve supplies the striated muscle that contributes to the rigidity of the erect penis. Parasympathetic activity increases blood flow through the penile corpora by dilatation of penile arteries and relaxation of trabecular smooth muscle. The peripheral neurotransmitter mechanisms controlling erection are still not fully known. It seems that transmission is mainly nonadrenergic and noncholinergic with vasoactive intestinal polypeptide (VIP) playing an important role. Other neuroeffector systems include the release of nitric oxide, a smooth muscle relaxant, from the vascular endothelium. The use of prostaglandin E1 in the treatment of erectile failure points to a role for vasodilatory prostacyclin in the physiology of erection.

Various studies have revealed the vulnerability of these pathways in diabetic neuropathy. Using animal models of diabetes, Italiano et al. *(10)* were able to demonstrate a significant decrease in myelinated fiber size in the cavernous and dorsal penile nerves, probably because of progressive axonal atrophy, suggesting that regionally specific structural changes occur in neuronal pathways serving erectile response. Saenz de Tejada et al. *(11)* studied cavernosal tissue from diabetic men and found a specific impairment of the endothelium-mediated release of nitrous oxide, implicating a failure of this mechanism in the high prevalence of erectile dysfunction in diabetes. Neurophysiological evaluations on human subjects *(7)* suggest that impaired urogenital sensation might also be significant.

### *Vascular Factors*

The production of a rigid erection depends on vascular changes that are under neural control. If the blood supply to the penis is compromised by generalized or microvascular disease, this will greatly compound the effect of any neuropathic changes. To maintain a full erection, it is also necessary to produce a compression of the penile venules, which decreases venous return. Occasionally a venous leakage is responsible for erectile problems and if this is suspected it must be investigated by cavernosography.

### *Drug Effects*

Many drugs are known to cause or exacerbate erectile failure, and some of these are quite commonly prescribed in the diabetic population, as summarized in Table 2. The most troublesome in clinical practice are the antihypertensives *(12)*.

Table 2
Drugs Associated with Erectile Dysfunction

| | |
|---|---|
| **Antihypertensives** | |
| | Thiazide diuretics |
| | Beta blockers (particularly propranolol) |
| | Methyldopa |
| | Spironolactone |
| | Reserpine and guanethidine |
| **Psychotropic drugs** | |
| | Phenothiazine antipsychotics (especially thioridazine) |
| | Haloperidol |
| | Tricyclic antidepressants |
| | Monoamine oxidase inhibitors |
| | Benzodiazepines |
| **Drugs with endocrine effects** | |
| | Antiepileptics |
| | Cimetidine |
| | Metoclopramide |
| | Clofibrate |
| **Other drugs or substances** | |
| | Alcohol, tobacco, heroin, methadone, amphetamine (at high doses) |

### *Psychological Effects*

Central neural mechanisms are also important in the erectile response, and psychogenic factors can be a powerful causal and complicating factor in sexual dysfunction. Sensory pathways from the genitalia provide feedback to cognitive centers in the cortex. This produces a response that can enhance or inhibit sexual arousal. Bancroft *(2)* has described this mechanism as the "psychosomatic circle of sex," a concept that explains the power of performance anxiety in sexual dysfunction. The man becomes aware that his erection is less firm than previously and he begins to worry about whether he will be able to sustain this for intercourse to take place. This anxiety produces an inhibitory response and the erection is lost. The anxiety increases with each failure, leading to complete inhibition of the erectile response in some cases or an understandable avoidance of sexual activity. The picture is further complicated by the effect that this can have on the sexual relationship *(13)*.

It can be seen from this that the distinction often drawn between "organic" and "psychogenic" impotence in diabetes is not very helpful in clinical practice, as many patients will have an inextricable combination of these factors. The effect of performance anxiety is very powerful in exacerbating and perpetuating erectile failure and can explain the cases in which profound sexual dysfunction is seen despite minimal evidence of neuropathy or vascular disease.

## ASSESSMENT

### *The History*

The presentation and progression of erectile problems in diabetes is very variable, as might be expected from the number of ways in which the diabetic process and psychological factors can affect sexual function. Fairburn *(14)* documented very detailed accounts from 27 men with diabetic erectile problems. Most of them first noticed a decline in the strength and duration of erections that was initially variable but became progressively more severe and consistent. Three of the group reported initial changes in ejaculation, including loss of ejaculatory control and of the pumping sensation usually associated with orgasm. Ejaculatory changes developed in half of the men, including orgasm without emission, though not all of these showed evidence of the retrograde ejaculation that can occur when innervation of the bladder neck is affected.

In most cases, any reported loss of libido can be understood as a response to the chronic erectile difficulties, but in men with significant renal impairment the uremia and other metabolic abnormalities are closely associated with impaired sexual interest *(15)*. In those men in whom psychological factors are important, there is often a clear history of anxiety and distress about the sexual dysfunction, reduced sexual interest, and sexual avoidance.

### *The Physical Examination*

Although the history may clearly suggest neuropathy or vascular disease, it is still important to exclude any conditions of the external genitalia that may contribute to erectile dysfunction. Painful phimosis (inability to retract the foreskin) may result from recurrent infections with *Candida albicans*. Peyronie's disease, in which bands of thickened tissue in the penile corpora lead to a bending of the erect penis, is also a fairly common finding, causing problems with penetration.

Basic examination of the cardiovascular system, including blood pressure, abdominal or femoral bruits, and absent peripheral pulses give a good indication of general vascular disease. The most helpful sign in the neurological examination is the loss of discrimination of temperature sensation in the feet *(16)*. Abnormal cardiovascular reflexes as an indicator of autonomic neuropathy are associated with aging and erectile dysfunction *(17)*.

### *Hormonal Investigations*

It is customary to screen serum testosterone in most cases, but a significantly low value is only found in 1% of patients without a clinical picture of hypogonadism *(18)*. Some endocrine abnormalities have been found in diabetes, including increased testosterone binding and abnormal response to stimulation with leuteinizing-hormone releasing hormone, but this is found in diabetic patients with or without sexual dysfunction. Although there is a such a small incidence of endocrine abnormality, the screening is probably worth undertaking for two reasons. Firstly, it avoids missing potentially serious and treatable endocrine conditions. Secondly, it helps the clinician to form a therapeutic alliance with the patient, who usually needs much reassurance that everything is being done to investigate his problem. It is sometimes possible to discuss psychological factors only if the man has been assured that his hormone levels are normal.

### *Specialist Investigations*

#### Intracavernous Injection

Intracavernous injecting into the corpus cavernosum can be used diagnostically as well as therapeutically *(19)*. A fully rigid erectile response to a standard dose excludes a significant vascular cause for the erectile failure. A partial response may be caused by vascular insufficiency or psychological inhibition *(20)*.

#### VASCULAR INVESTIGATIONS

The ratio of penile blood pressure to brachial blood pressure indicates vascular pathology, and can be measured with a penile cuff. However, Doppler ultrasound gives a much more accurate picture of the penile vasculature.

#### NOCTURNAL PENILE TUMESCENCE

Healthy young males usually have four episodes of nocturnal penile tumescence (NPT) each night, a pattern that diminishes with age. An intact cycle of nocturnal erections is usually interpreted as evidence a significant neurological or vascular problem is unlikely, and that psychological factors may be more important. However, recent studies *(21,22)* have indicated that even diabetic men with normal sexual function when awake often show abnormally reduced nocturnal penile tumescence, so this should not be taken as evidence of irreversible sexual dysfunction in the diabetic population.

#### AUTONOMIC NERVE TESTING

These investigations, reviewed by Pryor and Dickinson *(19)*, are more frequently used in research to elucidate the mechanisms of erectile failure than in a clinical setting, but they can provide the most direct evidence of neuropathic deficit.

**Bulbocavernosus Latency** This test is based on the bulbocavernosus latency reflex in which squeezing the glans penis causes a contraction of the anal sphincter. The latency time between electrical stimulation of the glans and detection of a response by an electromyographical needle placed in the bulbocavernosus muscle is a measure of the integrity of the sacral cord segment and its associated fibers.

**Sacral-Evoked Response** This test also demonstrates the integrity of the autonomic afferent fibers and depends on the urethro-anal reflex. Delayed latency times between stimulation of the posterior urethra and contraction of the anal sphincter have been found in men with impaired NPT.

**Pudendal Motor-Evoked Potential** This is a noninvasive test in which the brain is stimulated magnetically. The latency time to contraction of the anal sphincter is compared to that when the sacral root is stimulated.

**Single Potential Analysis of Cavernous Electrical Activity.** This is the most direct measurement of cavernous muscular activity, using needle electrodes.

### *Psychological Assessment*

#### AIMS

The clinical interview gives an opportunity to assess significant psychological factors. Firstly, any treatable psychiatric illnesses such as depression and anxiety states must be detected and managed appropriately. Next, the patient may give a history of increasing worry and despondency about his failing erections, indicating that performance anxiety may be a significant causal or complicating factor. The patient's attitudes about sexuality and masculinity affect the impact of erectile dysfunction on his self-esteem *(23)*. This can vary from emotional devastation to relief at being able to retire honorably from sexual activity. It is important to make an assessment of these issues as they will affect the man's expectations of and motivation for treatment.

If at all possible, it is invaluable to involve the man's sexual partner in this stage of the assessment. This allows the clinician to observe and inquire about interpersonal factors that may be of great importance in the etiology, maintenance, and future treatment of the problem *(13)*. It also provides another informant who may give additional information about life events and lifestyle that the patient may be reluctant or embarrassed to discuss (e.g., alcohol intake).

#### The Interview Setting

There are still major taboos and sensitivities surrounding the discussion of sexuality and especially sexual dysfunction. This needs to be appreciated by all personnel in the clinic including receptionists, so that it is not made obvious to all in the waiting area that the man is attending a consultation for a sexual problem. The interview room should afford privacy and be reasonably sound-proof. There must be facilities for uninterrupted and relatively unhurried discussion with individuals or couples. The clinicians involved in this stage of the assessment must be experienced, relaxed, and confident in speaking with patients about intimate sexual and relationship matters. There is nothing more inhibiting for the patient than the realization that the doctor he is speaking to is inwardly squirming with embarrassment. If necessary, extra training in the relevant interview skills should be sought for clinicians working in this field.

#### Rating Scales and Questionnaires

Standardized and validated instruments, reviewed by Gregoire *(24)*, are available for the assessment of both psychological and physical aspects of sexual dysfunction (*see* Table 3). These do not usually add much of practical value to the routine clinical assessment, but they are of great methodological importance in defining sample populations and measuring outcome in research.

## TREATMENT

With a good assessment of the relative contributions of neuropathy, vascular disease, psychological, and other factors, it should be possible to devise and recommend a rational treatment option for most patients with erectile dysfunction. However, this logical view does not take into account the vagaries of human nature. The prejudices and preferences of the man and his partner sometimes play a major role in treatment choice and the clinician must sometimes find a compromise between a management plan that is rational and one that is acceptable. Review of the currently available options shows why some patients may be reluctant to embark on possibly invasive procedures, none of which offer the cure that they are seeking.

### *Oral Medication*

It is frequently necessary to intervene to change a regular prescription of a drug that is adversely affecting sexual function (*see* Table 2). This should be done and the outcome assessed before trying any other measures. Sometimes sexual function returns to a satisfactory level, but problems can persist because of secondary psychological and relationship factors.

Many patients are understandably hoping for a tablet that they can take that will enhance their erections and restore their potency. Yohimbine hydrochloride has been used in the past *(25)* but has not gained acceptance due to its extensive side-effects. There have been encouraging reports from clinical trials (mainly on patients with no organic cause for their impotence) of s1ldenafil.

Sildenafil, a novel orally active phosphodiesterase inhibitor, has been shown to enhance the erectile response, including duration and rigidity of erection, in such

Table 3
Questionnaires and Rating Scales

| | |
|---|---|
| **For quantifying sexual dysfunctions** | |
| | Sexual Interaction Inventory (SII) |
| | Derogatis Sexual Functioning Inventory (DSFI) |
| | Golombok and Rust Inventory of Sexual Satisfaction (GRISS) |
| **To assess marital disharmony** | |
| | Locke-Wallis Marital Adjustment Test |
| | Golombok and Rust Inventory of Marital State (GRIMS) |

patients. The drug is well tolerated with mild and transient adverse events such as headache, dyspepsia, and pelvic musculoskeletal. Sildenafil is the first of this class of drugs to be approved by the FDA for use in the United States and may eventually be able to add an effective oral agent to our treatment options for diabetic patients. This would undoubtedly be popular with patients, as would further work on the possibility of topical preparations *(27)*.

### *Intracavernosal Injections*

The use of vasodilator intracavernosal injections of drugs directly into the corpus cavernosum, first described by Virag in 1982 *(28)*, has revolutionized the treatment of erectile problems. The initial work was done with the drugs papaverine and phentolamine, but the most commonly used preparation is now prostaglandin E1 (PGE1), as the incidence of potentially serious side effects is significantly less with this drug *(29)*.

#### The Procedure

A test dose is usually given in a clinic setting, using a 15-mm needle to inject into one of the corpora towards the base of the penis, using a lateral site that avoids major blood vessels and the urethra. The full effect may take up to 15 min to develop, and if the resulting erection is still not firm enough for intercourse, the dose of drug can be adjusted appropriately. The patient must be instructed in the technique of self-injection, so that the treatment can be used at home. This has recently been simplified by the development of single-dose injector pens that may be useful for patients with poor sight or limited manual dexterity.

#### Complications

**Prolonged Erections** The erection produced by the injection is generally defined as prolonged if there is no detumescence after 4 h or longer. As the erection is hemostatic, anoxic tissue damage *(30)* leading to necrosis may ensue. This potentially disastrous complication is less likely using PGE1 than papaverine *(29)*. If it does occur, patients must be warned to seek rapid treatment. This might mean aspiration of blood from the corpora, careful use of a vasoconstrictor drug, or even construction of a surgical shunt in the few cases that do not respond. Most clinics that offer intracavernosal injections issue written instructions that clearly inform patients how, where, and when to seek help in the event of a prolonged erection *(31)*, as the potential damage in the worst cases is severe and permanent.

**Pain** This occurs on insertion of the needle and from the effect of the drug in the tissues. This can lead to discontinuation of the treatment method in approx 10% of those who try it *(32)*.

**Local Complications** Infection at the injection site is a possible problem, but with adequate sterile technique it is rare in practice. Bruising can occur in up to 47% of patients *(33)*, but this can be minimized using good injection technique and is as little as 3% in other studies *(34)*. The formation of fibrotic plaques or nodules is a more serious complication that occurs in approx 6% of patients *(35)* and is one reason to discontinue the treatment. This is thought to be associated with long-term use, but there are case reports of scarring resulting from a single dose *(36)*. This implies that patients should be warned of this possibility before consenting to undergo a test dose. The manufacturers generally recommend that the injections should not be used more often than three times a week in the case of PGE1.

#### Outcome

There is no doubt that in suitable patients this method is highly effective in producing an adequate erection, with over 80% of men responding well *(37)*. However, there are some groups in which the technique is less useful. Patients with moderately severe vascular disease may show a partial or absent response, as the blood supply to the genital region is insufficient for local dilatation of vessels to be effective. There is also a subgroup of patients who do not respond because of psychological inhibition *(20)*. It has been assumed that the mechanism for this involves the anxiety and embarrassment associated with the procedure, especially in a clinic setting, but researchers have found that men who use the psychological defense mechanisms of dissociation and denial experience this inhibitory effect *(38)*.

#### Acceptability and Long-Term Use

Some patients and their partners will choose not to try this method, as they feel it is too clinical and will interfere with the spontaneity of lovemaking. Men who are nervous or even phobic of needles will have great difficulty initiating this technique, and it is possible that those who already have experience of self-injection with insulin take to it more easily *(39)*.

There is now a body of evidence emerging that a significant number of men choose not to use intracavernosal injections on a long-term basis, despite getting an adequate erectile response. The reasons for this are not simple, as Weiss et al. *(32)* found in their investigation of 140 patients beginning injection therapy. At the end of 6 mo, 80% had discontinued the treatment, though only 10% of these dropped out because of side-effects. Over 70% had lost interest in the method or changed to another form of treatment. Factors involving the sexual partner were cited by a further 10% of men. An improvement in the natural erectile response was the reason in 8% of the group. The large discontinuation rate therefore may reflect the realization that although this method is effective in achieving erections, it does not restore the natural and spontaneous sexual function that many men are seeking. Those men who experience a return of potency are likely to have overcome performance anxiety using the injections, which are then no longer needed.

### *Vacuum-Assisted Erection Devices*

These devices *(40)* can be effective even in patients who do not respond well to intracavernosal injections because of severe vascular problems.

#### Mechanism of Action

The vacuum-assisted erection device is supplied as a kit including a clear plastic cylinder, a pump attachment that can be hand or battery operated, and constriction rings.

Most manufacturers also supply an instruction video demonstrating the correct use of the device. The cylinder is placed over the penis, which should be well lubricated. When the pump unit is attached and activated, negative pressure is produced within the cylinder. This causes blood to be drawn into the corpora cavernosa and, after a few minutes, the penis becomes rigid. Tumescence is maintained by a constriction band that is slipped off the cylinder to grip the base of the penis. The pump and cylinder can then be removed, and intercourse can take place with the constriction ring *in situ*. This method produces a satisfactory quality of erection in over 70% *(41)* of diabetic men who try the pump, though there are some differences from the physiological erection that patients may notice. The erect penis produced by the pump method feels cool to the touch, as the blood within is relatively static. Also, the erectile tissue proximal to the ring is unaffected and still flaccid, so the angle of the erect penis is less upright and it is more difficult to direct accurately for penetration. However, most patients are able to adjust to these changes, and high levels of satisfaction with the method have been reported *(42)*. Men who can achieve a satisfactory erection but cannot sustain it can often successfully use the constriction ring without needing the vacuum pump, an option that is cheaper and less intrusive.

#### Contraindications

The constriction ring must be removed after 30 min to allow the penile circulation of blood to return to normal. It is therefore recommended that patients should not use the device after drinking alcohol because of the risk of falling asleep and forgetting to remove the ring, as anoxic tissue damage could occur. The operation of the device requires some manual dexterity and may prove difficult if the patient is vision-impaired or has poor manual coordination. Patients on anticoagulant medication should probably be advised against this method as the negative pressure required to produce the erection is likely to cause hemorrhage from small vessels in the penis. Care should also be taken if the patient has a phimosis or scarring leading to a tight or fragile foreskin, as this could split as the device is being operated. Ejaculation usually occurs normally, but if the constriction ring is too tight, it may be impeded. The patient should use the largest size ring that maintains tumescence, and some patients become adept at loosening the ring manually just before ejaculation.

#### Acceptability

There are a number of different devices available that work on the vacuum principle, and from patient surveys *(43)* it seems that the type of system described above is generally preferred to the alternative, in the form of a rigid synthetic condom that remains in place during intercourse. The most common complaints from patients and their partners about the use of vacuum devices are that they are cumbersome and intrusive. They can also be quite expensive for the patient, especially when they are not available on prescription or through insurance schemes. This does not make sense in health economic terms, as the cheapest vacuum device is equivalent in cost to only 12 injections of PGE1.

## *Surgical Approaches*

#### Revascularization Techniques

Various procedures have been used to increase the blood supply to the penis, with very variable degrees of success *(44)*. The absence of diabetes is often quoted as one of the criteria of suitability for such vascular reconstructive surgery.

### Penile Prostheses

Surgical approaches can restore potency effectively in some patients, but with this method a successful outcome depends even more on careful selection of patients who do not have unrealistic expectations.

**Indications** As most men with neuropathic erectile dysfunction respond well to intracavernosal injections and as those whose problems are complicated by vascular disease can successfully use a vacuum device, it should only be a minority of patients who need to consider surgery. The implantation of the prosthesis destroys the corpus cavernosum, so return to physiological erectile function is impossible thereafter. This must be explained clearly to patients, especially those with a large psychogenic component that makes their dysfunction potentially reversible. Men with irreversible organic erectile dysfunction who have found less invasive methods unsuitable and those with long-standing psychological causes that have not responded to appropriate treatment might benefit from a prosthesis. In a large series of 3884 men who have undergone this operation *(45)*, diabetes was the most common etiological factor, accounting for over 25% of the total.

**Acceptability** The simplest type of prostheses commonly offered to patients consists of malleable or mechanically hinged pairs of rods. These provide sufficient rigidity for penetration, but no increase in penile girth and the penis can not return to a flaccid state. The inflatable prosthesis, consisting of a pair of cylinders with a pump and reservoir that are sited within the scrotum, provides an erection that better approximates normal. This is generally preferred by patients *(46)*, but the simpler devices have the advantage of being cheaper and more reliable. It is vitally important that patients are clearly informed about what they can realistically expect a prosthesis to achieve for them, as they may have been given an over-optimistic view by media reports that surgery will restore normal potency. After careful assessment and explanation, Cumming and Pryor *(47)* found that only 16% of patients enquiring about the possibility of a prosthesis decided to proceed with implantation.

**Outcome** Successful outcome is marred by a complication rate as high as 36% in some series *(48)*. Complications include penile necrosis *(49)* perforation of the tunica albuginea or urethra, protrusion of the prosthesis through the glans, and urinary retention. However, the major complication leading to failure of the prosthesis and subsequent removal is infection. There is some evidence that this is more likely in diabetic patients *(47)*. In a study of 130 implants, the prosthesis needed to be removed for infection or was extruded in 30% of the diabetic patients, compared with 17% of the patients with nondiabetic vascular disease and 7% with nondiabetic neurogenic causes. Despite this, most men who undergo the procedure are satisfied with the outcome. Steege *(50)* found that 90% of patients did not regret the operation, despite recognizing that it did not fully restore sexual function or satisfaction. It is also important to take the partner's feelings into account when considering a prosthesis. One of the few studies to look at partner satisfaction *(51)* found that 42% were totally satisfied with the implant. Those who had not been involved in the decision were more likely to be dissatisfied, and only 20% of partners had been interviewed preoperatively.

## *Psychological Treatments*

Despite the proven efficacy of the pharmacological, mechanical, and surgical approaches, there is still a useful place for psychological therapies. In cases where psychogenic factors are the main cause of the dysfunction, where they are affecting the success of physical treatments, or where relationship issues are important, it is essential to be able to offer a range of appropriate psychological interventions as part of the treatment plan.

### Performance Anxiety

This is most effectively treated using modifications of the Masters and Johnson sensate focus therapy *(52)* as summarized by Bancroft *(2)*. This is a cognitive-behavioral treatment program in which couples are given "homework" assignments designed to overcome performance anxiety. The first stage entails nongenital touching, caressing, massage, and communication. This progresses to a stage including genital stimulation, still without any attempt or pressure to achieve intercourse. In this way, confidence is built up until the stage in which vaginal containment of the penis without movement is possible. If this is successful, intercourse can be re-established. This program can be highly effective *(53)* in patients in whom the organic component of the dysfunction is mild, but its success is much more limited in those with moderate or severe neuropathy or vascular disease.

### Cognitive Factors

The success of both physical and psychological treatments can be affected by the patient's thoughts, attitudes, and beliefs about their sexual function. Techniques of cognitive therapy *(54)* can be used to help the patient identify, challenge, and change the negative cognitions that undermine his attempts to tackle the situation. Sometimes the psychological stressors involved in chronic illness need to be addressed. Bullard *(55)* identified altered body image, adopting the "patient" role, fears of rejection by a partner, guilt, anxiety, depression, and anger as some of the common issues that patients face in adapting to their illness. All of these can be significant in the causation and perpetuation of sexual dysfunction, and need to be dealt with in the process of counselling the patient and his partner.

### Couple Therapies

Where there is significant conflict and hostility in the relationship it is unlikely that either physical or simple psychological treatments will restore harmonious sexual function to the couple without some attention to the underlying interpersonal difficulties. Couples may need a form of therapy that takes into account the altered balance in a relationship between the sick and the healthy partner, with all the fears and resentments that may arise in dealing with chronic illness.

## SEXUAL PROBLEMS IN WOMEN WITH DIABETES

The sexual problems of women with diabetes have attracted much less attention than those of men *(56)*, possibly because impaired arousal in women does not preclude intercourse as definitely as erectile failure does in men. The female equivalent of neuropathic erectile dysfunction would be impaired arousal, with reduction in vaginal lubrication and vulval tumescence. Many women who suffer from mild degrees of these symptoms do not consult their doctors, but use self-administered treatment with vaginal lubricants.

Some controlled studies have found evidence of impaired arousal in diabetic women *(57,58)*, but not to such a degree that caused problems. There is also some evidence that

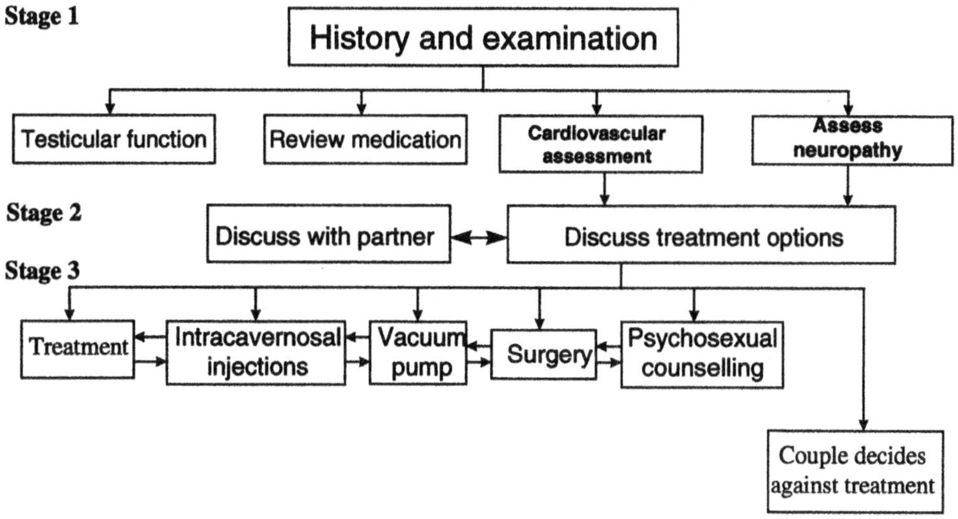


**Fig. 2.** Investigation and treatment of sexual problems in diabetic patients.

women with autonomic neuropathy are more likely to suffer from vaginal dryness *(58)*, but other studies have not found this *(57)*.

More global and nonspecific sexual dysfunctions in diabetic women, including low libido and dissatisfaction with the sexual relationship were reported by Schreiner-Engel *(59)*. These were more commonly seen in type II, non-insulin dependent patients and were related to factors such as menopausal status and relationship quality rather than to complications of the diabetes. Leedom et al. *(60)* also found that sexual dysfunction in women with diabetes was more closely linked to depression than to factors directly attributable to the disease processes of diabetes.

In the assessment of sexual dysfunction in women with diabetes, it is therefore important to take a wide view of the many factors that may be involved, not forgetting a review of the drug history, as women may also be subject to side effects including impairment of arousal caused by commonly used drugs such as beta blockers.

## SUMMARY AND CONCLUSIONS

The assessment and treatment process can be summarized in Fig. 2 *(61)*. It is clearly important to integrate medical, psychological, and surgical expertise to give diabetic men with erectile dysfunction the best possible service. How this can be achieved in a busy diabetes clinic has been addressed by Alexander *(62)*, but there is still reluctance in some services to even include an enquiry about sexual function in the routine review of possible diabetic complications *(63)*. Diabetes physicians and specialist nurses may still feel that such inquiries are intrusive and embarrassing, or may not be aware of the rapidly growing range of treatment options. In services that need to be ever more aware of the costs of treatment, there may be some reluctance to uncover symptoms of sexual dysfunction that patients might not mention spontaneously. This is unfortunate, because most patients benefit from at least discussing the options for treatment, even if they decide not to proceed. Some couples find that they can evolve an enjoyable range of nonpenetrative sexual activities, where mutual orgasm is possible despite the absence of erections. The skill involved in the management of sexual dysfunction in diabetes lies in helping the patient and his partner to choose a treatment option that they find acceptable for their circumstances and that takes into account the underlying pathology.

## REFERENCES


1. Fairburn CG, McCulloch DK, Wu FC. The effects of diabetes on male sexual function. Clin Endocrinol Metab 1982;11:749–768.
2. Bancroft J. Human Sexuality and its Problems, 2nd ed. Churchill Livingstone, London, 1989.
3. McCulloch DK, Campbell IW, Wu FC, Prescott RJ, Clarke BF. The prevalence of diabetic impotence. Diabetologia 1980;18:279–283.
4. Kinsey AC, Pomeroy WB, Martin, CF. Sexual Behaviour in the Human Male. Saunders, Philadelphia, 1948.
5. Feldman HA, Goldstein I, Hatzichristou DG, Krane RJ, McKinley JB. Impotence and its medical and psychosocial correlates: results of the Massachusetts Male Aging Study. J Urol 1994;151:54–61.
6. McCulloch DK, Young RJ, Prescott RJ, Campbell IW, Clarke BF. The natural history of impotence in diabetic men. Diabetologia 1984;26:437–440.
7. Bemelmans BL, Meuleman EJ, Doesburg WH, Notermans SL, Debruyne FM. Erectile dysfunction in diabetic men: the neurological factor revisited. J Urol 1994;151:884–889.
8. Veves A, Webster L, Chen TF, Payne S, Boulton AJM. Aetiopathogenesis and management of impotence in diabetic males: four years experience in a combined clinic. Diabetic Med 1995;12:77–82.
9. Lehman TP, Jacobs JA. Etiology of diabetic impotence. J Urol 1983;129:291–294.
10. Italiano G, Marin A, Pescatori ES, Calabro A, Artibani W, Pagano F, Triban C. Effect of streptozotocin-induced diabetes on electrically evoked erection in the rat. Int J Impotence Res 1993;5:27–35.
11. Saenz de Tejada I, Goldstein I, Azadzoi K, Krane RJ, Cohen RA. Impaired neurogenic and endothelium-mediated relaxation of penile smooth muscle from diabetic men with impotence. N Engl J Med 1989;320:1025–1030.
12. Huws R. Antihypertensive medication and sexual problems. In: Riley AJ, Peet M, Wilson C, eds. Sexual Pharmacology. Oxford University Press, Oxford, UK, 1993, pp. 146–158.
13. Webster L. Working with couples in a diabetes clinic: the role of the therapist in a medical setting. Sexual Marital Ther 1992;7:191–198.
14. Fairburn, CG, Wu, FCW, McCulloch, DK. The clinical features of diabetic impotence: a preliminary study. Br J Psychiatr 1982;140:447–452.
15. Kolodny RC, Masters WH, Johnson VE. Textbook of Sexual Medicine. Little, Brown, Boston, 1979.
16. Fowler CJ, Ali Z, Kirby RS, Pryor JP. The value of testing for unmyelinated fibre sensory neuropathy in diabetic impotence. Br J Urol 1988;61:63–67.
17. Nisen HO, Larsen A, Lindstrom BL, Ruutu ML, Virtanen, JM, Alfthan OS. Cardiovascular reflexes in the neurological evaluation of impotence. Br J Urol 1993;71:199–203.
18. Freidman DE, Clare AW, Rees LH, Grossman A. Should impotent males who have no clinical evidence of hypogonadism have routine endocrine screening? Lancet 1986;i:1041.
19. Pryor JP, Dickinson IK. Special investigations. In: Gregoire A, Pryor JP, eds. Impotence. An Integrated Approach to Clinical Practice. Churchill Livingstone, Edinburgh, 1993, pp. 115–126.
20. Buvat J, Lemaire A, Marcolin G, Dehaene JL, Buvat- Herbaut M. Intracavernous injection of papaverine (ICIP): assessment of its diagnostic and therapeutic value in 100 impotent patients. World J Urol 1987;5:150–155.
21. Nofzinger EA, Reynolds CF. 3d, Jennings JR, Thase ME, Frank E, Yeager A, Kupfer DJ. Results of nocturnal penile tumescence studies are abnormal in sexually functional diabetic men. Arch Int Med 1992;152:114–118.
22. Schiavi RC, Stimmel BB, Mandeli J, Rayfield EJ. Diabetes, sleep disorders and male sexual function. Biol Psychiatry 1993;34:171–177.
23. Schiavi RC, Stimmel BB, Mandeli J, Schreiner-Engel P, Ghizzani A. Diabetes, psychological function and male sexuality. J Psychosom Res 1995;39:305–314.
24. Gregoire A. Questionnaires and rating scales. In: Gregoire A, Pryor JP, eds. Impotence. An Integrated Approach to Clinical Practice. Churchill Livingstone, Edinburgh, 1993, pp. 97–104.
25. Riley AJ, Goodman RE, Kellett JM, Orr R. Double blind trial of yohimbine hydrochloride in the treatment of erection inadequacy. Sexual Marital Ther 1989;4:17–26.

26. Boolell M, Gepi-Attee S, Gingell JC, Allen MJ. Sildenafil, a novel oral therapy for male erectile dysfunction. Br J Urol 1996;78:257–261.
27. Gomaa A, Shalby M, Osman M, Eissa M, Eizat A, Mahmoud M, Mikhail N. Topical treatment of erectile dysfunction: randomised double blind placebo controlled trial of cream containing aminophylline, isosorbide dinitrate and codergocine mesylate. Br Med J 1996;312:1512–1515.
28. Virag R. Intracavernous injection of papaverine for erectile failure. Lancet 1982;ii:938.
29. Stackl W, Hasun R, Marberger M. Intracavernous injection of prostaglandin E1 in impotent men. J Urol 1988;140:66–68.
30. Virag R. About pharmacologically induced prolonged erection. Lancet 1985;1:519.
31. Crowe MJ, Qureshi MJH. Pharmacologically induced penile erection (PIPE) as a maintenance treatment for erectile impotence: a report of 41 cases. Sexual Marital Ther 1991;6:273–285.
32. Wiess JN, Badlani GH, Ravalli R, Brettschneider N. Reasons for high drop-out rate with self-injection therapy for impotence. Int J Impotence Res 1994;6:171–174.
33. Girdley FM, Bruskewitz RC, Feyzi J, Graversen PH, Gasser TC. Intracavernous self-injection for impotence; a long-term therapeutic option? Experience in 78 patients. J Urol 1988;140:972–974.
34. Sidi AA, Cameron JS, Duffy LM, Lange PH. Intracavernous drug-induced erections in the management of male erectile dysfunction: experience with 100 patients. J Urol 1986;135:704–706.
35. Valdevenito R, Melman A. Intracavernous self-injection pharmacotherapy program: analysis of results and complications. Int J Impotence Res 1994;6:81–91.
36. Brough R, Betts C, Payne S. Curvature of the penis following an injection of papaverine. Br J Sexual Med 1995;22:26–27.
37. Brindley GS. Maintenance treatment of erectile impotence by cavernosal unstriated muscle relaxant injection. Br J Psychiatr 1986;149:210–215.
38. Van der Borght W, Vanderschueren D, Demyttenaere K. The effects of stress and coping upon the diagnostic intracavernous injection in men with erectile dysfunction. J Psychosom Res 1995;39:865–873.
39. Bancroft J, Gutierrez P. Erectile dysfunction in men with and without diabetes mellitus: a comparative study. Diabetic Med 1996;13:84–89.
40. Webster L. Vacuum devices for erectile problems. Br J Sexual Med 1994;21:6–7.
41. Famuyiwa OO, Al-Jasser, SJ, Ahmad AS, Al-Nuaim AA, Yaqub B, Sulimani RA. Experience with the vacuum-enhanced tumescence ErecAid system in the treatment of erectile impotence among diabetic patients in Saudi Arabia. Pract Diabetes 1992;9:141–144.
42. Bodansky HJ. Treatment of male erectile dysfunction using the active vacuum assist device. Diabetic Med 1994;11:410–412.
43. Ryder REJ, Close CF, Moriarty KT, Moore KTH, Hardisty CA. Impotence in diabetes: aetiology, implications for treatment and preferred vacuum device. Diabetic Med 1992;9:893–898.
44. Pryor JP. Surgical procedures to correct erectile dysfunction. In: Gregoire A, Pryor JP, eds. Impotence. An Integrated Approach to Clinical Practice Churchill Livingstone, Edinburgh, 1993, pp. 191–200.
45. Pryor JP. Penile prostheses. In: Gregoire A, Pryor JP, eds. Impotence. An Integrated Approach to Clinical Practice Churchill Livingstone, Edinburgh, 1993, pp. 201–214.
46. Beutler LE, Scott FB, Rogers RR, Karacan I, Baer PE, Gaines JA. Inflatable and non inflatable penile prostheses: comparative follow-up evaluation. Urology 1986;27:136–143.
47. Cumming J, Pryor JP. Treatment of organic impotence. Br J Urol 1991;67:640–643.
48. Kabalin JN, Kessler R. Penile prosthesis surgery: review of 10 years experience and examination of reoperations. Urology 1989;23:17–19.
49. Bour J, Steinhardt G. Penile necrosis in patients with diabetes mellitus and end stage renal disease. J Urol 1984;132:560–561.
50. Steege JF, Stout AL, Carsen CC. Patient satisfaction in Scot and Small-Carrion penile implant recipients: a study of 52 patients. Arch Sexual Behav 1986;15:393–399.
51. Kramarsky-Binkhorst S. Female partner perception of Small-Carrion implant. Urology 1978;12:545.
52. Masters WH, Johnson VE. Human Sexual Inadequacy. Churchill, London, 1970.
53. Hawton K. Treatment of sexual dysfunctions by sex therapy and other approaches. Br J Psychiatr 1995;167:307–314.
54. Hawton K. Sexual dysfunction. In: Hawton K, Salkovskis PM, Kirk J, Clark D, eds. Cognitive Behaviour Therapy for Psychiatric Problems. Oxford University Press, Oxford, 1993, pp. 370–405.
55. Bullard DG. The treatment of desire disorders in the medically ill and physically disabled. In: Leiblum SR, Rosen R, eds. Sexual Desire Disorders. Guilford Press, New York, 1988, pp. 348–384.
56. Kolodny RC. Sexual dysfunction in diabetic females. Diabetes 1971;20:557–559.

57. Tyrer G, Steel JM, Ewing DJ, Bancroft J, Clark BF. Sexual responsiveness in diabetic women. Diabetologia 1983;24:166–171.
58. Schreiner-Engel P, Schiavi RC, Vietorisz D, Eichel J deS., Smith H. Diabetes and female sexuality: a comparative study of women in relationships. J Sexual Marital Ther 1985;11:165–175.
59. Schreiner-Engel P, Schiavi RC, Vietorisz D, Smith H. The differential impact of diabetes type on female sexuality. J Psychosom Res 1986;31:23–33.
60. Leedom L, Meehan WP, Procci W, Zeidler A. Symptoms of depression in patients with type II diabetes mellitus. Psychosomatics 1991;32:26–28.
61. Webster L. Management of sexual problems in diabetic patients. Br J Hosp Med 1994;51:465–468.
62. Alexander WD. The diabetes physician and an assessment and treatment programme for male erectile impotence. Diabetic Med 1990;9:540–543.
63. Price DE, O'Malley BP, James MA, Roshan M, Hearnshaw JR. Why are impotent diabetic men not being treated? Pract Diabetes 1991;8:10–11.

# 15 Gastrointestinal Disorders

*Juan-R. Malagelada,* MD

***Contents***



## INTRODUCTION

Gastrointestinal symptoms are common among diabetic patients *(1)*, although this is also true for the general population. In fact, it is not established by appropriate population studies whether the prevalence of gastrointestinal symptoms in diabetic patients is actually increased. What is clear is that a segment of the diabetic population presents gastrointestinal symptoms that can be related to specific physiologic gut dysfunctions. Interestingly, some diabetic patients without gastrointestinal symptoms may sometimes evidence physiological abnormalities (such as gastric stasis or anorectal dysfunction) at the subclinical level *(2)*. One reason why it is so difficult to ascertain whether diabetic patients have more symptoms referable to the digestive tract than the general population is because the nature of the symptomatology, which coincides with that of individuals with common functional-type abdominal disorders. Only when gastrointestinal symptoms in a diabetic can be attached to a specific physiological abnormality caused by neuromuscular dysfunction is the clinician reasonably certain that he or she is dealing with a gut diabetic syndrome. Unfortunately this is not usually the case for most diabetic patients complaining about gastrointestinal symptoms in whom the relation between the diabetes and their digestive ailment remains presumptive at best, since physiological studies are only undertaken in patients with severe and disabling symptoms. Clinicians should, therefore, refrain from ascribing digestive symptoms to diabetes without further evidence than simple association.

For the purpose of the present analysis, I will separately review symptoms that appear to arise from specific segments of the gastrointestinal tract. However, it should be clear that abnormalities and symptoms in diabetic patients are often diffuse or multifocal. Thus, although in a given patient an esophageal syndrome, for example, may be the most apparent manifestation, a detailed history may elicit other evidence of gas-

From: *Contemporary Endocrinology: Clinical Management of Diabetic Neuropathy*
Edited by: A. Veves © Humana Press Inc., Totowa, NJ

Table 1
Diabetic Gut Motility Disturbances

| *Region* | *Motor Disorder* | *Typical Clinical Manifestation* |
|---|---|---|
| Esophagus | Weak peristaltic waves<br>Uncoordinated contractions<br>Reduced clearance | Dysphagia<br>Reflux-like symptoms |
| Stomach | Postprandial antral hypomobility<br>Gastro-pyloro-duodenal incoordination | Nausea/vomiting<br>Gastric stasis |
| Small bowel | Neurogenic-type dysmobility | Abdominal pain and distention<br>Diarrhea |
| Colon/anorectum | Incoordination | Constipation or diarrhea<br>Incontinence<br>"Low volume" diarrhea |

trointestinal dysfunction elsewhere such as incontinence, or alterations in bowel habit, and so on (Table 1).

The nature of gastrointestinal symptoms in diabetic patients is also likely to evolve over time. It is not unusual for a given patient to focus the complaints on a certain region of the gut and replace it sometime later by symptoms that appear to arise from another part of the gastrointestinal tract. The reason for this "moving pattern" of symptoms is unknown, but it may well be because of the evolving nature of the neuromuscular abnormalities secondary to the diabetes. Thus, as visceral neuropathy and associated abnormalities progress, different regions of the gut become affected and also, as different neural fibers are damaged, the type of dysfunction in one given region also changes over time.

The mechanism of gut disturbances in diabetic patients has been the subject of extensive investigation for the last several decades but remains largely unelucidated. Visceral neuropathy was recognized very early as a key factor, and it continues to be considered (largely based on its analogy to peripheral neuropathy) the main pathogenic disturbance. It is probably responsible for alterations in gut motility, absorptive function, and visceral sensation *(3,4)*. Experimental models of diabetes in rats also show neuropathic changes *(5)*. However, other factors may also be involved. In recent years, metabolic and hormonal disturbances, chiefly hyperglycemia, and variations in insulin and glucagon release have been shown to be important. In addition, there may be secondary metabolic changes, such as dehydration, hypokalemia, long-term vascular changes of the gut itself (microangiopathy), whereas secondary disturbances to physiological derangement, such as small-bowel bacterial overgrowth, may develop.

One aspect still uncertain is the participation of smooth-muscle abnormalities. Electrophysiological studies of smooth-muscle tissue obtained from diabetic patients with gut dysmotility have shown normal morphology and function. These findings would suggest that muscle dysfunction is caused by abnormalities in control mechanisms rather than to muscle-cell dystrophy. Moreover, these patients are likely to respond to prokinetic drugs (at least acutely), which would seem to further corroborate the integrity of the smooth-muscle tissue. However, other investigators have described damage to smooth-muscle cells or replacement by connective tissue, perhaps as a result of long-term ischemic changes.

## ESOPHAGEAL SYMPTOMS

Severe esophageal symptoms are relatively uncommon among diabetic patients and yet, esophageal motor dysfunction is demonstrable in a substantial number of diabetic patients. Esophageal symptoms may be grouped around two key complaints: heartburn and dysphagia. Heartburn is considered to be a fairly specific symptom for gastroesophageal reflux, although sometimes it may be produced by motor disturbances in the body of the esophagus rather than by acid. Dysfunction of the lower esophageal sphincter (LES), either reduced basal pressure or increased transient esophageal relaxations, or both, has not been documented as a complication of diabetes. Therefore, there is no specific mechanism for increased reflux except in patients with concomitant gastroparesis. The latter would result in gastric stasis, and indirectly favor esophageal reflux. Given the high prevalence of symptomatic esophageal reflux in the general population, the symptom of heartburn in most diabetic patients may just be coincidental. In certain patients it may caused by medications such as anticolinergics or calcium-channel blockers used for other medical problems.

Dysphagia in the absence of mechanical impediment is usually caused by a motor dysfunction in the esophagus. However, as indicated earlier, most manometric abnormalities found in diabetic patients are, in fact, asymptomatic. The esophageal dysmotility observed at manometry usually consists of multiple wave complexes associated with sporadic tertiary contractions, absence of primary peristaltic waves, and delayed esophageal clearance *(6,7)*. These abnormalities should be regarded mostly as nonspecific and it has been even suggested that they may have psychosomatic origin *(8)*. In general, the lack of specificity and the poor correlation with symptomatic expression, casts doubt over their actual significance.

It should be apparent from the above discussion that in-depth investigation of esophageal function should be reserved either for patients with protracted reflux-type symptoms or clear-cut dysphagia (Fig. 1). In such patients, particularly if there is associated peripheral neuropathy or other signs of visceral neuropathy *(9)*, it may be appropriate to conduct an evaluation to establish whether symptoms and disturbances are interrelated. For this purpose, a radiographic study with barium may be too insensitive and therefore not particularly helpful. It may be more appropriate to perform, first, an endoscopic examination to exclude the presence of a structural lesion or mucosal disease. In patients with predominant symptom dysphagia, if endoscopy is negative or only minimal changes are observed, it would be pertinent to perform an esophageal manometry, to assess motor activity of the esophagus, and perhaps also a scintigraphic study to measure esophageal transit and residual clearance. Patients with the primary symptom heartburn would require first, an endoscopic examination and then, either a trial with a potent antisecretor (a proton-pump inhibitor or high-dose $H_2$ blocker) or, in more complex clinical situations, a 24-hr pHmetry to establish the presence of excessive gastroesophageal reflux.

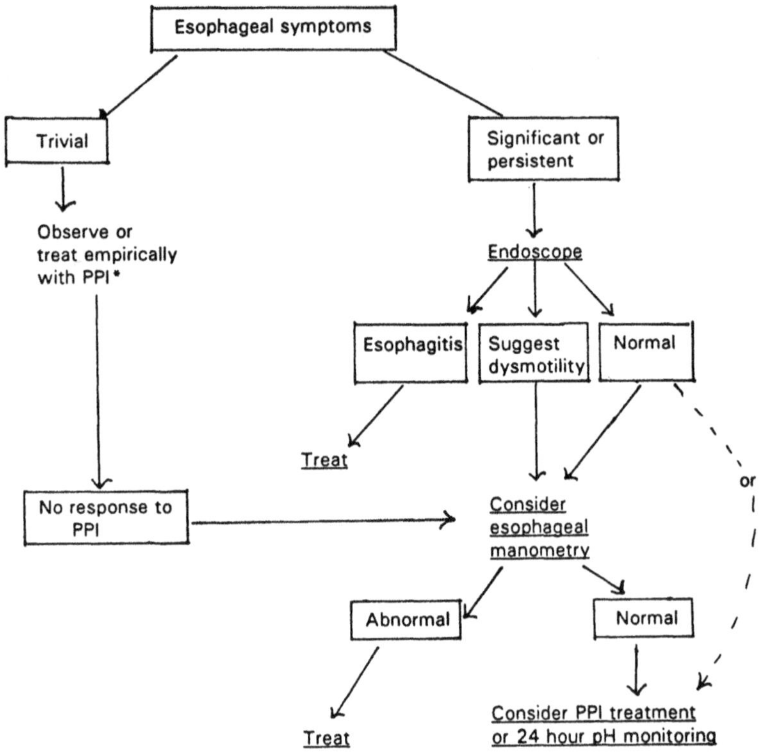


**Fig. 1.** Proton pump inhibitor.

## DIABETIC GASTROPARESIS

Diabetic gastroparesis was recognized very early as a prevalent disorder among diabetic patients, even asymptomatic *(2,10)*. Later studies indicate that up to one fifth of the symptomatic diabetic patients have radiological evidence of stasis *(1)*. On the other hand, others have not been able to confirm this high prevalence and, on the contrary, claim that the overall incidence of clinically significant gastroparesis among unselected diabetic patients is less than 1% *(11)*. Therefore, it is apparent that the correlation between physiologic abnormalities and symptoms is quite variable.

Diabetic gastroparesis must be regarded not only as a disorder of gastric motility but also of small-bowel motility *(12)*. Indeed, physiological studies show that the duodenum and the proximal small bowel play an important function in the regulation of gastric emptying. From this perspective, diabetic gastroparesis would represent a multifocal gut motility disorder involving decreased gastric tone, decreased antral propulsive activity, pyloric-gate dysfunction and disorganized motor activity in the proximal duodenum and small bowel *(10,13,14)*. In brief, it represents a combination of decreased pump activity and increased outlet resistance. The motility abnormalities may be evident both during fasting and postprandially. Gastric activity is normally associated with the interdigestive migrating motor complex and its absence may be responsible for accumulation of undigestible debris in the stomach and formation of bezoars, which is not uncommon in diabetic gastroparesis. Impaired or uncoordinated postprandial motility may be responsible for the typical delay in gastric evacuation of a meal and gastric stasis. Manometrically, the most common abnormalities encountered are antral hypomotility and a disorganized fed pattern in the small bowel. Phasic and tonic motor abnormalities may be responsible for the wider antrum observed ultrasonographically after ingestion of a meal *(15)*.

The pathogenesis of the above abnormalities in the diabetic gut are still unclear, but autonomic neuropathy definitely plays a major role *(16)*. Vagal dysfunction, both afferent and efferent, may be involved *(15)*, and there is some anatomic pathologic evidence of neuropathic vagal lesion. However, loss of sympathetic inhibitory break may also be responsible, particularly for the uncoordinated bursts of nonpropagated activity often observed in the small bowel *(12)*. There is also evidence that gastric dysrhythmia is common in the stomach of patients with diabetic gastroparesis, but we do not know whether these myoelectrical disturbances are primary or secondary. There is even the possibility that gastric dysrhythmia may be caused by central efferent activity brought about by nausea *(17)*. Hormonal abnormalities may also be involved. Motilin, in particular, is receiving attention because of the effectivity of motilin agonists in acutely stimulating gastric emptying in patients with diabetic gastroparesis. However, no clear evidence of motilin receptor downregulation or impaired motilin release has been obtained so far. Hyperglycemia is another factor that has been intensely studied in recent times. It appears that even small elevations in glycemia may decrease gastric propulsive activity, but again whether this is a direct effect of elevated glucose levels or caused by associated neurohormonal changes is unknown *(18)*.

The symptomatic expression of diabetic gastroparesis typically consists of episodes of nausea and vomiting that may occur either during fasting or postprandially. Diabetic gastroparetic patients often experience intense bouts of nausea and retching with expulsion of mucoid or bilious material in the morning before ingesting any food. These bouts are sometimes associated with epigastric pain. Other patients present manifestations of postcibal gastric stasis and their symptoms are exacerbated by eating, whereas vomiting of large quantities of retained food and secretions are also present. Rarely, there is vomiting of food ingested a day or more previously. At the other end of the spectrum, patients with milder manifestations of the gastroparesis syndrome manifest only dyspeptic-like symptoms such as frequent belching, early satiety, and epigastric fullness. Physical examination in diabetic gastroparesis usually does not reveal any abdominal sign. Occasionally, a gastric splash may be detected in patients with profound gastric stasis, but this is quite exceptional.

The episodes of nausea and vomiting that characterize typical diabetic gastroparesis tend to follow a variable course. In some patients the symptoms may be self limited after a few days or weeks, whereas in others the symptoms are unrelenting, and still in others, the symptoms follow a recurrent path. The manifestations of the gastroparesis syndrome may be aggravated by poorly controlled diabetes and episodes of diabetic discompensation associated with acidosis. Given the etiology of gut disturbances, it is not surprising that peripheral neuropathy, severe retinopathy, nephropathy, and signs of autonomic dysfunction such as orthostatic hypotension and sweating defects are often present in severe gastroparetics. Occasionally, however, relatively mild adult-onset diabetic patients without any evidence of systemic complications present with gastroparesis syndrome.

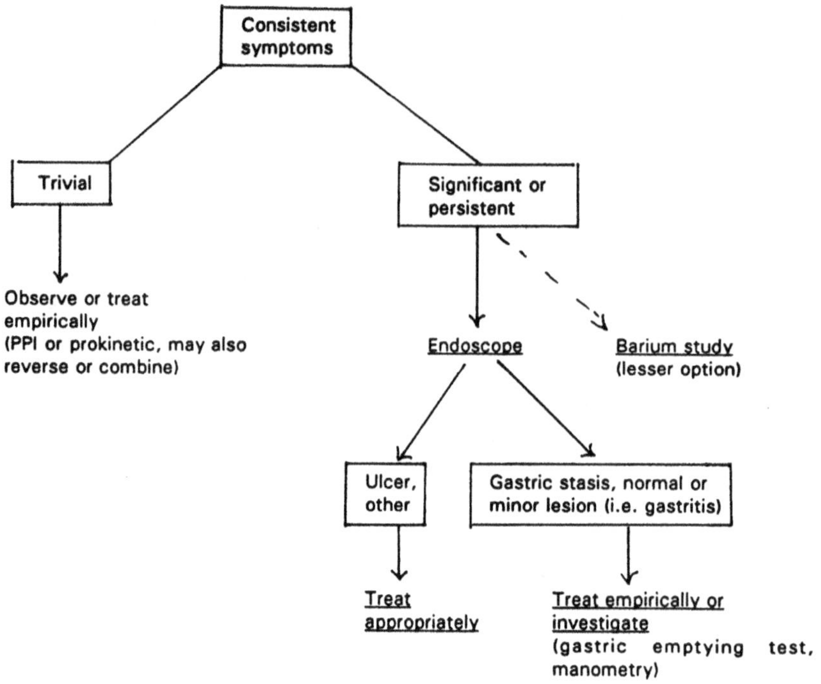


**Fig 2.**

The consequences of severe gastroparesis are important. They include dehydration and electrolyte abnormalities because of vomiting and, in protracted cases, malnutrition and poor control of the diabetes. It is also pendent to take into account the possibility of focal gut complications, most typically Mallory-Wise tears or severe erosive esophagitis, brought about by recurrent vomiting and retching.

The evaluation of the diabetic patient with suspected gastroparesis should follow a pre-established plan (Fig. 2). First, it is important to establish that the symptomatology is not caused by associated mucosal disease (for instance peptic ulcer) or mechanical impediment to gastric emptying. Upper gastrointestinal radiology may be an effective method to pick up obvious gastroparesis in a symptomatic patient by showing gastric dilatation and stasis, thus precluding the need to perform a more complex physiological assessment of gastric motor function. However, upper gastrointestinal endoscopy is also mandatory and, in most instances, the first choice test. It can detect relevant abnormalities that may have been overlooked by barium studies, such as a small pyloric-channel ulcer. In a sense, therefore, both imaging methods are complementary, but of the two, in my opinion, endoscopy cannot be dispensed with. Most sophisticated imaging methods, such as nuclear magnetic resonance or computerized tomography of the abdomen may be appropriate in doubtful cases, particularly when there is suspicion of a retroperitoneal lesion or thickening of the gastrointestinal wall. Along the same lines, endoscopic ultrasonography may also be helpful when there are doubts as to the presence of a submucosal lesion.

Once it has been established that the symptoms are not caused by obstructive or inflammatory process, it is important to consider obtaining physiological assessment. One reason for taking this instrumental approach is that unlike, for instance, gastroesophageal reflux symptoms, there are no consistently effective drugs that could be used for a therapeutic trial of gastroparesis. Therefore, if symptoms are attributed to a physiological derangement secondary to diabetes, motor activity will have to be measured to support the contention.

Which should be the first specific test to perform requires individual consideration. In symptomatic patients with gross evidence of stasis (such as radiological evidence of contrast pooling in the stomach or the finding of food retention at endoscopy after prolonged fasting), there is probably no need to measure gastric emptying. By contrast, in those patients in whom there is no apparent abnormality, it may be important to establish first whether there is or not a delay in gastric emptying. For this purpose, radioscintigraphic gastric emptying tests continue to be the most reliable and well contrasted. A single-isotope semisolid or liquid meal test may suffice but, if the technology is available, a dual-marker solid- and liquid-test is more informative and accurate *(19)*. A subtle and potentially useful sign of diabetic gastroparesis is the loss of normal discrimination between solids and liquids. In general, solid emptying is impaired to a greater extent than liquid emptying. In fact, liquid emptying may be faster than normal in some patients *(20)*. Therefore, if a single-marker technique is to be used, a solid marker should be preferred *(21)*. Ultrasonographic methods for measuring gastric emptying have also been described, but they are limited to liquid-test meals. Radiographically opaque solid pellets are another possible approach, and this technique may be particularly valuable in its simplicity, but it is also unlikely to have comparable sensitivity to the test-meal radioscintigraphic test. Interestingly, in some diabetic patients who are asymptomatic and present no clinical evidence of autonomic neuropathy, gastric emptying of solids has been found to be accelerated rather than delayed *(22)*.

Manometry is a useful diagnostic method in the context of diabetes with clinical suspicion of gastroparesis, but it is restricted to specialized centers. It is usually performed by an intubation with a multitube perfusion assembly provided with several pressure-sensitive ports. A group of closely spaced openings is located across the pylorus for measurement of distal antral, pyloric, and proximal duodenal activity *(13,14)*. In addition, there should be additional ports in the duodenum and proximal jejunum for assessment of intestinal motor responses. The test ideally should combine fasting and postprandial observation periods. During fasting, the test evaluates the presence and configuration of interdigestive migrating motor complexes. As indicated earlier, absence of phase-three activity appears to be a sign of impaired evacuation of indigestible solids from the stomach. However, it is also true that reliable evaluation of interdigestive motor activity requires very long recording sessions. These are best performed at night or, alternatively, employing an ambulatory, nonperfused manometric system. In any case, the most sensitive feature of the manometric test is the demonstration of antral hypomotility after ingestion of a solid-test meal. The hypomotility is characterized by decreased frequency of phasic pressure waves and, in some instances, there is also reduced wave amplitude or absence of waves.

Additional evidence of upper-gut dysmotility includes abnormalities in pyloric function ("pyloric spasm") and the presence of a disorganized motility pattern in the proximal small bowel either during fasting, postprandially, or both *(13)*. These intestinal abnormalities may be important in deciding whether gastric surgery is to be considered for a patient particularly resistant to medical therapy, because anastomosing a residual gastric stump to a neuropathic small bowel poses evident dysfunctional risks.

Whether electrogastrography adds to the diagnostic assessment of gastroparetic patients is questionable. Gastric dysrhythmias have been demonstrated in many patients with diabetic gastroparesis, but these have tended to be severely symptomatic cases *(23)*. Again there are doubts as to whether nausea could have induced the dysrhythmia because direct central stimulation, for instance, via gyroscopic exposure may induce both nausea and dysrhythmia in healthy volunteers. Thus, electrogastrography at present may not be a reliable enough method to establish a diagnosis, even though its non-invasiveness makes it clinically attractive. Moreover, there is no known benefits of attempting to reverse gastric myoelectrical disturbances with antiarythmic drugs.

## DIABETIC DIARRHEA

Chronic diarrhea associated with diabetic mellitus has been long recognized as a potential complication of the disease, although as commented for other gastrointestinal symptoms in diabetic patients, there is also the possibility of fortuitous and unrelated coincidence. Typically, diabetic diarrhea is watery, tends to occur in sudden bursts, and it is often preceded by abdominal cramps. It also has a preference for nocturnal episodes that may be accompanied by urgency and even incontinence (*see* later). The diarrhea, when it is reported to a referring physician, is usually severe and disabling, and common antidiarrheal remedies have usually been tried beforehand.

Similarly to the gastroparesis syndrome, symptoms of diabetic diarrhea may be self-limited and disappear after days or weeks. On the contrary, they may also become chronic or relapsing, and last for years, causing significant disability. As in functional gut disease, it is not uncommon for the episodes of diarrhea to alternate with constipation or to be combined with other manifestations of gut diabetic involvement, such as gastroparesis or dysphagia. Exceptionally, diabetic diarrhea may present as a malabsorption syndrome with steatorrheic stools and malnutrition.

The pathophysiology of diabetic diarrhea is no better understood than the pathophysiology of other diabetic gut disturbances. Although undoubtedly multifactorial, visceral neuropathy appears to be a key factor. Indeed, neuropathologic alterations in splanchnic nerves and ganglia have been described *(24,25)*. Moreover, altered intestinal motility associated to diabetic diarrhea, produces patterns that are similar to those observed in patients with postganglionic sympathetic lesions. However, it is unlikely that neuropathic changes are limited to sympathetic structures. Other anatopathologists have observed alterations in the myenteric plexus and, in a model of experimental diabetes in rats, diarrhea appears to be related to alteration in both the cholinergic and adrenergic innervation of the bowel *(26)*. Adrenergic dysfunction may be responsible for altered fluid absorption and, indeed, the secretory component, in addition to the motor disturbance, is an important element of diabetic diarrhea in the rat model and probably in humans as well. This feature is also consistent with reports of effective use of alpha-adrenergic agonists in diabetic diarrhoea (*see* subheading entitled "Treatment"). Another relevant factor may be diabetic microangiopathy of the intestinal wall *(27)*, which would alter the normal vascular flow to the gut and induce secondary mucosal-ischemic abnormalities.

Secondary disturbances brought about by intestinal dismotility may play a prominent role in diabetic diarrhea. Bacterial overgrowth in the small bowel is a relevant abnormality that appears to result from both alteration of intestinal transit and impairment of defensive factors. The contribution of bacterial overgrowth to diabetic diarrhea, how-

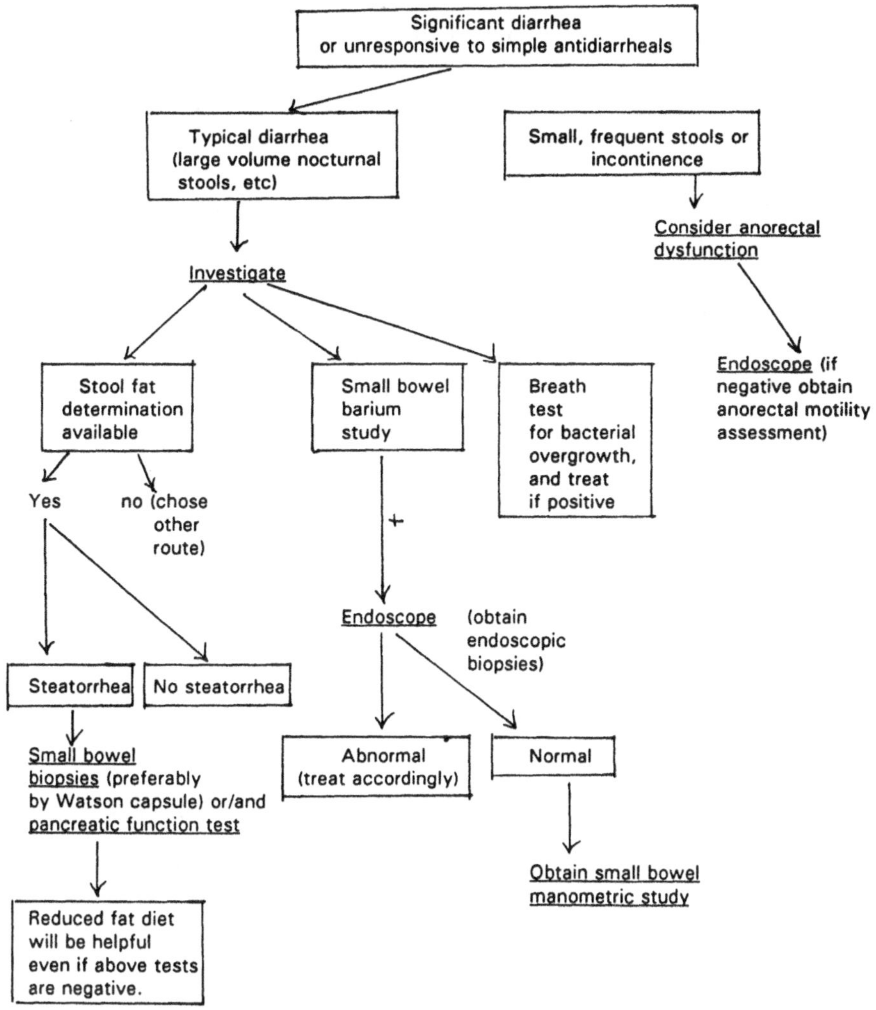


**Fig 3.**

ever, is very variable and only some patients experience symptomatic relief when treated with the appropriate antibiotics. Bile-acid malabsorption is another secondary factor, but again, response to bile-acid-binding agents is somewhat erratic. Finally, exocrine pancreatic insufficiency may be associated to diabetes mellitus, although the magnitude of the exocrine defect in most patients is not sufficient to be clinically relevant. It is known that, because of the large pancreatic exocrine reserve, only a profound diminution (90–95%) of pancreatic lipase secretion will result in significant steatorrhea.

The diagnostic process to follow in suspected diabetic diarrhea must be cautious and restrained, especially with regard to selection of appropriate diagnostic tests, to achieve a reasonable cost-benefit balance (Fig. 3). Currently, we favor a combination of diagnostic procedures and short therapeutic trials. As in any other instance of chronic diarrhea, it is important to first exclude structural abnormalities by the appropriate radiographic and endoscopic studies. The latter are particularly suited to evaluation of the distal small bowel, which is difficult to access by standard endoscopy. On the other hand, endoscopy is preferable to X-ray techniques in that it may allow one to obtain small bowel or colonic biopsies, sometimes useful in elucidating challenging cases. If the above imaging tests are unrevealing, a sensible therapeutic trial would be to administer a short course of antibiotics (tetracyclin, clarithromycin, or metronidazole) to eliminate potential bacterial overgrowth and to assess the clinical response. If negative, at this point it would be advisable to proceed with a 72-hr stool collection for determination of stool volume and fat content *(28)*. Frank steatorrhea should be further investigated by obtaining a small-bowel mucosal biopsy (if not done previously at endoscopy, and/or a pancreatic exocrine function test. The latter may sometimes be obviated by performing a therapeutic trial with pancreatic enzymes, which is simpler than conducting a formal pancreatic function test that may not be available at all institutions. Nevertheless, a number of noninvasive pancreatic tests have become commercially available, and these tend to be more commonly accessible than the traditional intubation tests.

In particularly resistant and severe cases of diarrhea, it may be appropriate to perform a small-bowel manometry test to determine whether there is disruption of normal motility patterns indicative of neuropathic dysmotility. Typical abnormal findings would be incoordination, disperse bursts of activity, or failure to convert a fasting into a fed pattern. All of these would be consistent with neuropathic pseudo-obstruction. Usually the amplitude of the waves is normal. Although effective pharmacologic therapy may not be available, evidence of profound disorganization in small-bowel motility may help inform both patient and physician that neuropathic dismotility is responsible for the bowel disturbances.

## CONSTIPATION ASSOCIATED WITH DIABETES

Even to a greater extent than for diarrhea, it is difficult to establish in a particular patient whether constipation is directly related to diabetes mellitus, because constipation is very prevalent among the general population. Nevertheless, in some reported series of patients with diabetic neuropathy, constipation was found to be a highly prevalent symptom. Moreover, there indeed appear to be some patients in whom, primarily as a result of autonomic dysfunction, there is a profound alteration in colonic motility resulting in delayed transit and the clinical feature of severe constipation *(1)*. One study has provided evidence that there is impaired gut-reflex activity (blunted postprandial gastrocolonic response) in diabetic patients with severe constipation *(29)*.

The usual clinical presentation is constipation severe enough to motivate physician consultation or referral to a subspecialist. In some patients, constipation may alternate with diarrhea, as it does typically in the irritable-bowel syndrome. More rarely, there are morphologic changes such as megacolon or megasigmoid, demonstrable by radiologic studies or at endoscopy *(30)*.

Diagnostic evaluation should be conducted judiciously and also the extent of the diagnostic work-up should be proportionate to the severity and clinical impact of the problem. Mild cases may be simply treated with appropriate corrective measures, without further investigation (Fig. 4).

For patients presenting with a relatively recent change in bowel-movement habit, standard procedures such as digital rectal examination, test stools for occult blood, proctocolonoscopy, or other imaging techniques, depending on availability and individual circumstances, are mandatory to exclude colonic neoplasia. Special procedures to consider include evaluation of colonic transit by radioscintigraphy or by radio-opacque

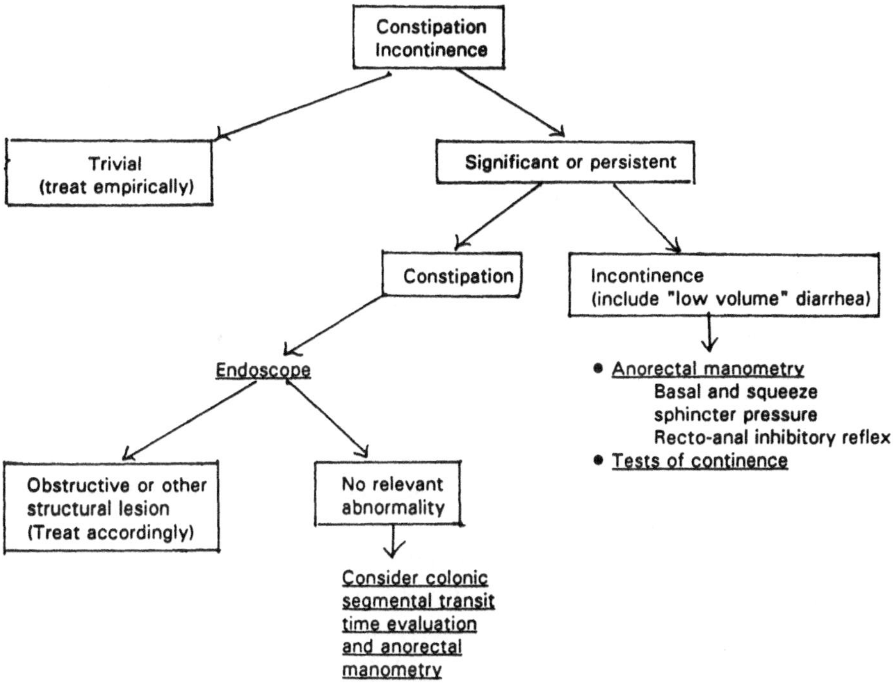


**Fig 4.**

pellet markers. Although these semiquantitative methods provide some information about regional colonic dysfunction, there are no data specifically relating to a diabetic population and we do not know the actual clinical usefulness of measuring colonic transit in this context.

## FECAL INCONTINENCE

This is a major and most bothersome complication of diabetic gut involvement *(1)*. As indicated earlier, incontinence may derive from significant diarrhea but, quite often, diabetic patients present independent anorectal motor dysfunction that is directly responsible for either fecal incontinence or "small volume" diarrhea. The latter is characterized by frequent expulsion of very small amounts of semi-liquid fecal material, which is quite typical of diabetic anorectal dysfunction.

The pathogenesis of anorectal dysfunction is, like other gut motor disorders in diabetic patients, causally related to autonomic neuropathy. In addition, to dysmotility there is evidence of impaired afferent nerve function, that produces a higher threshold for conscious rectal sensation to distension. This may lead to brain-bowel discoordination, and aggravates the problem *(3)*.

Physiological investigation may reveal disturbed external sphincter function and decreased basal- and squeeze-pressure generated by the anus. Incontinent diabetic patients tend to show abnormal levels in basal pressure, suggesting an abnormal internal anal sphincter function *(31)*. They also manifest impaired continence to either solid or liquid material infused intrarectaly.

In the clinical evaluation of diabetic incontinent patients it is most important to establish the differential diagnosis between diarrhea-associated incontinence and the previous described "low volume" or "false" diarrhea. In true diarrhoea, 24-h stool weights are higher than normal, whereas in the latter they are within normal limits *(31)*. A rectal manometric study combined with a test of continence can be quite useful in the evaluation of these patients with suspected anorectal dysfunction. Manometry provides data about basal-sphincter pressure and squeeze-sphincter pressure. It is also appropriate to test for adequacy of the recto-anal inhibitory reflex and for conscious rectal sensitivity to balloon distension. Continence can be directly assessed by techniques employing standard solid spheres or liquids placed intrarectaly *(32)*. Such physiological assessment will often provide information about the mechanism of incontinence, but it cannot guarantee a predictive value in terms of therapeutic response to biofeedback or drugs *(33)*.

## TREATMENT

The treatment of clinical gut syndromes associated with diabetes mellitus is largely symptomatic and palliative, since gut dysfunction derives primarily from the neuromuscular complications of diabetes mellitus.

The only truly effective etiologic treatment would be to cure the diabetes. Short of this ideal and mostly unattainable goal, a good metabolic control should be a priority target, particularly in light of physiological studies suggesting that hyperglycemia and associated systemic neurohormonal disturbances may aggravate gastrointestinal dysmotility.

In upper-gut motor disorders, both prokinetics and gastric antisecretory agents have a therapeutic place. Antisecretors, particularly the potent proton-pump inhibitors, are helpful to treat both the symptoms and esophageal lesions derived from pathological gastroesophageal reflux (as well as esophagitis secondary to retching and vomiting). They may also be used appropriately in gastroparesis with vomiting as adjuvant agents to prokinetics, because they reduce the volume of gastric juice and help prevent gastric overexpansion.

In the setting of acute gastroparesis with retracted vomiting and severe stasis, nasogastric suction may be needed to attain symptomatic control. At the same time, iv drug treatment should be started. Metoclopramide may be helpful in this acute setting because of its central antiemetic effects, although care should be taken not to administer it too rapidly as a bolus, because it may induce abrupt restlessness and anxiety. Erythromycin is a macrolide antibiotic with strong upper-gastrointestinal prokinetic effects when given iv in repeat boluses of 100 to 200 mg every few hours *(34)*. It acts as a motilin agonist and induces potent activity fronts that help clear the stomach of retained content. This drug seems to be less helpful when used chronically in oral form, although a number of macrolide derivatives, deprived of antibiotic action but retaining prokinetic effect, are currently under development.

Cisapride is a prokinetic benzamide active in oral form at a daily dose of 30 to 40 mg, which has a sustained therapeutic action and scarce side effects *(10)*. Antidopaminergic agents, such as metoclopramide and levosulpride, may also be helpful because of their central antinausea effects and because the inhibitory action of hyperglycemia on gastric motility may be partially mediated via dopamine receptors *(35)*. In refractory gastroparesis, surgical placement of a jejunostomy tube to bypass the gastric reservoir and deliver fluid and nutrients directly into the intestine may help overcome disability and improve subjective appreciation of overall health status *(36)*.

Treatment of intestinal disorders depends largely on correcting specific defects. In diabetic diarrhea, I have already alluded to the practical value of certain empiric trials with antibiotics (for bacterial overgrowth) and/or pancreatic enzymes (for pancreatic exocrine insufficiency). Obviously these therapies need to be applied long term (cyclically in the case of antibiotics) when there is confirmation of efficacy. Whenever there is a component of steatorrhea, a low fat diet is a useful adjuvant measure.

Otherwise, treatment of diabetic diarrhea is based on the empiric use of antidiarrheal agents chiefly loperamide, an opioid agonist that poorly crosses the blood–brain barrier and, therefore, has a predominantly peripheral action. Doses need to be adjusted depending on response. From 2 to 8 mg daily is the most common dosage range. When abdominal cramping and distension are associated with irregular bowel-movement pattern, it may be necessary to associate antispasmodic agents (unfortunately of limited value on account of their unpleasant anticholinergic side effects and somewhat unpredictable efficacy) and even prokinetics, such as cisapride, in an attempt to restore coordinated propulsive activity in the small bowel.

Severe constipation is managed empirically for the most part with bulk, stool softeners, and so on. Fecal incontinence can be a challenging management problem. Sometimes correction of either excessively fluid stools or constipation (with fecal impaction) is sufficient to bring reasonable symptomatic relief. However, when there is markedly uncoordinated anorectal motility, incontinence may be refractory to pharmacological modification of transit and physical characteristics of stools. A trial of feedback therapy at a specialized center should then be considered, but clinical success cannot be guaranteed.

## REFERENCES


1. Feldman M, Schiller LR. Disorders of gastrointestinal motility associated with diabetes mellitus. Ann Intern Med 1983;98:378.
2. Kassander P. Asymptomatic gastric retention in diabetes (gastroparesis diabeticorum). Ann Intern Med 1958;48:797.
3. Wald A, Tunuguntla AK. Anorectal sensorimotor dysfunction in fecal incontinence and diabetes mellitus. Modification with biofeedback therapy. N Engl J Med 1984;310:1282.
4. Whalen GE, Soergel KH, Geenen JE. Diabetic diarrhoea. A clinical and pathological study. Gastroenterology 1969;56:1021.
5. Lincoln J, Bokor JT, Crowe R, Griffith SG, Haven AJ, Burnstock G. Myenteric plexus in streptozotocin-treated rats. Neurochemical and histochemical evidence for diabetic neuropathy in the gut. Gastroenterology 1984;86:654.
6. Russell COH, Gannon R, Coatsworth J, et al. Relationship among esophageal dysfunction, diabetic gastroenteropathy, and peripheral neuropathy. Dig Dis Sci 1983;28:289.
7. Stewart IM, Hosking DG, Preston BJ, Atkinson M. Esophageal motor changes in diabetes mellitus. Thorax 1976;31:278.
8. Clouse RE, Reidel WL, Lustman PJ. Correlation of esophageal motility abnormalities with neuropsychiatric states in diabetic patients (abstract). Gastroenterology 1985;88:1351.
9. Hollis JB, Castell DO, Braddom RL. Esophageal function in diabetes mellitus and its relation to peripheral neuropathy. Gastroenterology 1977;73:1098.
10. Abrahamsson H. Gastrointestinal motility disorders in patients with diabetes mellitus. J Intern Med 1995;237(4):403–409.
11. Zitomer BR, Gramm HF, Kozak GP. Gastric neuropathy in diabetes mellitus: clinical and radiologic observations. Metabolism 1968;17:199.
12. Camilleri M, Malagelada J-R. Abnormal intestinal motility in diabetic patients with the gastroparesis syndrome. Eur J Clin Invest 1984;14:420.

13. Malagelada J-R, Rees WDR, Mazzotta LJ, Go VLW. Gastric motor abnormalities in diabetic and post-vagotomy gastroparesis: effect of metoclopramide and bethanechol. Gastroenterology 1980;78:286.
14. Malagelada J-R, Stanghellini V. Manometric evaluation of upper gut symptoms. Gastroenterology 1985;88:1223.
15. Undeland KA, Hausken T, Svebak S, Aanderud S, Berstad A. Wide gastric antrum and low vagal tone in patients with diabetes mellitus type I compared to patients with functional dyspepsia and healthy individuals. Dig Dis Sci 1996;41(1):9–16.
16. Jenkinson KM, Reid JJ. Effect of diabetes on relaxations to nonadrenergic, noncholinergic nerve stimulation in longitudinal muscle of the rat gastric fundus. Br J Pharmacol 1995;116(1):1551–1556.
17. Jebbink HJA, Bruijs PPM, Bravenboer B, Akkermans LMA, Vanberge-Henegouwen, GP, Smout AJPM. Gastric myoelectrical activity in patients with type I diabetes mellitus and autonomic neuropathy. Dig Dis Sci 1994;39(11):2376–2383.
18. Samson M, Salet GAM, Roelofs JMM, Akkermans LMA, Vanberge-Henegouwen GP, Smout AJPM. Compliance of the proximal stomach and dyspeptic symptoms in patients with type I diabetes mellitus. Dig Dis Sci 1995;40(9):2037–2042.
19. Thomforde GM, Brown ML, Malagelada J-R. Practical solid and liquid phase markers for studying gastric emptying in man. J Nucl Med Technol 1985;13:11.
20. Frank JW, Saslow SB, Camilleri M, Thomforde GM, Dinnen S, Rizza, RA. Mechanism of accelerated gastric emptying of liquids and hyperglycemia in patients with type II diabetes mellitus. Gastroenterology 1995;109(3):755–765.
21. Wright RA, Clemente R, Wathen R. Diabetic gastroparesis: an abnormality of gastric emptying of solids. Am J Med Sci 1985;289:240.
22. Nowak TV, Johnson CP, Kalbfleisch JH, Roza AM, Wood CM, Weisbruch JP, Soergel KH. Highly variable gastric emptying in patients with insulin dependent diabetes mellitus. Gut 1995;37(1):23–29.
23. Abell TL, Camilleri M, Malagelada J-R. High prevalence of gastric electrical dysrhythmias in diabetic gastroparesis (abstract). Gastroenterology 1985;88:1299.
24. Low PA, Walsh JC, Huang CY, McLeod JC. The sympathetic nervous system in diabetic neuropathy: a clinical and pathological study. Brain 1975;98:341.
25. Hensley GT, Soergel KH. Neuropathologic findings in diabetic diarrhoea. Arch Pathol 1968;85:587.
26. Schmidt RE, Nelson JS, Johnson EM. Experimental diabetic autonomic neuropathy. Am J Pathol 1981;103:210.
27. Schmidt H, Riemann JF, Schmid A, Sailer D. Ultrastructure of diabetic microangiopathy and autonomic neuropathy of the gut (abstract). Gastroenterology 1984;86:1236.
28. Bo-Linn G, Fordtran JS. Fecal fat concentration in patients with steatorrhea. Gastroenterology 1984;87:319.
29. Battle WM, Snape WJ, Alavi A, Cohen S, Braunstein S. Colonic dysfunction in diabetes mellitus. Gastroenterology 1980;79:1217.
30. Katz LA, Spiro HM. Gastrointestinal manifestations of diabetes. N Engl J Med 1966;275:1350.
31. Schiller LR, Santa Ana CA, Schmulen AC, Hendler RS, Harford WV, Fordtran, JS. Pathogenesis of fecal incontinence in diabetes mellitus. Evidence for internal anal sphincter dysfunction. N Engl J Med 1982;307:1666.
32. Read NW, Haynes WG, Bartolo DCC, et al. Use of anorectal manometry during rectal infusion of saline to investigate sphincteric function in incontinent patients. Gastroenterology 85:105.
33. Wald A. Biofeedback therapy for fecal incontinence. Ann Intern Med 1981;95:146.
34. Desautels SG, Hutson WR, Christian PE, Moore JG, Datz FL. Gastric emptying response to variable oral erythromycin dosing in diabetic gastroparesis. Dig Dis Sci 1995;40(1):141–146.
35. Mansi C, Savarino V, Vigneri S, Perilli D, Melga P, Sciabè L, De Martini D, Mela GS. Gastrokinetic effects of levosulpiride in dyspeptic patients with diabetic gastroparesis. Am J Gastroenterol 1995;90(11):1989–1993.
36. Fontana RJ, Barnett JL. Jejunostomy tube placement in refractory diabetic gastroparesis: a retrospective review. Am J Gastroenterol 1996;91(10):2174–2178.

# 16 Exercise and Diabetic Neuropathy

## *Implications for Exercise Participation and Prescription for Patients with Insulin-Dependent and Non-Insulin-Dependent Diabetes Mellitus*

*Nathan K. LeBrasseur*, MSPT
*and Roger A. Fielding*, PHD

**CONTENTS**



## INTRODUCTION

Diabetes mellitus affects nearly 15 million Americans and is associated with debilitating complications that include, retinopathy, coronary artery disease, peripheral vascular disease, nephropathy, and autonomic and peripheral neuropathy *(1)*. Recent evidence suggests that programs designed to increase physical activity may be useful in the treatment and prevention of diabetes and diabetic complications. In addition, all of the resultant complications of diabetes may have effects on exercise capacity and physical function. The purpose of the present chapter will be to review the metabolic effects of exercise and physical activity on carbohydrate metabolism and insulin sensitivity with specific reference to the metabolic responses to exercise in patients with insulin-dependent (IDDM) and non-insulin dependent diabetes mellitus (NIDDM). Secondly, peripheral and autonomic neuropathy in diabetes will be discussed in reference to their influence on exercise capacity and function. The final section of this review will concentrate on exercise recommendations for the diabetic patient (with and without neuropathy) to promote health and encourage an active lifestyle.

## METABOLIC RESPONSE TO EXERCISE

Physical exercise presents the most profound challenge to fuel homeostasis in normal humans. Whole-body energy expenditure can increase 10-fold from rest to maximal

From: *Contemporary Endocrinology: Clinical Management of Diabetic Neuropathy*
Edited by: A. Veves © Humana Press Inc., Totowa, NJ

Table 1
Fuel Reserves and Rates of Utilization Under Different Conditions in Humans

| | *Approximate Total Fuel Reserve* | | *Estimated Period for Which Fuel Store Would Provide Energy* |
|---|---|---|---|
| *Tissue* | *g* | *kcal* | *Minutes of Marathon Running* |
| Adipose tissue triacylglycerol | 16,000 | 144,000 | 7143 |
| Liver glycogen | 90 | 360 | 18 |
| Muscle glycogen | 350 | 1400 | 71 |
| Blood and extra | 20 | 80 | 4 |

Adapted from Newsholme and Start *(9)*.

exercise *(2)*. To maintain this increased rate of energy expenditure, the performance of physical activity is associated with a marked increase in the fuel and oxygen needs of working muscles. Since the available quantities of high-energy phosphate compounds such as creatine phosphate (CP) and adenosine triphosphate (ATP) within muscle are relatively limited (26 mmol/kg wet wt CP, and 8 mmol/kg wet wt ATP), the availability of the necessary metabolic machinery and oxidizable substrate is a necessity for sustained muscular activity. In order to meet these requirements and at the same time maintain the fuel and energy supply to other vital organs, major metabolic, hormonal, and cardiovascular adjustments are essential (*see* Table 1).

Under resting conditions, glucose production matches glucose utilization, resulting in euglycemia as the stimulatory effects of catecholamines, glucagon, cortisol, and growth hormone on hepatic glucose production balance the stimulatory action of insulin on glucose uptake *(3)*. However, with the onset of exercise, skeletal muscle glucose uptake can increase up to 28-fold depending on the intensity of the exercise *(4)*, despite a decrease in insulin secretion by the beta cell. It appears that catecholamines released from the adrenal medulla and/or nerve endings in the liver and the pancreas may be involved in the suppression of insulin secretion and the activation of hepatic glucose production *(5,6)*. In addition to the effects of sympathetic nerve endings in the liver, a state of hypoinsulinemia coupled with a relative state of hyperglucagonemia in the portal blood facilitates an increase in hepatic glucose output during exercise *(7)*. The resultant effect of these hormonal alterations is that blood-glucose levels remain unchanged during exercise of relatively short duration (Fig. 1).

Similar to blood-glucose supply, intramuscular stores of glycogen are broken down to enable resynthesis of high-energy phosphate compounds. Muscle glycogen's direct availability to the contractile tissue eliminates the need for a circulatory response for its mobilization. Muscle glycogen utilization appears to be greatest at the onset of exercise and then as other substrates become available the rate of muscle glycogen utilization slows *(8)* (Fig. 2). As with blood-glucose uptake, the rate of muscle glycogen utilization will increase with increasing exercise intensity reaching maximal rates well above the maximal oxygen uptake *(8)*.

Furthermore, skeletal muscle possesses the capacity to derive energy from blood–borne nonesterified fatty acids and intramuscular stores of triglyceride. It has been estimated that in an individual of normal body mass and composition, the total

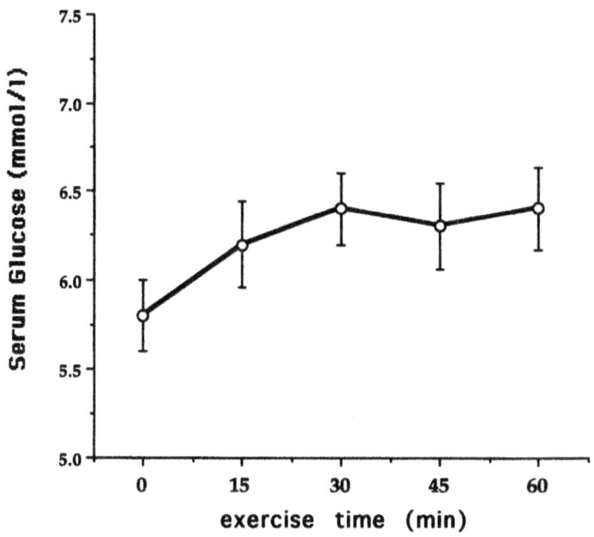


**Fig. 1.** Plot of change in blood glucose during 60 min of exercise at 70% of $VO_2max$ in well-conditioned runners. Note the early rise in glucose that results from the slight mismatch between hepatic glucose output and skeletal-muscle glucose uptake. Adapted from Fielding et al. *(93)*.

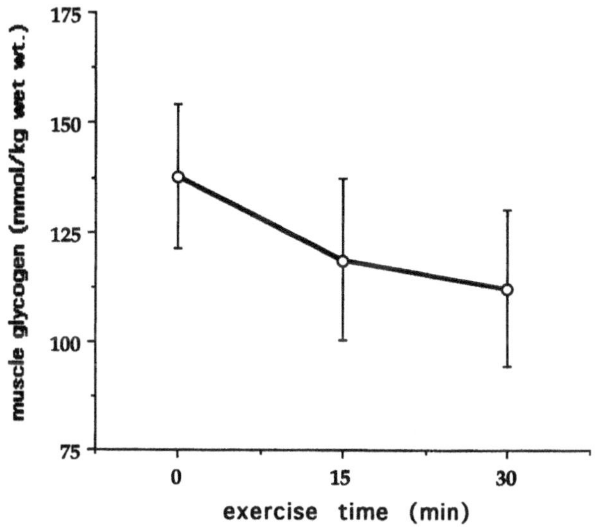


**Fig. 2.** Plot of the change in muscle glycogen during 30 min of exercise at 70% of $VO_2max$ in well-conditioned runners. Note the greater rate of glycogen utilization during the first 15 min compared to the last 15 min during this bout of exercise. Adapted from Fielding et al. *(93)*.

body stores of carbohydrate and fat account for 2000 and 140,000 kcal of energy, respectively *(9)*. Because of the enormous difference in the amounts of these substrates available for energy metabolism, the coordinated process of carbohydrate and fat metabolism is essential for the performance of prolonged muscular activity. During prolonged exercise and the resultant hypoinsulinemia and increased catecholamine release,

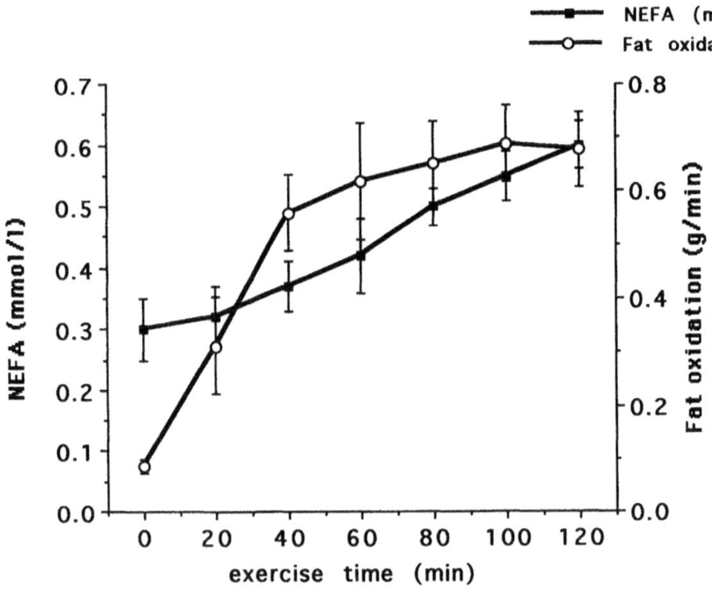


**Fig. 3.** Plot of change in the serum concentrations of nonesterified fatty acids (NEFA) (open circles) during 120 min of submaximal cycling exercise and calculated rates of whole-body fat oxidation from indirect calorimetry measurement (filled squares). Fielding et al. (unpublished observations).

free fatty acids (FFA) mobilized from adipose tissue become a more important energy-yielding substrate. The process of lipolysis occurring in adipose tissue results in the breakdown of triglyceride to FFA and glycerol. Epinephrine further stimulates lypolysis in an effort to preserve circulating glucose in addition to its effect on liver-glucose production *(10)*. Transported in the plasma bound to albumin, FFAs are then taken up by contractile tissue independent of insulin, but not necessarily by simple diffusion *(11)*. Sorrentino and coworkers and Stremmel have isolated FFA-binding proteins from plasma membranes of adipocytes, hepatocytes, and cardiac myocytes, and because antibodies raised against these proteins inhibit FFA uptake, it has been hypothesized that FFA transport across the plasma membrane is in fact carrier-mediated *(12,13)*.

Oxidation of specific amino acids such as the branched-chain amino acids leucine, isoleucine, and valine can also be increased during exercise to a smaller extent than fat and carbohydrate (10–15% of total oxidized substrate) assist in ATP resynthesis *(14)*. Several studies have reported that the increased amino acid oxidation during prolonged exercise results in an increased dietary requirement for protein in physically active individuals *(15,16)*.

The sequence of metabolic-fuel mobilization as outlined above can be significantly modified by several variables including the duration of exercise, the intensity of exercise, the fitness of the individual performing the exercise, and the previous nutritional state.

## ACUTE EXERCISE RESPONSE IN IDDM AND NIDDM

Changes in glucose homeostasis in patients with IDDM in response to exercise are quite complex, variable, and depend upon a number of additional factors, including the degree of insulinization, the type of insulin used, the injection site, prior metabolic control, the presence or absence of autonomic neuropathy, and recent food intake *(17,18)*. The method of insulin replacement in patients with IDDM does not duplicate the normal secretion of insulin from the pancreas. Insulin and contractile activity constitute the two most instrumental stimulators for membrane transport of glucose in skeletal muscle *(19,20)*. The mechanism by which these two stimuli increase the rate of glucose entry into the cell is difficult to determine. Insulin stimulation in skeletal muscle induces an increase in the number of tissue-specific glucose transporter proteins at the plasma membrane and a corresponding decrease in the number of transporters in an intracellular pool *(21–24)*. Similarly, contractile activity gives rise to an increased permeability of muscle to glucose. Thus, in addition to an increased number of transport molecules at the plasma membrane, muscle contraction seems to induce an increase in the intrinsic activity of the transporters *(25,26)*. Studies by Wallberg-Henricskson et al. indicate that diabetes affects both the insulin- and exercise-stimulated glucose transport, but that the insulin-induced transport is affected to a greater degree *(27)*. The fact that both insulin- and contraction-dependent glucose transport are affected is somewhat surprising because there is a considerable amount of evidence suggesting that insulin and contractile activity stimulate muscle glucose transport by two independent mechanisms *(28,29)*.

Despite the dramatic increase in glucose uptake by active muscle, plasma glucose concentration remains notably level in normal humans during exercise of low-to-moderate intensity. Feedback signals from plasma-glucose sensors appear to elicit changes in neuroendocrine function so that hepatic-glucose production increases *(11)*. Also, decreases in plasma glucose may directly stimulate hepatic-glucose production. Feedback mechanisms are less involved during intense exercise as plasma-glucose concentrations increase initially, then fall as hepatic-glycogen stores are depleted *(11)*. Instead, the glycemic response during periods of intense exercise may be subject to a feed-forward regulation elicited by the central command that changes neuroendocrine function, and subsequently causes an initial overshoot in hepatic-glucose production. For example, at the onset of exercise, impulses from the working muscles and motor centers increase neuroendocrine activity in an intensity-dependent manner *(30)*.

Consequently, diabetic patients commonly oscillate between states of insulin excess and insulin deficiency. As a result, the metabolic responses to exercise have been shown to correlate with the metabolic state at the onset of exercise *(31–35)*. The most familiar disturbance of glucose homeostasis during exercise in IDDM is hypoglycemia. Hypoglycemia most often occurs during a relatively prolonged session of moderately intense exercise when hepatic-glucose production cannot keep pace with the increased use of glucose by exercising muscle. This is because of unrestrained peripheral glucose utilization while portal hyperinsulinemia suppresses an appropriate rise in hepatic-glucose output *(32,10)*. Conversely, patients experiencing a state of chronic insulin deficiency of moderate degree have decreased glycogen stores in the liver and, to a lesser extent, in skeletal muscle *(36)*. Insulin deficiency results in impaired aerobic exercise endurance, a more rapid switch of fuels during prolonged activity to the utilization of free fatty acids, hyperglycemia, and accelerated ketone-body formation by the liver *(36)*. Increased levels of plasma glucose are further elevated by an exaggerated increase in hepatic-glucose production caused by insulin deficiency *(7,31)*. Elevated muscle-glycogen concentrations and a rapid rate of glycogen breakdown lead to high intramuscular concentrations of glucose-6-phosphate, which inhibit hexokinase

*(37)*. As intracellular muscle-glucose concentrations increase, the gradient of glucose from the interstitial space to the cytoplasm decreases and in turn reduces net glucose uptake by the cell *(36,39)*. Furthermore, when glycogen concentrations are elevated, lactate production is higher than when glycogen stores are low. A relationship has been suggested between muscle glycogen concentrations and muscle-membrane permeability based on the intracellular pH. The lowered pH levels have been implicated in decreasing muscle-membrane vesicle rate of glucose transport *(40)*. Thus, the metabolic profile of an exercising individual with hyperglycemia after 40 min mirrors that of a normal human who has been performing aerobic exercise for 4 h, the so-called accelerated adaptation to exercise *(41)*.

In NIDDM, the diabetic state (i.e., hyperglycemia concomitant with either insulin deficiency or hyperinsulinemia) gives rise to metabolic alterations that affect skeletal muscle glucose transport *(42)*. Changes in glucose homeostasis in patients with NIDDM in response to exercise result from the positive impact on peripheral-insulin action. Insulin resistance in the periphery primarily occurs in the skeletal muscle as it represents the body's largest insulin-sensitive tissue, and therefore, has a significant impact on overall glucose homeostasis in type II diabetic patients *(43)*. Muscle strips from a group of lean type II diabetic patients demonstrated a 50% decrease in insulin responsiveness for glucose transport when compared with nondiabetic subjects. These results suggest the presence of postreceptor defects in type II diabetic skeletal muscle *(44)*. Muscle contraction during physical activity has shown to increase both the number of glucose transporters at the plasma membrane *(23,45–47)*, and the activity of the transporters at the plasma membrane *(47)*. Thus, in the presence of insulin resistance, it appears physical exercise improves peripheral-glucose disposal.

During the first 2 h postexercise, the highest rate of skeletal-muscle-glycogen resynthesis occurs leading to complete reparation after 24 h. Evidence suggests glucose transport and glycogen synthase activation are coordinated in an effort to increase the rate of glycogen synthesis following glycogen-depleting exercise *(48)*. Furthermore, Maehlum et al. observed a similar rate of muscle-glycogen synthesis following prolonged heavy exercise in muscles of diabetic patients compared to normal subjects when administered adequate amounts of carbohydrates and subcutaneous insulin *(49)*. This may explain the reported increase in hypoglycemia in diabetic individuals following exercise and also may play a role in the need for diabetic individuals to adjust their meal scheduling and insulin doses.

In nondiabetic populations, the improvements in peripheral-insulin action induced by exercise training is balanced by a reduced insulin secretory response to a glucose challenge *(50)*. An increase in both insulin-receptor number and affinity following physical training have been well demonstrated, however, little support exists that such adaptations occur during exercise itself *(17)*. Both young and older nondiabetic exercise-trained individuals have demonstrated improvements in oral-glucose tolerance *(51)*. Trained individuals demonstrate the same overall insulin secretion and average plasma-glucose concentration as untrained persons despite a higher caloric intake *(52)*. Thus, during training the pancreas and insulin-sensitive tissues adapt to allow the necessary increase in caloric intake without causing hyperglycemia or overstimulation of β cells.

Similarly, in patients with IDDM, increased insulin sensitivity resulting from physical training has failed to demonstrate a positive influence on glycohemoglobin levels. Despite improvements in maximum oxygen uptake, improved lean body mass, increased insulin sensitivity, and possible improvements in cardiovascular risk factors, research has failed to support that exercise in the absence of adjustments in insulin and diet will improve overall glycemic control *(53,54)*.

On the other hand, physical training programs have been shown to significantly improve fasting plasma glucose and $A_{1c}$ in NIDDM subjects. This has been attributed to an improvement in skeletal-muscle insulin sensitivity and a subsequent increase in nonoxidative muscle-glucose disposal for glycogen resynthesis following exercise *(54)*. Physical activity appears to benefit NIDDM patients the most early in the disease while β-cell function may still be relatively intact *(55,56)*. Furthermore, physical activity may play a significant role in the primary prevention of the development of NIDDM in addition to obesity, and several chronic diseases, especially coronary heart disease *(57)*.

## DIABETIC NEUROPATHY AND EXERCISE

Several studies have demonstrated that the exercise capacity of people with diabetes without neuropathy or serious long-term complications of diabetes is comparable to nondiabetic subjects with similar habitual activity *(58,59)*. However, in diabetic patients with autonomic neuropathy, an abnormal pattern of hormonal responses, an elevated resting work product, a below normal increase in work product, and a reduced physical work capacity during exercise have been observed *(60,61)*.

### *Metabolic and Hormonal Effects of Diabetic Neuropathy*

Metabolic and hormonal effects of diabetic neuropathy result in major disturbances of the normal pattern of hormonal responses to exercise. The responses of norepinephrine, epinephrine, growth hormone, cortisol, and pancreatic polypeptide to exercise are blunted in diabetic patients with autonomic neuropathy *(62)*, suggesting an impaired metabolic response to exercise. However, in studies examining plasma-metabolite concentrations during exercise, no differences were noted between diabetic patients with and without autonomic neuropathy *(33,63)*. One may speculate that this occurs secondary to either a negligible effect of the measured hormones on the metabolic response to physical activity, or because of a heightened sensitivity of adipose tissue and glycogen stores to the action of glucoregulatory hormones in patients with neuropathy compared to nonneuropathic diabetic patients *(35)*. Similar to diabetic patients without neuropathy, neuropathic diabetic patients with insulin deficiency demonstrate exaggerated metabolic responses to exercise compared to healthy subjects *(33)*. Again, the metabolic state prior to the commencement of exercise governs the metabolic response during the course of physical activity. In insulin-deficient neuropathic patients, the impaired muscle uptake of plasma glucose in combination with ongoing hepatic glycogenolysis and gluconeogenesis, and the inappropriate gut delivery of glucose in the presence of gastroparesis, can result in extreme elevations in serum-glucose levels *(64)*. Hypoglycemia is more frequently encountered in autonomic neuropathy during exercise as insulin suppresses hepatic glucose output in the absence of counterregulation, and also following exercise because of irregular gut-fuel delivery, impaired counterregulatory hormone responses, and as muscle continues to take up increased amounts of plasma glucose for up to 24 h *(18,65)*. Hypoglycemia may range from very mild lowering of glycemia with minimal or no symptoms, to severe hypoglycemia with very low levels of glucose and neurologic impairment. Neuropathic patients may be unaware of the hypoglycemic state because of a deficient autonomic response (initial bradycardia and mild hypotension), and diminished or absent symptoms (associated to catecholamine release with cutaneous vasoconstriction, sweating, and a sense of anxiety) *(66)*. Finally, patients with symptomatic autonomic neuropathy are at high risk for developing complications during exercise. Sudden death and silent myocardial infarction, a condition in which the heart becomes unresponsive to nerve impulses, are attributed to severe autonomic neuropathy in diabetes *(67)*.

### *Cardiovascular Effects of Diabetic Neuropathy*

People with cardiovascular effects of diabetic neuropathy who also have autonomic neuropathy may exhibit an elevated resting heart rate or even pronounced tachycardia compared to diabetic patients without neuropathy and nondiabetic individuals *(61,68)*. This findings suggests a cardiac vagal defect in neuropathic patients *(61)*. In normal subjects and diabetic patients without neuropathy, increase in heart rate during low-intensity exercise is caused by withdrawal of vagal tone, and increases in heart rate in response to higher work loads are mediated through increased sympathetic activity *(69–71)*. In comparison, diabetic patients with autonomic neuropathy demonstrate a diminished increase in heart rate at low work intensities, indicating a cardiac vagal defect *(33)*. Furthermore, in neuropathic subjects, a lower sympathetic tone on the heart increases during exercise in intensity and is reflected by a lower heart rate compared to individuals without neuropathy at all relative work loads *(58)*. Finally, at maximal effort, diabetic patients with neuropathy attain significantly lower maximal heart rates compared to nondiabetic and diabetic patients without neuropathy *(59,61)*.

Meanwhile, individuals with diabetes and autonomic neuropathy not only have reduced heart-rate responses to exercise, but have lower resting blood pressure and reduced blood pressure responses to physical activity compared to nondiabetic and diabetic patients without neuropathy *(58,72,73)*. In nonneuropathic individuals, autonomic reflexes and endocrine mechanisms regulate blood pressure *(72)*, and sympathetic control of circulation is a major determinant of blood pressure during exercise *(74)*. In diabetic patients with neuropathy, a reduced blood pressure response to increasing work loads suggests a decrease in the sympathetic outflow to the heart and resistance vessels *(61)*.

Furthermore, increasing cardiac output and reducing hepatosplanchnic blood flow during exercise appear to be impaired by diabetic neuropathy. Impaired myocardial contractility resulting from either diminished adrenergic stimulation of the heart, because of autonomic neuropathy, or diabetic cardiomyopathy, or both, lowers cardiac output *(35,75)*. Failure to increase hepatosplanchnic vascular resistance during exercise because of sympathetic neuropathy in the splanchnic vascular bed hinders redistribution of blood flow to the periphery *(33)*. This may have a negative impact on blood pressure response and thermoregulation during physical activity.

Finally, maximal aerobic capacity is significantly impaired in patients with diabetic neuropathy compared to nondiabetic and nonneuropathic diabetic patients *(59,61)*. This may be caused by the reduced maximal heart rate and/or cardiac output, however, impaired redistribution of blood flow and volume as well as impaired lung function and decreased oxidative metabolic capacity of muscle fibers may cause a reduction in maximal oxygen uptake *(59,61)*.

### *Exercise and Risk Factors for Foot Problems*

Foot problems are common in diabetic patients despite being the most preventable long-term complications of diabetes *(76)*. Neuropathy and peripheral vascular disease

Table 2
Disuse Syndrome

| *Physiologic and Biochemical Changes* | |
|---|---|
| Decreased physical work capacity | Renal lithiasis |
| Muscle atrophy | Cardiovascular deconditioning |
| Negative nitrogen and protein balance | Pulmonary restrictions |
| Contracture of connective tissue | Decubitus ulcers |
| Osteoporosis | Mental depression |

Adapted from ref. *92*.

are the main etiopathogenic factors, whereas other risk factors include high foot pressures, limited joint mobility, history of previous foot problems, and reduced resistance to ischemia *(77)*.

Motor neuropathy in the diabetic foot leads to atrophy of the small muscles of the foot with an imbalance between flexors and extensors. This results in clawing of the toes, prominent metatarsal heads, and moving of the footpad forward *(78)*. As a result of these deformities, high pressures develop under the metatarsal heads both during standing and walking. Limited subtalar joint mobility, related to increased collagen glycation, affects the biomechanics of the foot and results in high foot pressures and foot ulceration *(79,80)*. High foot pressures in the presence of sensory neuropathy have been shown to be highly predictive for foot ulceration *(86,81)*. Charcot joint disease related to painless joint injury and subsequent foot deformity, mainly in the form of rocker-bottom foot with newly developed areas of high pressures in the midfoot is another serious complication of diabetic neuropathy and is mainly present in patients with good vascular function *(82)*. Patient education accompanied by proper footwear are the main strategies employed today in an effort to reduce foot ulceration in the at-risk patients *(83,84)*.

Diabetes also poses a risk factor for the development of peripheral vascular disease, which increases the susceptibility to ischemic ulcers and gangrene *(64,87)*. For the patient with peripheral vascular disease, exercise precedes and aggravates intermittent claudication, which induces pain as a result of insufficient blood flow to exercising skeletal muscle *(88)*. Nevertheless, moderate exercise can be beneficial even in patients with claudication, as it is known to slow down the progression of the disease.

There is no information available regarding the risk factors for foot problems and the rate of foot injuries in diabetic endurance athletes or in diabetic patients who exercise regularly. In nondiabetic endurance athletes the most common foot problems include stress fractures, tendonitis, and ankle sprains *(85)*. It would therefore be reasonable to suggest that diabetic exercises are similarly at risk for such problems and that neuropathic patients have a greater risk for foot ulceration and Charcot arthropathy. On the other hand, a decrease in the physical activity and fitness of the individual with diabetic neuropathy may result in a further deterioration of the blood-glucose control and more advanced impairment of the autonomic function, and ultimately, a more extensive decrease in the work capacity *(60)*. Although exercise cannot prevent the occurrence of peripheral neuropathy, it can slow it down and prevent a further loss of function and fitness because of disuse *(64)*. Disuse syndrome (Table 2) negatively impacts our overall state of health, which includes social, emotional, mental, and physical attributes. Multiple clinical manifestations of disuse syndrome affect most organs and systems of the body bringing forth both physiologic and biochemical changes *(89)*.

## PRACTICAL GUIDELINES FOR EXERCISE PRESCRIPTION

With the influence of exercise on management of IDDM and NIDDM not well understood among healthcare professionals, when complications present secondary to the disease, the role of exercise is often overlooked. The remainder of this chapter will discuss exercise options for persons with autonomic neuropathy followed by persons with sensory or motor peripheral neuropathy.

Prior to exercise participation, it is recommended that all persons with IDDM and NIDDM undergo an assessment, reviewing patient history and noting contraindications to exercise such as cardiopulmonary or orthopedic limitations, other metabolic dysfunction, medications, prior activity level, and laboratory data *(89)*. The American College of Sports Medicine recommends an exercise stress test prior to beginning an exercise program for healthy adults over the age of 45 *(90)*, and most experts recommend the same protocol for individuals with diabetes over the age of 35, or who have had diabetes for greater than 10 yr. These are important and prudent steps because of the high incidence of occult cardiovascular disease and manifestations of secondary complications in patients with diabetes, and they allow the professional to assess the functional capacity on which to base exercise prescription. In addition, instruction on proper care of the diabetic foot should be performed and reviewed. Clearly, diabetic patients who wish to begin a program of increased physical activity should consult with their primary-care physician about any necessary alterations in their insulin therapy and/or dietary intake.

In the presence of autonomic neuropathy, the defective sympathetic and parasympathetic coordination cause poor control of cardiac output and inability to redirect peripheral-blood flow to working muscles. Therefore, standard measures of exercise intensity, namely heart rate and blood pressure, are unreliable. Subjective measures of perceived exertion, such as the Borg scale, provide a useful tool for assessing exercise intensity. The Borg scale is a subjective rating scale from 6 to 20 which has been widely used to gage the perception of effort during physical exercise (Table 3) *(91)*. Aerobic exercise gradually targeted at moderate-to-heavy exertion generally equates to 60–85% maximum heart rate in nonneuropaths *(90)*.

Furthermore, appropriate responses in heart rate and blood pressure cannot be made during activities requiring rapid changes in body position. Sitting or recumbent exercises are beneficial for maintaining or increasing muscular strength without requiring rapid responses in blood pressure. Water therapy is a viable option as the pressure of the water helps maintain blood pressure during dynamic exercise. Donning full-length supportive garments such as body stockings will enhance venous return during physical activity. In addition, diabetic patients with autonomic neuropathy also have a predisposition to dehydration during exercise in the heat, and poor tolerance for activity in the cold. Therefore, adequate hydration should be emphasized, while avoiding exercise in temperature extremes.

Regardless of the severity of complications, or the mode of activity, a conservative approach based on subjective feedback is the best way to determine the appropriateness of a training regimen for diabetic patients with autonomic neuropathy. Regarding the patient with peripheral neuropathy, the loss of proprioception and touch in the extremities results in a dependence on vision when performing motor tasks. The following

Table 3
RPE Scale (Rate of Perceived Exertion)

| | |
|---|---|
| 6 | |
| 7 | Very, very light |
| 8 | |
| 9 | Very light |
| 10 | |
| 11 | Fairly light |
| 12 | |
| 13 | Somewhat hard |
| 14 | |
| 15 | Hard |
| 16 | |
| 17 | Very hard |
| 18 | |
| 19 | Very, very hard |
| 20 | |

Adapted from Borg *(8)*.

strategies to facilitate movement in patients with peripheral neuropathy are recommended by Graham et al. With impaired sensation and/or proprioception in the lower extremities, the use of mirrors facilitates body awareness without forcing the patient to focus down at the feet. Providing visual cues, such as footprints on the walking surface during gait activities, will further enhance proprioception. Furthermore, applying resistance manually or with therapeutic equipment through the range of movement stimulates joint reflexes and proprioception. Facilitation techniques such as rubbing or tapping may elicit muscle recruitment and contraction. Patients with limited muscle function or range of motion can independently perform stretches with props *(89)*.

Certain precautions should be implemented by the diabetic with peripheral neuropathy while exercising. Patients with impaired balance caused by peripheral neuropathy should learn basic principles of equilibrium and utilize external support during balance activities. Furthermore, loss of sensation creates a risk for overstitching in muscle and connective tissue. Patients should be taught gentle, pain free range-of-motion exercises, and that quivering of a muscle on stretch, or increasing pain as a stretch is held, indicate over-stretching of a muscle. Moreover, range-of-motion activities for the major joints are important for preventing or minimizing contractures. Limiting weight-bearing activities and encouraging activities such as arm exercises, swimming, and bicycling, in addition to frequent inspection of feet and not wearing shoes more than 5 h at a time, are important measures to include in an exercise routine for a diabetic with impaired sensation of feet or Charcot's foot. Appropriate footwear can provide redistribution of the diabetic's weight away form pressure points secondary to the deformities *(89)*. Finally, in the instance of impaired sensation in the fingers, palpation of the radial pulse is an inaccurate assessment of exercise intensity. Therefore, use of the Borg scale for perceived exertion is a more reliable estimate.

## SUMMARY AND CONCLUSIONS

Nearly all persons with diabetes, even those with severe complications, can receive benefits from properly prescribed exercise programs. The consequences of physical inactivity and a sedentary lifestyle take a significantly longer time to reverse than to develop. Therefore, diabetes health-care professionals need to encourage patients to take the preventive measures offered through various modes of exercise to avoid the complications associated with a sedentary lifestyle. Both IDDM and NIDDM patients can safely realize the improved cardiorespiratory and functional benefits of regular exercise training. In patients with IDDM, specific care must be taken in monitoring blood-glucose concentrations, insulin dosage, and carbohydrate intake to ensure euglycemia before, during, and after exercise. In diabetic patients with autonomic neuropathy, the exercise prescription must be further tailored to accommodate their altered cardiovascular response to exercise. In summary, education of persons with diabetes must promote increased physical activity in their daily lives with the goal of improving health and restoring optimal physical function.

## REFERENCES


1. National Institutes of Health. Diabetes in America, 2nd ed. National Institutes of Health, Bethesda, 1995.
2. Taylor HL, Buskirk E, Henschel A. Maximal oxygen uptake as an objective measure of cardiorespiratory performance. Am J Physiol 1955;8:73–80.
3. Kemmer F, Berger M. Therapy and better quality of life: the dichotomous role of exercise in diabetes mellitus. Diabetes/Metab Rev 1986;2:53–68.
4. Katz A, Broberg S, Sahlin K, Wahren J. Leg glucose uptake during maximal dynamic exercise in humans. Am J Physiol 1986;251:E65–E70.
5. Galbo H, Richter E, Hilsted J, Holst J, Christensen N, Henrickson J. Hormonal regulation during prolonged exercise. Ann NY Acad Sci 1977;301:72–80.
6. Wasserman DH. Control of glucose fluxes in the post-absorptive state. Ann Rev Physiol 1995;191–218.
7. Vranic M, Kawamori R, Pek S, Kovacevic N, Wrenshall GA. The essentially of insulin and the role of glucagon in regulating glucose utilization and production during strenuous exercise in dogs. J Clin Invest 1976;57:245–255.
8. Hermansen L, Hultman E, Saltin B. Muscle glycogen during prolonged severe exercise. Acta Physiol Scand 1967;71:129–137.
9. Newsholme EA, Start C. In: Regulation in Metabolism. Wiley, New York, 1979, pp. 255.
10. Zinman B, Murray F, Vranic M, Albisser A, Leibel B. McLean P, Marliss E. Glucoregulation during moderate exercise in insulin treated diabetics. J Clin Endocrinol 1977;45:641–652.
11. Richter E, Turcotte L, Hespel P, Kiens B. Metabolic responses to exercise: effects of endurance training and implications for diabetes. Diabetes Care 1992;15:1767–1776.
12. Sorrentino E, Stump D, Potter BJ, et al. Oleate uptake by cardiac myocytes is carrier mediated and involves a 40-kD plasma membrane fatty acid binding protein similar to that of liver, adipose tissue, and gut. J Clin Invest 1988;82:928–935.
13. Stremmel W. Fatty acid uptake by isolated rat heart myocytes represents a carrier-mediated transport process. J Clin Invest 1988;81:844–852.
14. Rennie MJ, Edwards RHT, Krywawych S, Davies CTM, Halliday D, Waterlow JC, Milward DJ. Effect of exercise on protein turnover in man. Clin Sci 1981;62:627–639.
15. Meredith CN, Zackin MJ, Frontera WR, Evans WJ. Dietary protein requirements and body protein metabolism in endurance-trained men. J Appl Physiol 1989;66:2850–2856.
16. Tarnopolsky MA, Atkinson SA, MacDougall JD, Chesley A, Phillips S, Schwarcz HP. Evaluation of protein requirements for trained strength athletes. J Appl Physiol 1992;73:1986–1995.
17. Vitug A, Schneider S, Ruderman N. Exercise and type I diabetes mellitus. 1988;16:285–304.
18. Zinman B, Zuniga-Guajardo S, Kelly D. Comparison of the acute and long term effects of exercise on glucose control in type I diabetes. Diabetes Care 1984;7:515–519.

19. Arvill A. Relationship between the effects of contraction and insulin on the metabolism of the isolated levator ani muscle of the rat. Acta Endocr 1967;56:27.
20. Helmreich E, Cori CF. The distribution of pentoses between plasma and muscle. J Biol Chem 1957;224:663.
21. Wallberg-Henriksson H. Interaction of exercise and insulin in type II diabetes mellitus. Diabetes Care 1992;15:1777–1782.
22. Douen AG, Ramlal T, Cartee GD, Klip A. Exercise modulates the insulin-induced translocation of glucose transporters in rat skeletal muscle. FEBS Lett 1990;261:256–260.
23. Fushiki T, Wells JA, Tapscott EB, Dohm GL. Changes in glucose transporters in muscle in response to exercise. Am J Physiol 1989;256:E580–E587.
24. Klip A, Ramlal T, Young DA, Holloszy JO. Insulin induced translocation of glucose transporters in rat hindlimb muscles. FEBS Lett 1987;224:224–230.
25. Holloszy JO, Constable SH, Young DA. Activation of glucose transport in muscle by exercise. Diabetes/Metab Rev 1986;1:409–423.
26. Ivy J. In: Pando KB, ed. Exercise and Sports Sciences Review, vol. 15, Macmillan, New York, 1987, pp. 29–51.
27. Wallberg-Henriksson H, Holloszy JO. Activation of glucose transport in diabetic muscle: responses to contraction and insulin. Am J Physiol 1985;249:C233–C237.
29. Constable SH, Favier RJ, Carter GD, Young DA, Holloszy JO. Muscle glucose transport: interactions of in vitro contractions, insulin, and exercise. J Appl Physiol 1988;64:2329–2332.
29. Wallberg-Henriksson H, Constable SH, Young DA, Holloszy JO. Glucose transport into rat skeletal muscle: interaction between exercise and insulin. J Appl Physiol 1988;65:909–913.
30. Galbo H. Hormonal and Metabolic Adaptations to Exercise. Thieme, New York, 1983, pp. 1–116.
31. Vranic M, Wrenshall G. Exercise, insulin and glucose turnover in dogs. Endocrinology 1969;85: 165–171.
32. Kawamori R, Vranic M. Mechanism of exercise-induced hypoglycemia in depancreatized dogs maintained on long-acting insulin. J Clin Invest 1977;59:331–337.
33. Hilsted J. Pathophysiology in diabetic autonomic neuropathy: cardiovascular, hormonal, and metabolic studies. Diabetes 1982;31:730–737.
34. Vranic M, Wasserman D, Bukowiecki L. Metabolic implications of exercise and physical fitness in physiology and diabetes. In: Rifkin HP, ed. Diabetes Mellitus: Theory and Practice. Elsevier, New York, 1990, pp. 198–219.
35. Giacca AM, Davidson J, Lickley H. In: Davidson J, ed. Clinical Diabetes Mellitus: A Problem Oriented Approach. Thieme-Stratton, New York, 1991; pp. 218–265.
35. Holloszy J, Schultz J, Kusnierkierkieweicz J, Hagberg J, Ehasani A. Effects of exercise on glucose tolerance and insulin resistance. Acta Med Scand 1986;711(Suppl.):55–65.
36. Wasserman D, Zinman B. In: Ruderman N, Devlin J. eds. Health Professionals Guide to Diabetes and Exercise. American Diabetes Association, Alexandria, VA, 1995, pp. 29–47.
37. Newsholme EA, Leech AR. In: Biochemistry for the Medical Sciences. Wiley, New York, 1983, pp. 339–346.
38. Hespel P, Richter EA. Glucose uptake and transport in contracting, perfused rat muscle with different pre-contraction glycogen concentrations. J Physiol 1990;427:347–359.
39. Richter EA, Galbo H. High glycogen levels enhance glycogen breakdown in isolated contracting skeletal muscle. J Appl Physiol 1986;61:827–831.
40. Richter EA, Hansen SA, Hansen BF. Mechanisms limiting glycogen storage in muscle during prolonged insulin stimulation. Am J Physiol 1988;255:E621–E628.
41. Wahren J, Sato Y, Ostman J, Hagenfeldt L, Felig P. Turnover and splanchnic metabolism of free fatty acids and ketones in insulin deficient diabetes at rest and in response to exercise. J Clin Invest 1984;73:1367–1376.
42. Olefsky JM, Garvey WT, Henry RR, Brillon D, Freidenberg MS. Cellular mechanisms of insulin resistance in non-insulin dependent (type II) diabetes. Am J Med 1988;85:86–105.
43. Wallberg-Henriksson H. Glucose transport into skeletal muscle. Influence of contractile activity, insulin, catecholamines an diabetes mellitus. Acta Physiol Scand 1987;131:1–80.
44. Andreasson K, Galuska D, Thorne A, Sonnenfeldt T, and Wallberg-Henriksson H. Decreased insulin stimulated 3-0-methylglucose transport in in vitro incubated muscle strips from type II diabetic patients. Acta Physiol Scand 1991;142:255–260.
45. Goodyear L, King P, Hirshman M, Thompson C, Horton ED, Horton ES. Contractile activity increases plasma membrane glucose transporters in the absence of insulin. Am J Physiol 1990;259:E667–672.

46. Hirshman M, Wallberg-Henriksson H, Wardzala L, Horton ED, Horton ES. Acute exercise increases the number of plasma membrane glucose transporters in rat skeletal muscle. FEBS Lett 1988;238:235–239.
47. King P, Hirshman M, Horton ED, Horton E. Glucose transport in skeletal muscle membrane vesicles from control and exercised rats. Am J Physiol 1989;257:C1128–1134.
48. Friedman J, Neufer P, Dohm GL. Regulation of glycogen resynthesis following exercise. Sports Medicine 1991;11:232–243.
49. Maehlum SH, Hostmark AT, Hermansen L. Synthesis of muscle glycogen during recovery after prolonged severe exercise in diabetic and non-diabetic subjects. Scand J Clin Lab Invest 1977;37:309–316.
50. King DS, Staten MA, Kohrt W, Clutter WE, Dalsky GP, Holloszy JO. Insulin secretory capacity in endurance trained and untrained young men. Am J Physiol 1990;259:E155–E161.
51. Seals DR, Hagberg JM, Allen WK, Hurley BF, Dalsky GP, Ehsani AH, Holloszy JA. Glucose tolerance in young and older athletes and sedentary men. J Appl Physiol 1984;56:1521–1525.
52. Dela F, Mikines KJ, Von-Listow M, Galbo H. Does training spare insulin secretion and diminish glucose levels in real life? Diabetes Care 1992;15:1712–1715.
53. Landt K, Campaigne B, James F, Serling M. Effects of exercise training on insulin sensitivity in adolescents with type I diabetes. Diabetes Care 1985;8:461–465.
54. Devlin J. Effects of exercise on insulin sensitivity in humans. Diabetes Care 1992;15:1690–1693.
56. Schneider S, Amorosa L, Khachadurian A, Ruderman N. Studies on the mechanism of improved glucose control during regular exercise in type 2 diabetes. Diabetologia 1984;26:355–360.
57. Helmrich, S, Ragland D, Leung R, Paffenbarger R. Physical activity and reduced occurrence of non-insulin-dependent diabetes mellitus. N Engl J Med 1991;325:147–152.
58. Hilsted J, Galbo H, Christensen N, Parving H, Benn J. Haemodynamic changes during graded exercise in patients with diabetic autonomic neuropathy. Diabetologia 1982;22:318–323.
59. Veves A, Saouaf R, Donaghue VM, Mullooly CA, Kistler JA, Giurini JM, Horton ES, Fielding RA. The relationship of regular exercise to maximal aerobic capacity and endothelial function in young insulin-dependent diabetic patients, in press.
60. Barkai L, Peja M, Vamosi I. Physical work capacity in diabetic children and adolescents with and without cardiovascular autonomic dysfunction. Diabetic Med 1996;13:254–258.
61. Hilsted J, Galbo H, Christensen N. Impaired cardiovascular responses to graded exercise in diabetic autonomic neuropathy. Diabetes 1979;28:313–319.
62. Hilsted J, Galbo H, Christensen N. Impaired responses of catecholamines, growth hormone, and cortisol to graded exercise in diabetic autonomic neuropathy. Diabetes 1980;29:257–262.
63. Hilsted J. Autonomic neuropathy: cardiovascular, hormonal and metabolic studies. Acta Endocrinologica 1980;94:139–144.
64. Vinik A, Milicevic Z. Preventive measures and treatment options for diabetic neuropathy. Cont Int Med 1994;6:41–55.
65. Berger M. Metabolic and hormonal effects of muscular exercise in juvenile type I diabetes. Diabetologia 1977;13:355–355–367.
66. Thomas PK, Eliasson SG. Diabetic Neuropathy. In: Dyck PJ, Thomas PK, Lambert EH, Burger R, eds. Peripheral Neuropathy, vol. 2. Saunders, Philadelphia, 1984, pp. 1773–1810.
67. Ewing DCB. Diagnosis and management of diabetic autonomic neuropathy. Br Med J 1982;285: 916–918.
68. Robinson BF, Epstein SE, Beiser GD, Braunwald E. Control of heart rate by the autonomic nervous system. Circ Res 1966;19:400–411.
69. Page M, Watkins P. The heart in diabetes: autonomic neuropathy and diabetes. Clin Endocrinol Metab 1977;6:377–389.
70. Freyschuss U. Cardiovascular adjustments to somatomotor activation. Acta Physiol Scand Suppl 1970;342:1–63.
71. Christensen NBO. The relationship between plasma catecholamine concentration and pulse rate during exercise and standing. Eur J Clin Invest 1977;3:299–306.
72. Hornung RS, Mahler RF, Raftery EB. Ambulatory blood pressure and heart rate in diabetic patients: an assessment of autonomic function. Diabetic Med 1989;6:579–585.
73. Radice M, Rocca A, Bendon E, Musacchio N, Morabito A, Segalini G. Abnormal response to exercise in middle-aged NIDDM patients with and without autonomic neuropathy. Diabetic Med 1996;13:259–265.

74. Clausen J. Circulatory adjustments to dynamic exercise and effect of physical training in normal subjects and in patients with coronary artery disease. Prog Cardiovasc Dis 1976;18:459–495.
75. Sanderson J, Brown DJ, Kovallese A, Kohner J. An echocardiac study of young diabetics. Br Med J 1978;6110:404–407.
76. Bessman AN. Foot problems in diabetes. Compr Ther 1982;8:32–37.
77. Young MJ, Veves A, Boulton AJM. The diabetic foot: aetiopathogenesis and management. Diabetes Metab Rev 1993;9:109–127.
78. Brand PW. Repetitive stress in the development of diabetic foot ulcers. In: Levin ME, O'Neal LW, eds. The Diabetic Foot. Mosby, St. Louis, 1988, pp. 83–90.
79. Delbridge L, Perry P, Marr S, Arnold N. Yue OK, Turtle JR, Reeves TS. Limited joint mobility in the diabetic foot: relationship to neuropathic ulceration. Diabetic Med 1988;5:333–337.
80. Fernando DJS, Masson EA, Veves A, Boulton AJM. Limited joint mobility: relationship to abnormal foot pressures and diabetic foot ulceration. Diabetes Care 1991;14:8–11.
81. Veves A, Murray HJ, Young MJ, Boulton AJM. The risk of foot ulcerationin diabetic patients with high foot pressure: a prospective study. Diabetologia 1992;35:660–663.
82. Sanders LJ, Frykberg RG. In: Levin ME, O'Neal LW, Bowker JH, eds. The Diabetic Foot. Mosby, St. Louis, 1993, pp. 149–180.
83. Assal JP, Mulhauser I, Permat A, Gfeller R, Jorgens V, Berger M. Patient education as the basis for diabetes care in clinical practice and research. Diabetologia 1985;28:602–613.
84. Veves A, Masson EA, Fernando DJS, Boulton AJM. The use of experimental hosiery to reduce plantar foot pressures in diabetic neuropathy. Diabetes Care 1989;9:653–655.
85. Coker TP. Sports injuries to the foot and ankle. In: Jahss MH, ed. Disorders of the Foot and Ankle. Medical and Surgical Management, 2nd ed. Saunders, Philadelphia, 1991, pp. 2415–2445.
86. Levin ME. Preventing amputation in the patient with diabetes. Diabetes Care 1995;18:1383–1394.
87. Janzon L, Bergent S, Ericsson B, Hanson M, Lindell S. Leg blood flow in intermittent claudication—a comparison between non-insulin dependent diabetics and non diabetics. Angiology 1984;36:724–728.
88. Boyd C, Bird P, Teates C, Wellons H, MacDougall M, Wolfe L. Pain-free physical training in intermittent claudication. J Sports Med 1984;24:24–28.
89. Graham CL-MP. Exercise options for persons with diabetic complications. Diabetes Educ 1990;16:212–220.
90. American College of Sports Medicine. Guidelines for Exercise Testing and Prescription, 5th ed. Lea and Febiger, Philadelphia, 1996.
91. Borg G. Perceived exertion as an indicator of somatic stress. Scand J Rehab Med 1970;2:92–98.
92. Valbona C. In: Kottke FS, Lehman G, eds. Krusen Handbook of Physical Medicine and Rehabilitation, 3rd ed. Saunders, Philadelphia, 1982, pp. 963–975.
93. Fielding RA, Costill DL, Fink WJ, King DS, Kovaleski JE, Kirwan JP. Effect of pre-exercise carbohydrate feedings on muscle glycogen use during exercise in well-trained runners. Eur J Appl Physiol 1986;56:225–229.

# 17 Epidemiology of the Diabetic Foot

## *Ulcerations and Amputations*

*Robert G. Frykberg,* DPM, MPH,
*Geoffrey M. Habershaw,* DPM,
*and James S. Chrzan,* DPM

CONTENTS



## INTRODUCTION

Of the 16 million people in the United States with diagnosed or undiagnosed diabetes, many will suffer the long-term complications of the disease affecting their lower extremities including peripheral neuropathy and vascular disease. When combined with physical or mechanical trauma, these important predisposing risk factors can frequently lead to infection, ulceration, or gangrene. In fact, each of these events are, in turn, major risk factors for diabetic lower-extremity amputation (LEA), perhaps the most feared of all complications attendant with diabetes mellitus.

Much of our understanding of the pathophysiology of the diabetic foot is derived from epidemiological data acquired from cross-sectional surveys and longitudinal or retrospective observational studies. These have been valuable instruments in elucidating potential risk factors for foot lesions as well as for determining the measures of association (odds ratios or risk ratios) for adverse outcomes. Nonetheless, the information obtained can only be considered as estimates of the true population values, since the entire diabetic population has not been sampled. To date, we do not even have reliable estimates of the true prevalence or incidence of foot infection and ulceration in the diabetic population, since many of these complications are treated in the outpatient setting. Our methods of data collection simply fail to capture the majority of these events because of the absence of a nationwide registry. Hence, the importance of large prospective studies of diabetic patient groups becomes apparent in elucidating the frequency and determinants of foot disease. Clinical trials have become important tools for testing hypotheses related to wound-healing methodologies or treatments (growth factors, dressings, total contact casting, and so on) as well as for assessing the values of

From: *Contemporary Endocrinology: Clinical Management of Diabetic Neuropathy*
Edited by: A. Veves © Humana Press Inc., Totowa, NJ

various preventive interventions (education, footwear, and so on). Although experimental studies in this area were infrequent only a few years ago, such investigations are being reported with increasing frequency as new treatments become available. The majority of epidemiological data concerning frequency of LEA (and of severe ulcerations) in the United States population comes from National Hospital Discharge Surveys (NHDS) which capture data from civilian (public and private) hospitals. Since this does not include data from 172 Veterans Affairs (VA) hospitals and the numerous military hospitals, such estimates actually underreport the true frequency of these complications *(1)*. Furthermore, the NHDS itself underreports diabetes-related LEA discharges in that diabetes is not even listed on the discharge record in approx 40% of such admissions *(2)*. The Centers for Disease Control and Prevention (CDC) maintains a surveillance system that systematically collects, analyzes, and disseminates national data on diabetes and its sequelae. Much of the national data presented in this chapter is derived from the CDC surveillance system, which utilizes data sources such as vital statistics, National Health Interview Surveys (NHIS), the NHDS, and Medicare claims data *(3)*. Lower-extremity diabetic ulcerations are identified by ICD (*International Classification of Diseases*, rev. 9) code 250 for diabetes and code 707 for ulcer *(1,4)*. Diabetic lower-extremity amputations are identified by ICD-9 codes 84.11–84.18, including toe (84.11), foot (84.12), leg (84.13–84.16), or thigh (84.17–84.18) with the additional code 250 for diabetes. Traumatic LEAs (codes 895–897) should be excluded from such analyses.

It is often difficult to directly compare rates of ulceration or amputation from one study to another because of differing methodologies, populations, and reporting techniques. For example, some reports of population-based studies may only use sex-specific or age-specific rates of disease that are indeed valid measures, but that are not summary measures across the entire population studied. Therefore, these specific rates cannot really be contrasted with other populations using population summary rates. Age-adjustment using a standard population to which age-specific rates are applied (direct method) combined with sex adjustment will control for variations over time and between population differences in age and sex distributions. Therefore, age- and sex-adjusted rates can be used to compare frequencies of these complications over time within one population or across populations. We must also, however, be concerned with ethnic differences in populations since there are distinct differences in rates of diabetic complications across racial backgrounds *(3)*. Since the United States population is quite heterogeneous compared to populations such as that in Germany or Pacific Islanders, these ethnic differences must be kept in mind when using comparisons of summary rates. Age-adjusted rates within the various ethnic populations (Black, Hispanic, Native American, and so on) are therefore most often used to compare rates of foot ulceration or LEA between groups. Generalizability also becomes an issue when analytical or experimental studies investigate disease frequency or predisposing risk factors in either defined or undefined cohorts. Readers must be particularly cognizant of the population at risk within each study when determining prevalence or incidence rates of disease. Does the population under study only consist of patients with diabetes or is it heterogeneous? Have all of the diabetic patients been included or just those with neuropathy? Have those with vascular disease been excluded or included? The denominator used for calculation of rates is therefore extremely important when generalizing the results of a given study to external populations *(1)*. Furthermore, are rates calculated using numerators on the basis of first-time ulcers or amputations, secondary events, or only the highest level of amputation upon hospital discharge? What is the particular time frame for the reported rates? Is the investigation dealing with a cumulative incidence of ulceration over 4 yr or only one year? In the former case, the total cumulative incidence would be divided by four to yield an annual incidence rate. An excellent example of the variability of rates, numerators, and denominators that can be used to explore various outcomes within this framework has been reported by Apelquist *(5)*. From the foregoing it is clear that when reviewing epidemiological literature, the reader must keep in mind the differences between study populations, the comparability of data, and the generalizability of rates or outcomes among the entire diabetic population.

This chapter will primarily focus on the two major complications of the diabetic foot, ulceration and amputation. In addition to presenting our current estimation of their prevalence, incidence, and natural history based on cross-sectional and analytical studies, a thorough discussion of risk factors will be equally important in our understanding of the pathophysiology leading to these outcomes. Through an appreciation of the underlying determinants of these complications, preventive strategies can be discussed in terms of education and appropriate foot care practices.

## ULCERATIONS

Foot ulceration with infection is one of the leading causes of hospitalization for patients with diabetes mellitus *(6–8)*. Approximately 15% of all patients with diabetes will develop a foot or leg ulceration at some time during the course of their disease *(9)*. However, solid data pertaining to the true incidence and prevalence of diabetic foot lesions is still lacking. Some of the information concerning such pathology is based upon hospital discharge data (NHDS) that does not capture the majority of ulcerations treated in the outpatient setting. Population based studies and cross-sectional surveys provide a general picture of their frequency and distribution, whereas case-control (retrospective) and prospective cohort studies are helpful in determining the associated risk factors for these disorders.

The recent comprehensive epidemiological review by Reiber et al. indicates that chronic ulcers were present in 2.7% of all diabetes-related hospitalizations and 46% of all hospitalizations listing any ulcer condition *(10)*. This NHDS survey data also indicates that the highest rates were found in individuals aged 45–64 yr with males having a higher ulcer rate than in females. The average length of stay (LOS) for diabetes discharges with ulcerations was 59% longer than in those without them, approx 14 and 8 d, respectively.

Several population-based studies report an annual incidence of diabetic foot ulceration in the range of 2–3% in both IDDM and NIDDM patients, whereas the prevalence varies between 4 and 10% *(11–17)*. In the 4-yr prospective cohort study reported by Moss (Wisconsin Epidemiologic Study of Diabetic Retinopathy) the 4-yr cumulative incidence of ulcers in younger-onset patients was 9.5 or 2.4% per year *(11)*. The corresponding 4-yr incidence in older-onset patients (diagnosed after age 30 yr) was 10.5 or 2.6% per year. In a 1984 cross-sectional study of 617 diabetic patients from Stockholm, Sweden the respondents to a self-administered questionnaire reported an ulcer/gangrene prevalence of 4.7% *(12)*. Limitations of this survey were that it included a stratified sample only of persons on registers of previously hospitalized patients and that results were not corroborated by medical record review. Another study from Sweden involving

Table 1
Diabetic Foot Ulcer Incidence and Prevalence: Selected Studies

| *Author(s)* | *Incidence (%)* | *Prevalence (%)* |
|---|---|---|
| Moss et al. (1992) | IDDM: 2.4<br>NIDDM: 2.6 | |
| Borssen (1990) | IDDM: 3 | IDDM: 10<br>NIDDM: 9 |
| Rosenquist (1984) | | 4.4 |
| Kumar (1994) | | 5.3 |
| Walters (1992) | | 7.4 |
| Smith (1994) | 5.6 | |

examinations of 380 diabetic patients aged 15–50 yr reported an ulcer prevalence of 3% *(13)*. Ten percent of the patients had a history of healed ulcers. A community-based study in the UK involving interviews and examinations of 1077 diabetic patients from 10 general practices revealed a prevalence of past or present foot ulcers of 7.4 compared to 2.6% in the 751 control subjects ($p < 0.001$) *(14)*. Thirty-three patients (3.3%) had active foot ulcers at the time of examination. There was no significant difference in ulcer prevalence between male and female subjects nor between Type 1 or Type 2 diabetes. There was a slightly higher frequency of active ulceration in the Oxford Community Diabetes Study, which found a 5% prevalence in all age groups and a 7% prevalence in those diabetic patients aged 60 yr or greater *(15)*. In yet another population study from the UK restricted to persons with Type 2 diabetes, 5.3% of the 811 patients had current or past foot ulcers *(16)*. There was a significant trend for higher prevalence of ulceration with both increasing age and duration of diabetes. Finally, a 3-yr prospective study of 754 diabetic outpatients in Seattle found an annual foot ulcer incidence of 5.6%, whereas the prevalence of prior foot lesions was 28% *(17,18)*. These findings are summarized in Table 1.

### *Risk Factors for Ulceration*

Numerous putative risk factors for diabetic foot ulceration have been ascertained *(6,10,16,17,19–25)*. Aside from the major factors neuropathy, ischemia, infection, and trauma (high pressure), multiple other contributory factors interact to produce foot lesions. Intrinsic risk factors include metabolic or biologic characteristics that may or may not be causally related to diabetes but do contribute to the etiology of ulceration. Such factors include duration of diabetes, glycosylated hemoglobin, peripheral neuropathy, peripheral vascular disease, limited joint mobility, structural deformity, nephropathy, obesity, and impaired visual acuity. Extrinsic risk factors are the result of the patient's interaction with the environment such as trauma, abnormal stress, occupational hazards, social considerations, and cigaret smoking. Table 2 lists these and additional risk factors that must be considered when attempting to identify those patients most susceptible to foot ulceration.

Several recent clinical studies have documented the importance of both neuropathy and vascular disease as predisposing risk factors for foot ulceration. Kumar found in his community survey that increasing Neuropathy Disability Scores (combined measure of

Table 2
Risk Factors for Diabetic Foot Ulceration

| *Intrinsic Factors* | *Extrinsic Factors* |
|---|---|
| Neuropathy | Minor trauma |
| Sensorimotor | High plantar pressures |
| Autonomic | Shoe pressure |
| Vascular disease | High impact |
| Structural deformity | Thermal injury |
| Immunopathy | Hot soaks |
| Limited joint mobility | Frostbite |
| Nephropathy | Chemical burns |
| Age | Bathroom surgery |
| Duration of diabetes | Occupational hazards |
| Blindness | Poor knowledge of diabetes |
| Previous ulceration | |

multiple neurologic deficits) were significantly related to development of foot ulceration after adjusting for both age and duration of diabetes (odds ratio [OR] = 1.3) *(16)*. Vascular disease, as measured by absence of 2 or more pulses or history of revascularization, was also a significant independent predictor of ulceration (OR = 2.6). These community-based findings were also corroborated by Walters wherein logistic regression analysis yielded significant associations with ulceration for both light touch (OR = 2.85) and impaired pain perception (OR = 3.58) *(14)*. An absent dorsalis pedis pulse increased the risk for ulceration sixfold (OR = 6.27). In these studies, as in most others, the majority of ulcerations were neuropathic or neuro-ischemic in origin.

In a clinical evaluation of 314 non-insulin dependent diabetic (NIDDM) patients, cutaneous monofilament pressure perception, vibration, and thermal thresholds were compared among those with and without a history of current or past ulceration *(23)*. Pressure perception thresholds were significantly higher in ulcerated patients and were highly predictive in distinguishing them from those without ulceration. Although not as predictive, vibration and thermal thresholds were also significantly higher in ulcerated patients. A case-control study from the Seattle VA Hospital also analyzed the association between neuropathy and risk of ulceration in comparing 46 ulcerated diabetic patients with 322 diabetic control subjects *(21)*. Significant independent risk factors for diabetic foot ulceration included an inability to sense a 10-g monofilament (OR = 18) *(42)* and absent ankle reflexes (OR = 6.48) after adjusting for age. Additionally, $TcPO_2 < 30$ mmHg imposed a very strong risk (OR = 57.87) when compared to patients with $TcPO_2 > 60$ mmHg. Prospective evidence of the etiologic role of impaired vibratory perception was obtained from Young's 4-yr study of a cohort of 469 diabetic outpatients without a history of ulceration at baseline *(24)*. For final analysis, the patients were stratified into three levels of vibration-perception thresholds (VPT) using biothesiometry. Those patients with VPT > 25 had an eightfold increased risk (OR = 7.99) of ulceration compared to those with VPT < 15, with a cumulative incidence of 19.8 vs 3.0%, respectively. After adjusting for diabetes duration, itself an important risk factor, the independent effect of VPT> 25 remained strong (OR = 6.8).

Table 3
Risk Factors for Diabetic Foot Ulcers

| *Author* | *Long DM Duration* | *Neuropathy (VPT or SW 5.07)* | *High Plantar Pressure* | *Low ABI or TcPO2 or Pulse Deficit* | *High HbA1c* | *Smoking* |
|---|---|---|---|---|---|---|
| Sosenko (1990) | + | + | | | | |
| Rith-Najarian (1992) | + | + | | + | | |
| Veves (1992) | | + | + | | | |
| Moss (1992) | + | | | | + | + |
| Walters (1992) | + | + | | + | | |
| Young (1994) | + | + | | | | |
| McNeely (1995) | | + | | + | | |

Modified from Reiber GE, Boyko EJ, Smith DG: Lower extremity foot ulcers and amputations in diabetes. In: Harris MI, Cowie C, Stern MP, eds. *Diabetes in America, 2nd ed.* NIH Publication No. 95-1468, 1995.

High plantar pressures are a frequent cause of mechanical trauma to the high-risk neuropathic or neuro-ischemic foot. As such, high foot pressures resulting from structural deformities, neuropathy, or inadequate foot wear have long been considered potential causes of plantar ulceration *(20)*. Veves and associates reported the first prospective study in this regard wherein a cohort of 86 diabetic patients were followed for a mean period of 30 mo *(25)*. Using an optical pedobarograph, all patients had baseline and follow-up foot pressure measurements with the intent to investigate its relationship with foot ulceration. At follow-up, 21 feet in 15 patients developed ulceration, all of whom had high pressures (12.3 kg/cm$^2$) at baseline. No ulcerations occurred in patients with normal pressures at baseline and all but one of the lesions occurred in patients with coexistent neuropathy. In concert with cross-sectional studies making similar suggestions, this study provides fairly convincing evidence for the role of high foot pressure in the etiology of plantar ulceration.

Table 3 summarizes the results of these clinical studies, indicating those factors independently associated with risk of ulceration. Figure 1 illustrates the numerous interactions between these risk factors that may lead to diabetic foot ulceration.

## AMPUTATIONS

Approximately 50% of all nontraumatic lower extremity amputations (LEA) in the United States occur in people with diabetes *(10,26–28)*. In 1990 there were 54,000 diabetes-related LEA discharges, accounting for 1.1 million days of hospital stay with an average length of stay (LOS) of 21 d *(3)*. This is an increase of 50% from 1980 when the number of LEAs was reported as 36,000. Depending on the study, the annual incidence of LEA can range between 37 to 137 per 10,000 people with diabetes, a rate 15–40 times higher than that found in nondiabetic individuals *(10,26–29)*. The 1990 age-adjusted rate based on hospital discharge data was 81 per 10,000 diabetic persons, a

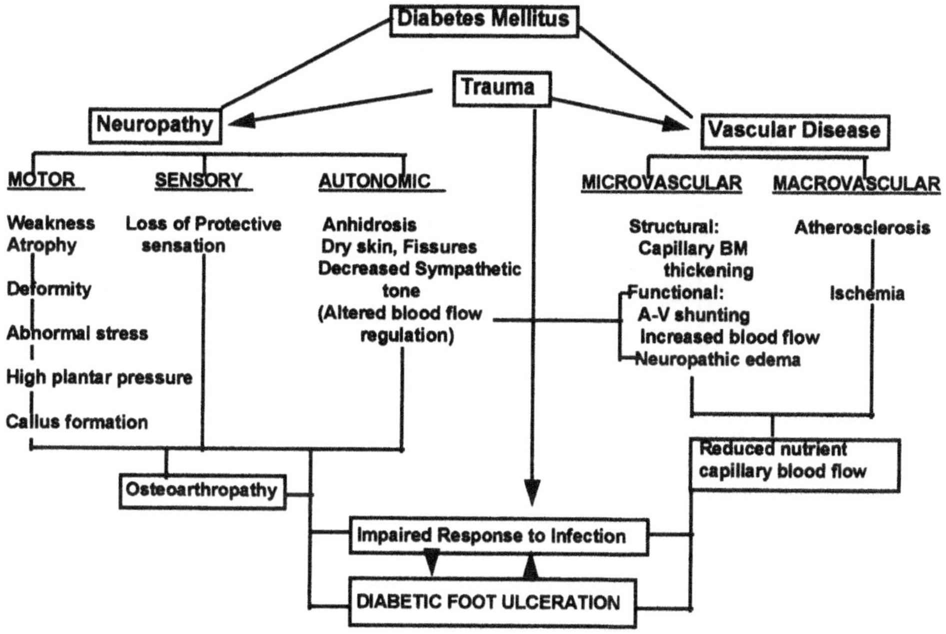


**Fig. 1.** Interactions between contributory factors for diabetic foot ulceration.

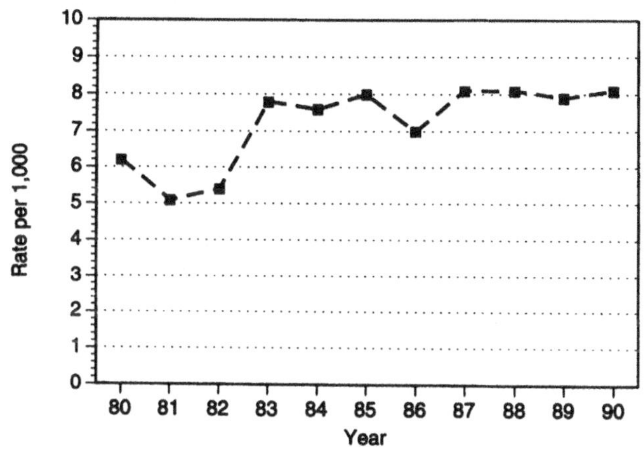


**Fig. 2.** Age-standardized rates for lower extremity amputation in United States per 1000 diabetic population by year. (From Centers for Disease Control and Prevention. *Diabetes Surveillance, 1993.* Atlanta, GA, US Dept. Health and Human Services, 1993, pp. 87–93.)

31% increase from 62 per 10,000 in 1980 *(3,10)* (Fig. 2). Averaging frequencies in the 1989–1992 NHDS, lower-limb amputations (toe, foot, and ankle) are more common in this population with toe amputations comprising approx 40% of all diabetes-related LEA *(10)*. In contrast, above-knee amputations are more frequent in nondiabetic persons, averaging approx 39% of the total amputations vs 16% in persons with diabetes. Below-knee amputations (BKA), comprising approx 21–23% of all LEAs, seem to occur with similar frequencies in both populations. According to the 1989 National

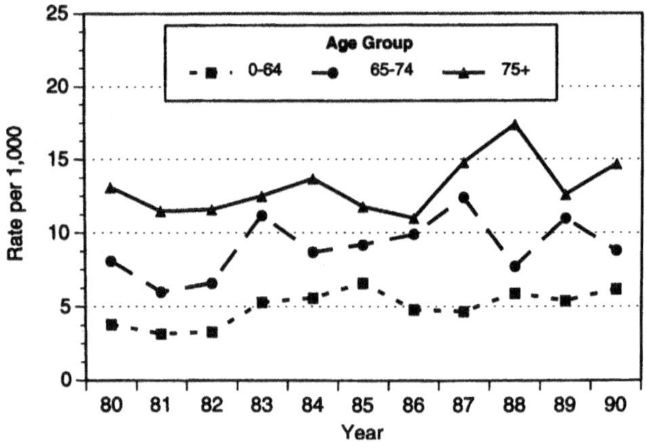


**Fig. 3.** Rates of lower extremity amputation in United State per 1000 diabetic population by age and year. (From Centers for Disease Control and Prevention. *Diabetes Surveillance, 1993.* Atlanta, GA, US Dept. Health and Human Services, 1993, pp. 87–93.)

Health Interview Survey, 2.8% of all diabetic persons surveyed reported a LEA compared with a prevalence of 0.29% in persons not diagnosed with diabetes *(27)*. This implies an overall tenfold risk in persons with known diabetes. LEA prevalence increased with advancing age in both groups, occurring in 3.6% of diabetic persons aged ≥65 yr. These prevalence rates are similar to those found in the Oxford, UK study *(15)*. Diabetic LEA rates also increased with age based on NHDS data, with the age-specific rates gradually increasing from 1980 to 1990 *(3)* (Fig. 3). The highest rate in 1990 was in the ≥75 category (14.7/1000) as opposed to the broad 0–64 category n which the rate was 6.2/1000. Amputation rates are consistently higher in males than in females *(10,13,17,26,29)*. Data from the State of Washington in 1988 indicate an overall relative risk (RR) of 48 for LEA in diabetic men and RR = 39.2 for diabetic women in comparison to persons without diabetes *(29)*. In 1990, the national age-standardized LEA rate was 10.3/1000 for males compared with 6.4/1000 for females, a 60% excess in men *(3)* (Fig. 4). Racial and ethnic differences in frequency of amputation are also readily apparent from recent data. The American Diabetes Association reports that African Americans with diabetes have LEA rates 1.5–2.5 times that of Caucasians, whereas Native Americans rates can reach 3–4 times higher than found in whites *(26)*. The 1990 age-adjusted rate in whites was 6.6/1000, whereas the rate in Blacks was 23% higher at 8.1/1000 with diabetes *(3)* (Fig. 5). A study of California discharge data from 1991 indicates somewhat higher rate distributions between blacks (95.3/10,000) and whites (56/10,000), but the incidence of diabetes-related LEA in Hispanics was approx 20% lower than that found in whites (44.4/10,000) *(31)*. However, diabetes accounted for 83% of all LEAs within the Hispanic population. Prospective data from several Native American populations reveal significantly higher rates of LEA than found in other ethnic groups *(32,33)*. The age-adjusted incidence rate of first LEA among diabetic (NIDDM) Pima Indians was 137/10,000 person-years at risk *(32)*. The rate of amputation in men was 2.6 that of women after controlling for age and diabetes duration. In Oklahoma Indians, first lower-extremity amputation occurred at an incidence rate of 180/10,000 person-years with males also having a rate twice as high as women

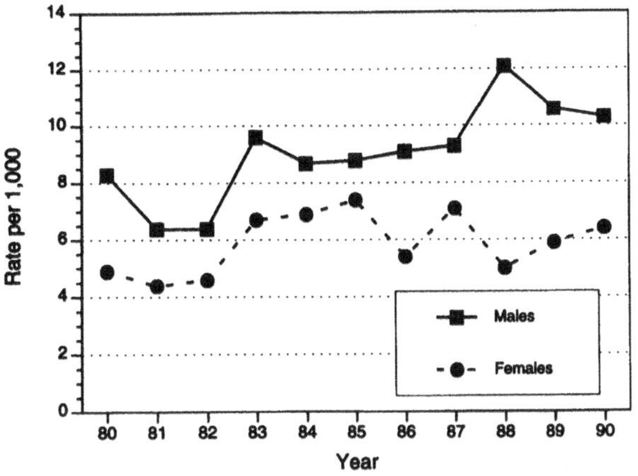


**Fig. 4.** Age-standardized rates for lower extremity amputation in United States per 1000 diabetic population by sex and year. (From Centers for Disease Control and Prevention. *Diabetes Surveillance, 1993*. Atlanta, GA, US Dept. Health and Human Services, 1993, pp. 87–93.)

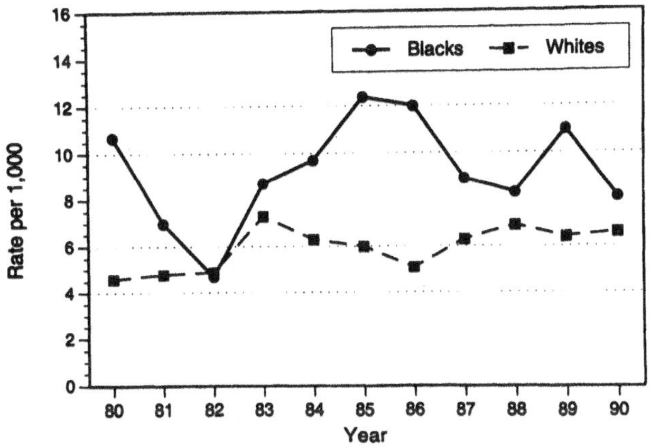


**Fig. 5.** Age-standardized rates for lower extremity amputation in United States per 1000 diabetic population by race and year. (From Centers for Disease Control and Prevention. *Diabetes Surveillance, 1993*. Atlanta, GA, US Dept. Health and Human Services, 1993, pp. 87–93.)

*(33)*. The variations in LEA rate across different populations and ethnic backgrounds are summarized in Table 4.

Several recent population-based studies illustrate both the differences in reported rates of amputation as well as differing methodologies used in determining these rates. The differing methods used to collect and analyze data often contribute to the discrepancies in rates and make direct comparisons somewhat difficult *(34,35)*. Regardless, trends in population are clearly evident, as are the aforementioned differences between sexes, age groups, and racial categories. As methodolgies improve and become more standardized, definitive comparisons between populations will be possible *(34)*.

The 4-yr population-based cohort study from Wisconsin reported the cumulative risk of LEA in both younger-onset and older-onset patients with diabetes to be 2.2% *(11)*. True population incidence rates were not determined nor was a comparison made with a

Table 4
Racial Variations in Incidence of LEA

| | *Lavery 1996 CA* | *CDC 1993 NHDS* | *Trautner 1996 Germany* | *Humphrey 1996 Nauru* | *Lee 1993 OK* | *Nelson 1988 Pima* |
|---|---|---|---|---|---|---|
| White | | | | | | |
| diabetes[a] | 55.98 | 66 | 20.92 | | | |
| no diabetes[a] | 2.01 | | .94 | | | |
| Relative risk | RR = 28 | | RR = 22.2 | | | |
| %LEA in DM | 57% | | 77.4% | | | |
| Black | | | | | | |
| diabetes[a] | 95.25 | 81 | | | | |
| no diabetes[a] | 6.78 | | | | | |
| Relative risk | RR = 14 | | | | | |
| %LEA in DM | 61.6% | | | | | |
| Hispanic | | | | | | |
| diabetes[a] | 44.43 | | | | | |
| no diabetes[a] | 1.74 | | | | | |
| Relative risk | RR = 25 | | | | | |
| %LEA in DM | 82.7% | | | | | |
| Natives | | | | | | |
| diabetes[a] | | | | 81 | 180 | 137 |
| no diabetes[a] | | | | 0 | | |
| Relative risk | | | | RR = ∞ | | |
| %LEA in DM | | | | 100 | | |

[a] Rates per 10,000 at risk.

nondiabetic population. In a retrospective cohort study from the UK, an annual cumulative incidence rate of 5.7/1000 persons with diabetes was estimated *(36)*. As in other retrospective studies, case ascertainment, quality of information, and population-estimation methodologies become problematic. In an older study from the University Group Diabetes Program, there was a 13-yr cumulative LEA incidence of 3%, translating into 2.4 LEA per 1000 patients per year *(37)*. The majority of cases were toe amputations, but the cumulative risk for major amputation (BKA or AKA) was 1.3% or 1/1000 patients per year. One of the more thorough population studies to date was a 25-yr retrospective open cohort study from Rochester, Minnesota *(38)*. All 2015 newly diagnosed patients with diabetes from 1945 through 1979 were entered into the cohort and followed until 1985 for the incidence of lower-limb amputations. The overall incidence of LEA in the diabetic cohort was 375/100,000 person-years (p-y). When age and sex adjusted to the 1980 white United States population, the rate was 167 per 100,000 p-y. In NIDDM the overall rate was 388/100,000 p-y, and for patients with IDDM the rate was 283/100,000 p-y (adjusted values were 162/100,000 p-y and 337/100,000 p-y, respectively). The 25-yr cumulative risk of first LEA for both diabetic groups was approx 11%, with a 17-fold risk of LEA in NIDDM patients in comparison to the non-diabetic population. Furthermore, over 60% of lower extremity amputations in the population at large were attributable to non-insulin dependent diabetes.

Several international studies further illustrate the disparities in rates and prevalence of LEA obtained when studying various populations. In eastern Finland, a population-based retrospective study determined the age-adjusted rate of LEA per year for diabetic men to be 34.9/10,000, whereas the rate for diabetic women was 23.9 per 10,000 *(39)*. When compared to the nondiabetic population, diabetic men and women had a 10.3- and 13.8-fold increased risk of amputation, respectively. A prospective cohort study of 1044 NIDDM patients from western Finland subsequently reported a cumulative incidence of 58 first LEA, 5.6% in men and 5.3% in women after 7 yr *(40)*. Amputated patients had a mean duration of diabetes greater than 9 yr at entry into the cohort. A recent population study from Germany investigated the incidence of LEA by a review of operating-room records over a 2-yr period *(41)*. Although complete case ascertainment questions and population estimations are potential limitations of the study, the reported age-adjusted incidence rate was 20.9 LEA per ten thousand persons with diabetes. Seventy-seven percent of the amputations were performed on diabetic patients yielding a 22-fold increased risk for LEA in diabetes (RR = 22.2) and a population attributable risk of 72%. Two further prevalence surveys from Europe have recently been reported and seem to agree in their estimation of amputation frequency. In an outpatient survey of 5843 diabetic patients from the Lombardia region of Italy, an overall LEA prevalence of 1.2% was found, whereas in England, a community-based survey and examination of 7820 persons with diabetes yielded an LEA prevalence of 1.25% *(42,43)*. Finally, in a study from the Central Pacific island of Nauru, the estimated annual age-adjusted incidence of LEA in NIDDM was reported to be 76 per 10,000 person-years nationally and 81 per 10,000 p-y in a retrospective cohort study *(44)*. These rates are comparable with those found in United States Pima Indians, especially when also stratified by duration of diabetes *(32)*. Although these contrasts are useful in describing incidence and prevalence of LEA in defined populations, it should be reiterated that cross comparisons are difficult because of discrepant methodologies and lack of standard reporting techniques *(34)*. Table 5 summarizes the rates reported in several of these studies.

### *Amputation Risk Factors*

Risk factors for diabetic LEA, are quite similar to those for foot ulceration. In fact, foot ulceration itself seems to be a major predisposing risk factor for LEA, preceding approx 85% of patients who go on to amputation *(5,10,45,46)*. Therefore, the aforementioned etiologic factors for foot ulceration should certainly be considered putative risk factors for LEA as is the prior occurrence of lower-limb amputation at any level. Most studies indicate that duration of diabetes, degree of glucose control, and various measures of neuropathy are independent predictors for amputation, as are blood pressure, retinopathy, nephropathy, and peripheral vascular disease or low $TcPO_2$ *(11,32,33,40, 44–48)*. Cigaret smoking is an inconsistent risk factor across a variety of study designs, perhaps because of a lack of power and inadequate samples of smokers. Table 6 summarizes the results of several studies investigating risk factors for diabetic LEA.

In their landmark paper, Pecoraro et al. determined the causal pathways responsible for lower-extremity amputations in a series of consecutive male diabetic patients *(46)*. Using the model established by Rothman, the causal sequence was defined by both component and sufficient causes *(49)*. *Component* causes are risk factors that are insufficient by themselves to cause the outcome of interest (LEA or ulceration) but are

Table 5
Summary of Incidence of Lower Extremity Amputations in Selected Studies

| | *Age-adjusted Number of LEAs Per 10,000 Persons Per Year* | | | *Diabetes-specific Findings* | | |
|---|---|---|---|---|---|---|
| *Study (year)* | *No Diabetes* | *Diabetes* | *RR* | *Diabetes Among LEA Cases (%)* | *Below-knee And Above-knee of Total LEA (%)* | *Mean Hospital LOS* |
| Nelson (1988) | 1.3[a] | 137[a] | 105 | 95 | 16 | |
| Washington (1991) | 1.0 | 52 | 52 | 50 | | |
| Newcastle (1992) | | 57 | | 42 | 63 | |
| CDC (1993) | | 81 | | 51 | 43 | 20.6 |
| Lee (1993) | | 180[a] | | | 41.7 | |
| Humphrey (1994) | | 16.7[a] | 17 | 61 | 68 | |
| Lavery (1996) | 3.5 | 54 | 15 | 62.6 | | |
| Lehto (1996) | | (5.5%) | | | 46 | |
| Humphrey (1996) | | 84[a] | | 100 | 61 | |
| Trautner (1996) | .94 | 21 | 22 | 77 | 44 | |

[a] Estimates given as incidence per 10,000 person-years.

Modified from Reiber GE, Boyko EJ, Smith DG. Lower extremity foot ulcers and amputations in diabetes. In: Harris MI, Cowie C, Stern MP, eds. *Diabetes in America, 2nd ed.* NIH Publication No. 95-1468, 1995.

Table 6
Risk Factors for Diabetic Lower Extremity Amputation

| *Author* | *Neuropathy* | *Duration* | *High HbA1c* | *High BP* | *Sex* | *Ulcer* | *PVD or $TcPO_2$* | *Smoking* |
|---|---|---|---|---|---|---|---|---|
| Nelson (1988) | + | + | + | | + | | | 0 |
| Reiber (1992) | + | | + | | | + | + | 0 |
| Moss (1992) | | + | + | | + | + | | + |
| Lee (1993) | | + | + | + | + | + | | |
| Selby (1995) | + | + | + | + | | | | 0 |
| Lehto (1996) | + | + | + | | | | + | 0 |
| Humphrey (1996) | | + | + | | + | | | 0 |

Modified from Reiber GE, Boyko EJ, Smith DG. Lower extremity foot ulcers and amputations in diabetes. In: Harris MI, Cowie C, Stern MP, eds. *Diabetes in America, 2nd ed.* NIH Publication No. 95-1468, 1995.

Table 7
Mortality Following LEA in DM

| *Selected studies by time period* | *Reference* | *%* |
|---|---|---|
| • **1-yr mortality** | | |
| —Lund, Sweden | *(5)* | 20 |
| —Newcastle, UK | *(36)* | 40 |
| • **2-yr mortality** | | |
| —Lund | *(5)* | 31 |
| —Newcastle | *(36)* | 50 |
| • **3-yr mortality** | | |
| —Lund | *(5)* | 41 |
| —Oklahoma Indians | *(33)* | 40 |
| • **5-yr mortality** | | |
| —Pima Indians | *(32)* | 39 |
| —Oklahoma Indians | *(33)* | 60 |
| —Lund | *(5)* | 73 |

required components of a complete causal pathway that is sufficient to produce the outcome. A *sufficient* cause is therefore a constellation or grouping of the minimal number of specific component causes that, in concert with each other, inevitably produce disease. There can be a number of sufficient causes with various combinations of component causes that produce the same outcome. However, removal of any component cause will block the completed pathway to the sufficient cause and thereby prevent disease through this specific pathway. Pecoraro found that the particular triad of minor trauma, cutaneous ulceration, and wound healing failure preceded 72% of amputations, often in combination with gangrene and infection *(46)*. Eighty-four percent of the amputations could in part be attributed to cutaneous ulceration, 81% to faulty wound healing, 81% to initial minor trauma, 46% to ischemia, 55% to gangrene, 59% to infection, and 61% to neuropathy. A pivotal triggering event was identifiable in 86% of the cases which led to the sequence of events completing the causal chain to amputation. Most of the pivotal events were minor trauma that caused ulceration and most could have been prevented.

## MORTALITY

Prevention or control of predisposing risk factors takes on immediate significance when one evaluates the survival data after lower-extremity amputation in diabetic patients. (Table 7). The 3- and 5-yr survival rates are approx 50 and 40%, respectively with the major cause of death being from cardiovascular disease *(26)*. Following one lower-extremity amputation, there is a 50% incidence of serious contralateral foot lesion within 2-yr and a 50% incidence of contralateral amputation within 2–5 yr *(50)*. The 30-d diabetic amputation mortality averaged 5.8% in the United States between 1989 and 1992 according to NHDS data *(10)*. A study from Lund, Sweden reported only a 27% 5-yr survival rate after amputation with a fourfold excess risk of mortality when compared to an age- and sex-matched Swedish population *(5)*. These authors also found a 3-yr cumulative additional amputation rate of 48% after undergoing an initial diabetic

LEA, indicating the significance of this event as a risk factor for further amputation. The higher mortality rates in diabetic patients were confirmed in a Finnish study that contrasted survival after first LEA between diabetic and nondiabetic subjects *(39)*. After adjusting for age, diabetes status *per se* did not contribute to mortality in men, but independently predicted mortality in women. In a study of LEA in the Netherlands, the perioperative age-adjusted death incidence after diabetes-related amputations was 36.3/1000, whereas the rate in nondiabetic LEA was 28.2/1000 *(51)*. Although 9% of the diabetic amputees died while in the hospital, nondiabetic amputees with peripheral vascular disease (PVD) had higher mortality rates than even the diabetic patients with PVD. In the diabetic population, both age and multiple amputations within one hospitalization were significant negative predictors for surviving the operation. In the retrospective survey from Newcastle, UK, the mortality within 30 d after amputation was 10% *(36)*. The median life expectancy was 22 mo after surgery and 19% of the patients underwent an additional amputation within the 36-mo follow-up period. Most of these patients had PVD and the majority of amputations were at or above the knee level. In the 12-yr Pima Indian study, 15% of all diabetic deaths occurred in amputees *(32)*. After controlling for age, sex, and diabetes duration, the death rate in amputees was 1.6 times greater than that of nonamputated diabetic persons. The estimated 5-yr survival was 61% in this population after first LEA, with the most common causes of death being cardiovascular disease. Also within the Native American population, the Oklahoma Indian Study reported a 66% increased mortality in those NIDDM patients with amputation compared to nonamputees *(33)*. There was also a trend for higher death rates with higher levels of amputations, as found in other mortality studies. The 3-yr survival rate after first LEA was 59.8%, whereas 40.4% survived after 5 yr. Diabetes and cardiovascular disease were the most common causes of death. In summary, it is apparent that survival rates after diabetic LEA vary depending on age, sex, level of amputation, and perhaps across populations. Notwithstanding these factors, diabetic amputees clearly suffer earlier mortality than their diabetic cohorts who have not undergone amputation.

## PREVENTION

Prevention is indeed the key element in reducing the incidence not only of lower-extremity amputation, but of diabetic foot ulcerations as well. Since approx 70–80% or more of amputations are preceded by ulceration, efforts aimed at preventing foot lesions can also have a major impact on the frequency of amputation *(5,46,52)*. This is best accomplished through the coordinated effort of multiple specialists working together as a foot-care team with a primary goal of limb preservation *(6,20,52,53,54)*. Regular podiatric examinations and foot care, proper footwear, pressure reduction, and patient education are the major facets of the prevention program *(53)*. When an acute lesion develops, the entire foot-care team is called into service to provide aggressive, early intervention to prevent progression of the lesion. As indicated, foot-sparing procedures are preferred to amputations, with an eye towards maintaining foot function and structure *(54)*. Once healed, attention is redirected to preventive foot care, appropriate shoeing, and preventive education. Figure 6 illustrates the composition of such a foot team that employs the services of a podiatrist, diabetologist, vascular surgeon, and numerous other multidisciplinary specialists.

The success of the multidisciplinary team approach has been amply demonstrated by Edmonds et al., who reported that 86% of neuropathic ulcers and 72% of ischemic

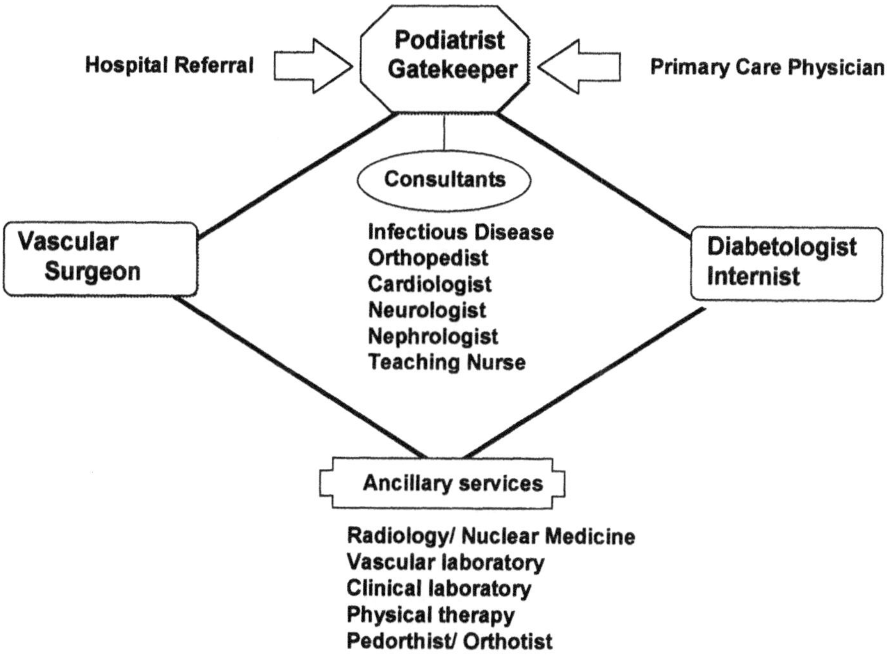


**Fig. 6.** Paradigm for multidisciplinary diabetic foot service.

ulcers healed through such a comprehensive management *(6)*. Those patients who wore appropriate footwear as recommended experienced one-third the relapse rate of ulceration as compared to those who wore their usual shoes. Notably, there was a 58% reduction in the number of annual amputations once the specialized foot clinic had been established. The Manchester program also relies heavily on podiatric care in providing prophylactic foot care, pressure reduction, and ulcer care *(55)*. Although achieving healing in 81% of their ulcer cases, they note a 42% reduction in amputation since the initiation of the multidisciplinary clinic. In the United States, a dramatic reduction in yearly amputations was reported from the Winnebago Indian Health Service Hospital *(56)*. After the implementation of a podiatric medical service to provide comprehensive foot care to this high-risk population, a 100% reduction in amputation rate was achieved within 1 yr. Averaging 16 lower-limb amputations annually before the program, no limbs had been reported lost in the 2 yr since its establishment. At the New England Deaconess Hospital in Boston, significant reductions in LEA and length of hospital stay have taken place since integrating podiatric services and local procedures into the limb-salvage strategy for ischemic diabetic foot ulcers and infections *(57,58)*. Finally, a 78% reduction in the incidence of major amputations was achieved in Sweden upon the establishment of a multidisciplinary program for the prevention and treatment of diabetic foot ulcers *(52)*.

As many of the cited studies suggest, the majority of amputations could be prevented through programs designed to prevent and treat foot ulcers and that recognize the essential role of patient education pertaining to diabetic foot care. The American Diabetes Association estimates that up to 50% of diabetic LEA can be prevented through aggressive treatment and education programs *(26)*. With an annual incidence of 80/10,000 people, they project that 15,000 amputations per year can be prevented should this target be achieved. Aside from morbidity, mortality, and disability associated with LEA, the cost savings attendant with prevention programs are quite significant. The total cost of an amputation is estimated to be between $24,000 and 40,000 with approx $1 billion spent on the 54,000 LEAs performed in 1990 *(10)*. If just 15,000 cases per year can be prevented as predicted by the ADA, a cost savings of $360 million annually could be realized. Clearly, this tragic outcome of diabetic foot lesions must be adequately addressed and controlled if we are to improve the quality of life of the 16 million people in the United States with this disease. Recognizing both the necessity and morbidity attendant with diabetic lower-extremity amputations, the United States Department of Health and Human Services has set a goal to reduce the incidence of such procedures by 40% by the year 2000 *(59)*.

## REFERENCES

1. Reiber GE. Epidemiology of the diabetic foot. In: Levin M, O'Neal L, Bowker J eds. The Diabetic Foot, 5th ed. Mosby Yearbook, St. Louis, 1993, pp. 1–15.
2. Aubert RE, Geiss LS, Ballard DJ, Cocanougher B, Herman WH. Diabetes related hospitalization and hospital utilization. In: Harris MI, Cowie C, Stern MP, Boyko EJ, Reiber GE, Bennett PH, eds. Diabetes in America, 2nd ed. NIH Publication No. 95-1468, 1995, pp. 553–569.
3. Centers for Disease Control and Prevention. Diabetes Surveillance, 1993. Atlanta, GA, U.S. Dept. Health and Human Services, 1993, pp. 87–93.
4. International Classification of Diseases, Ninth Revision: Clinical Modifications (ICD 9 CM), vol. 3, ed. 2. DHHS publ. no. (PHS) 80-1260. Rockville, MD, 1980, U.S. Gov. Printing Office, p. 235.
5. Apelquist J, Larsson J, Agardh C-D. Long term prognosis for patients with foot ulcers. J Int Med 1993;233:485–491.
6. Edmonds ME, Blundell MP, Morris ME, et al. Improved survival of the diabetic foot: the role of a specialized foot clinic. Q J Med 1986;232:763.
7. Gibbons GW, Eliopoulos GM. Infection of the diabetic foot. In: Kozak GP, Campbell DR, Frykberg RG, Habershaw GM eds. Management of Diabetic Foot Problems. WB Saunders, Philadelphia, 1995, p. 121.
8. Sussman KE, Reiber G, Albert SF. The diabetic foot problem—a failed system of health care? Diabetes Res Clin Pract 1992;17:1.
9. Palumbo PJ, Melton LJ. Peripheral vascular disease and diabetes. In: Diabetes in America: Data compiled 1984. (NIH publ. no. 85-1468). US Government Printing Office, Washington, DC, 1985, p. 1.
10. Reiber GE, Boyko EJ, Smith DG. Lower extremity foot ulcers and amputations in diabetes. In: Harris MI, Cowie C, Stern MP, eds. Diabetes in America, 2nd ed. NIH Publication No. 95-1468, 1995.
11. Moss SE, Klein R, Klein B. The prevalence and incidence of lower extremity amputation in a diabetic population. Arch Internal Med 1992;152:610–616.
12. Rosenqvist U. An epidemiological survey of diabetic foot problems in the Stockholm County 1982. Acta Med Scand 1984;(Suppl)687:55.
13. Borssen B, Bergenheim T, Lithner F. The epidemiology of foot lesions in diabetic patients aged 15–50 years. Diabetic Med 1990;7:438–444.
14. Walters DP, Gatling W, Mullee MA, Hill RD. The distribution and severity of diabetic foot disease: a community study with comparison to a non-diabetic group. Diabetic Med 1992;9:354–358.
15. Neil HAW, Thompson AV, Thorogood M, Fowler GH, Mann JI. Diabetes in the elderly: the Oxford Community Diabetes Study. Diabetic Med 1989;6:608–613.
16. Kumar S, Ashe HA, Parnell LN, Fernando DJS, Tsigos C, Young RJ, Ward JD, Boulton AJM. The prevalence of foot ulceration and its correlates in Type 2 diabetic patients: a population-based study. Diabetic Med 1994;11:480–484.
17. Reiber G. The epidemiology of diabetic foot problems. Diabetic Med 1996;13:S6–S11.
18. Smith DG, Boyko E, Ahroni JH. Prospective evaluation of the risk factors for foot ulceration in diabetes—early results. American Orthopedic Foot and Ankle Society, New Orleans, LA, 1994.
19. Sims DS, Cavanagh PR, Ulbrecht JS. Risk factors in the diabetic foot; recognition and management. Physical Ther 1988;68:1887.

20. Frykberg RG. Diabetic foot ulcerations. In: Frykberg RG, ed. The High Risk Foot in Diabetes Mellitus. Churchill Livingstone, New York, 1991, p. 151.
21. McNeely MJ, Boyko E, Ahroni JH. The independent contributions of diabetic neuropathy and vasculopathy in foot ulceration: how great are the risks? Diabetes Care 1995;18:216–219.
22. Boulton AJM. The pathogenesis of diabetic foot problems: an overview. Diabetic Medicine 1996;13:S12–S16.
23. Sosenko JM, Kato M, Soto R, Bild DE. Comparison of quantitative sensory threshold measures for their association with foot ulceration in diabetic patients. Diabetes Care 1990;13:1057–1061.
24. Young MJ, Breddy JL, Veves A, Boulton AJM. The prediction of diabetic neuropathic foot ulceration using vibration perception thresholds: a prospective study. Diabetes Care 1994;17:557–560.
25. Veves A, Murray HJ, Young MJ, Boulton AJM. The risk of foot ulceration in diabetic patients with high foot pressure: a prospective study. Diabetologia 1992;35:660–663.
26. American Diabetes Association. Diabetes 1996 Vital Statistics. American Diabetes Association, Alexandria, VA, 1996, p. 31.
27. Most RS, Sinnock P. The epidemiology of lower extremity amputations in diabetic individuals. Diabetes Care 1983;6:87–91.
28. Bild DE, Selby JV, Sinnock P, Browner WS, Braveman P, Showstack JA. Lower extremity amputation in people with diabetes: epidemiology and prevention. Diabetes Care 1989;12:24–31.
29. Anonymous. Lower extremity amputations among persons with diabetes mellitus—Washington, 1988. MMWR 1991;40:737–739.
30. National Center for Health Statistics. Current estimates from the National Health Interview Survey, 1989. Vital and Health Statistics Series 10, no. 176, 1990.
31. Lavery LA, Ashry HR, van Houtum W, Pugh JA, Harkless LB, Basu S. Variation in the incidence and proportion of diabetes-related amputations in minorities. Diabetes Care 1996;19:48–52.
32. Nelson RG, Gohdes DM, Everhart JE, Hartner JA, Zwemer FL, Pettit DJ, Knowler WC. Lower extremity amputations in NIDDM: 12-yr follow-up study in Pima Indians. Diabetes Care 1988;11:8–16.
33. Lee JS, Lu M, Lee VS, Russel D, Bahr C, Lee ET. Lower-extremity amputation: incidence, risk factors, and mortality in the Oklahoma Indian Diabetes Study. Diabetes 1993;42:876–882.
34. LEA Study Group. Comparing the incidence of lower extremity amputations across the world: the Global Lower Extremity Amputation Study. Diabetic Med 1995;12:14–18.
35. Edmonds M, Boulton A, Buckenham T, Every N, Foster A, Freeman D, Gadsby R, Gibby O, Knowles A, Pooke M, Tovey F, Unwin N, Wolfe J. Report of the Diabetic Foot and Amputation Group. Diabetic Med 1996;13:S27–S42.
36. Deerochanawong C, Home PD, Alberti K. A survey of lower limb amputation in diabetic patients. Diabetic Med 1992;9:942–946.
37. Kreines K, Johnson E, Albrink M, Knatterud G, Levin M, Lewitan A, Newberry W, Rose F. The course of peripheral vascular disease in Non-insulin dependent diabetes. Diabetes Care 1985;8:235–243.
38. Humphrey LL, Palumbo PJ, Butters MA, Hallet JW, Chu C, O'Fallon WM, Ballard DJ. The contribution of non-insulin dependent diabetes to lower extremity amputation in the community. Arch Intern Med 1994;154:885–892.
39. Sittonen O, Niskanen L, Laakso M, Sittonen J, Pyorala K. Lower extremity amputations in diabetic and nondiabetic patients: a population-based study in eastern Finland. Diabetes Care 1993;16:16–20.
40. Lehto S, Ronnemaa T, Pyorala K, Laakso M. Risk factors predicting lower extremity amputations in patients with NIDDM. Diabetes Care 1996;19:607–612.
41. Trautner C, Haasert B, Giani G, Berger M. Incidence of lower limb amputations and diabetes. Diabetes Care 1996;19:1006–1009.
42. Segalini G, Aldeghi A, Morabito A, Radici M. Prevalence of lower extremity amputations and ulcers in the Lombardia region diabetic out-patients population. (abstract). Diabetes 1996;45(Suppl 2):108A.
43. Carrington A, Abbott C, Kulkarni J, Van Ross E, Boulton A. Prevalence and prevention of foot ulceration and amputation in North Western England. Diabetes 1996;45(Suppl 2):26A.
44. Humphrey A, Dowse G, Thoma K, Zimmet P. Diabetes and nontraumatic lower extremity amputations: incidence, risk factors, and prevention—a 12 year follow-up study in Nauru. Diabetes Care 1996;19:710–714.
45. Reiber GE, Pecoraro RE, Koepsell TD. Risk factors for amputation in patients with diabetes mellitus: a case-control study. Ann Int Med 1992;117:97–105.

46. Pecoraro RE, Reiber G, Burgess EM. Pathways to diabetic limb amputation; basis for prevention. Diabetes Care 1990;13:513.
47. Selby JV, Zhang D. Risk factors for lower extremity amputation in persons with diabetes. Diabetes Care 1995;18:509–516.
48. Rith-Najarian S, Stolusky T, Gohdes D. Identifying diabetic patients at high risk for lower extremity amputation in a primary health care setting: a prospective evaluation of simple screening criteria. Diabetes Care 1992;15:1386–1389.
49. Rothman KJ. Modern Epidemiology. Little, Brown, Boston, MA, 1986.
50. Goldner MG. The fate of the second leg in the diabetic amputee. Diabetes 1960;9:100–103.
51. Lavery L, van Houtum W, Harkless L. In-hospital mortality and disposition of diabetic amputees in the Netherlands. Diabetic Med 1996;13:192–197.
52. Larsson J, Apelqvist J, Agardh C-D, Stenstrom A. Decreasing incidence of major amputation in diabetic patients: a consequence of a multidisciplinary foot care team approach? Diabetic Med 1995;12:770–776.
53. Frykberg RG. Podiatrist's role in the care and treatment of the diabetic foot. In: Baba S, Kaneko T, eds. Diabetes 1994. Elsevier, Amsterdam, 1995, pp. 734–743.
54. Caputo GM, Cavanagh PR, Ulbrecht JS, Gibbons GW, Karchmer AW. Assessment and management of foot disease in patients with diabetes. N Engl J Med 1994;331:854–860.
55. Thomson FJ, Veves A, Ashe H, Knowles EA, Gem J, Walker MG, Hirst P, Boulton A. A team approach to diabetic foot care—the Manchester experience. The Foot 1991;2:75–82.
56. Levy LA, Ung KV. Unusual prevalence of diabetes mellitus among Native Americans and the podiatric medical implications. Lower Extremity 1994;1:3–8.
57. Logerfo FW, Gibbons GW, Pompselli FB, Campbell DR, Miller A, Freeman D, Quist W. Trends in the care of the diabetic foot: expanded role of arterial reconstruction. Arch Surg 1992;127:617–621.
58. Gibbons GW, Marcaccio EJ, Burgess AM, Pomposelli FB, Freeman D, Campbell DR, Miller A, Logerfo F. Improved quality of diabetic foot care, 1984 vs 1990: reduced length of stay and costs, insufficient reimbursement. Arch Surg 1993;128:576–581.
59. Diabetes and Chronic Disabling Conditions. In: Healthy People 2000. US Department of Health and Human Services, Public Health Service. DHHS publ. no. PHS 91–50212, 1991, p. 442.

# 18 The Pathogenesis of Foot Problems

*Jonathan E. Shaw*, MRCP
*and Andrew J. M. Boulton*, MD, FRCP

*CONTENTS*



## INTRODUCTION

The diabetic foot can present with many different problems, but the most important clinically are ulceration, amputation, and Charcot neuroarthropathy. These will be the focus of this chapter. Many diabetic complications have a great impact on the foot and it is therefore not surprising that diabetic foot problems account for more hospital inpatient days than any other diabetic problem *(1)*. Diabetic neuropathy and peripheral vascular disease are the main etiological factors in foot ulceration, and may act alone, together, or in combination with other factors such as microvascular disease, biomechanical abnormalities, limited joint mobility, and increased susceptibility to infection. A thorough understanding of the contributory factors that lead to foot ulceration and amputation is essential for successful treatment of established pathology. Perhaps more importantly, as the role of education and appropriate footwear in preventing ulceration and amputation is now established, accurate identification of high-risk patients on whom these services can be focused is vital.

## PERIPHERAL VASCULAR DISEASE

Atherosclerotic vascular disease is probably present (at least in a subclinical form) in most patients with long-duration diabetes. The basic pathophysiology of atherosclerosis is no different in diabetic than nondiabetic patients and is characterized by endothelial damage followed by platelet aggregation, lipid deposition, and smooth muscle proliferation with plaque formation. The same risk factors also operate and include smoking, hypertension, dyslipidaemia, abnormal fibrinolysis, and altered platelet function *(2)*. These classical risk factors, however, do not fully explain the huge excess of vascular disease in diabetes, and attention has recently focused on endothelial dysfunction and

From: *Contemporary Endocrinology: Clinical Management of Diabetic Neuropathy*
Edited by: A. Veves © Humana Press Inc., Totowa, NJ

particularly adhesion molecules. Binding of monocytes, leukocytes, and platelets to the endothelium is one of the earliest steps in the pathogenesis of the atherosclerotic plaque and is promoted by adhesion molecules, such as intercellular adhesion molecule-1 and vascular cell adhesion molecule-1. Such molecules have now been found to be elevated in diabetes *(3)* and especially so in patients with microalbuminuria *(4)*, a group known to be at particularly high risk of vascular disease.

Like other forms of macrovascular disease, peripheral vascular disease (PVD) is more common in diabetes. The Framingham study found a 50% excess of absent foot pulses in diabetic females and a nonsignificant 23% excess in diabetic males *(5)*. In another population-based study using Doppler pressures, PVD (diagnosed as ankle brachial pressure index less than or equal to 0.9) was found to be 2.5 to 3 times more common in diabetic than nondiabetic subjects *(6)*. Only in females with type 1 diabetes was the excess of PVD over controls not statistically significant, but this was probably related to the small number of cases. The distribution of vascular disease in the lower limb is thought to be different in diabetes, with more frequent involvement of vessels below the knee. Surprisingly, however, there are few good studies available to support this widely held belief. In diabetic patients with known vascular disease, Strandness reported two thirds of the patients having infrapopliteal disease *(7)* on the basis of clinical findings, and King found involvement of the profunda femoris was increased in diabetes *(8)*. A recent detailed study of angiograms *(9)* demonstrated that among patients requiring angiography for clinical purposes, proximal disease was equally common in diabetic and nondiabetic subjects, but calf-vessel stenoses were about twice as frequent in diabetic subjects. Although PVD is more prevalent among the diabetic population, once established, it does not progress any more rapidly than does PVD in the nondiabetic population *(10)*. The difficulties posed by the distribution may be further complicated by a reduced ability to develop a collateral supply, but despite these problems, revascularization procedures are frequently successful, although may require a more distal anastomosis.

In the pathogenesis of ulcers, ischemia is a major factor in 38 to 52% of cases *(11,12)*, and Pecoraro attributed 46% of amputations to ischemia *(13)*. Unlike nondiabetic patients with PVD, who usually present with intermittent claudication, the first presentation among diabetic patients is often with ischemic ulceration or even gangrene. This is probably because of a combination of concomitant neuropathy and a more distal pattern of involvement, but means that the disease is more advanced at presentation, and less amenable to revascularization either by angioplasty or bypass. Spontaneous ischemic ulceration is rare and the usual trigger is minor trauma. Injury leads to increased demands on the circulation that cannot be met, and ischemic ulceration with the risk of amputation follow.

## DIABETIC NEUROPATHY

### *Somatic Neuropathy*

Chronic sensorimotor peripheral neuropathy, as detailed in other chapters, is one of the commonest long-term complications of diabetes. It was found in at least one third of older diabetic hospital outpatients *(14)*, in 28% of IDDM subjects in the large EURODIAB study *(15)* and in 16% of a population-based sample from the south of England *(16)*. Peripheral somatic neuropathy has been associated with foot ulceration in several cross-sectional studies *(17,18)*, and its central role in ulceration has been confirmed by a recent prospective study. Young et al. showed that in a population free of significant peripheral vascular disease, peripheral neuropathy as measured by vibration perception using a biothesiometer was associated with a sevenfold increase in the risk of foot ulceration during a 4-yr follow-up period *(19)*. Similarly, using pressure perception thresholds—another large fiber function—in a 32-mo prospective study of American Indians, insensitivity to the 10-g monofilament predicted a 10-fold increase in plantar ulceration *(20)*. The onset of neuropathy is insidious and data from the Rochester study suggest that only 28 to 29% of patients with objective evidence of neuropathy have any related symptoms *(21)*. Thus, progression to the insensitive foot at high risk of ulceration can occur without the patient being aware of any disorder. Identification of the neuropathic foot at risk of ulceration therefore relies on careful and regular examination. The presence of neuropathic pain does not of course mean that sensation is intact; usually the opposite applies and positive neuropathic symptoms are accompanied by reduced or absent sensation rendering the foot at high risk of ulceration. The high-risk foot typically has reduced or absent sensation to painful, thermal, and vibration modalities. Moreover, the motor component leads to wasting of the small intrinsic muscles of the foot with a consequent imbalance of flexor and extensor muscles leading to clawing of the toes and prominence of the metatarsal heads. This alters the biomechanical function of the foot, and is discussed later in this chapter.

### *Autonomic Neuropathy*

Sympathetic dysfunction affecting the lower limbs leads to reduced sweating and results in dry skin that is prone to crack and fissure. This can be an initiating event in foot ulceration, and can act as a portal of entry for microorganisms. Sympathetic failure also increases blood flow to the foot (in the absence of large vessel PVD) as a result of opening of arteriovenous shunts. The insensitive foot is therefore often warm, resulting in a false sense of security, as the patient (and unfortunately sometimes the physician) perceives that because the circulation is intact, the risk is minimal. Autonomic neuropathy can also markedly reduce toe blood pressure *(22)*—an important observation, as toe pressures are sometimes used to assess PVD in an attempt to overcome the problems of the false elevation of ankle pressures caused by medial arterial calcification.

It must be pointed out, however, that the neuropathic foot does not ulcerate spontaneously: It is the combination of neuropathy and trauma, whether extrinsic from, for example, ill-fitting footwear or intrinsic from repetitive pressure on the plantar surface of the foot during walking that results in tissue breakdown. Thus, the dorsum of the toes, where tight shoes usually rub, and the metatarsal heads, where dynamic plantar pressures are highest, are the most frequent sites of neuropathic ulceration.

## OTHER RISK FACTORS FOR FOOT ULCERS

### *Biomechanical Aspects*

The trauma required to ulcerate the neuropathic foot can take several different forms. Sometimes it is a single event such as standing on a nail, but more frequently it occurs as repeated minor trauma such as unperceived shoe rubbing to the toes or increased pressure beneath the metatarsal heads during walking. A number of studies have clearly demonstrated that vertical dynamic plantar foot pressures are elevated in diabetic neuropathy and especially in patients with a history of plantar ulceration *(23,24)*. More importantly, a prospective study has shown that elevated plantar pressures are predictive of ulceration, with 17% of patients with high foot pressures developing plantar ulcers during a 30-mo follow-up period, whereas no plantar ulcers developed in patients with normal pressures *(25)*. The presence of callus (hypertrophy and excessive keratinization of the stratum corneum in response to pressure) may exacerbate the problem both by acting as a foreign body and by increasing plantar pressures. The presence of callus has been shown among patients with neuropathy and high pressures to be a strong predictor of plantar ulceration *(26)*, and its removal significantly reduces foot pressures *(27)*. Interestingly, callus was a better predictor of ulceration than was foot pressure *(26)*, and there are a number of possible explanations for this. Firstly, callus may provide a real measure of long-term exposure to high pressure (mainly while wearing footwear), whereas foot pressures in this study measured only the barefoot condition. Secondly, the variability of foot-pressure measurements probably reduces their predictive power. Thirdly, the pressure required to produce callus may vary between individuals, but the development of callus may represent an abnormal response to pressure, which is part of the same process that leads to ulceration. Finally, foot-pressure systems measure only vertical pressure, but callus and ulceration develop in response to vertical and horizontal forces, and callus may represent a better measure of "total pressure."

The main cause of increased pressure is thought to be the alteration in foot shape resulting in prominent metatarsal heads. The distal nature of diabetic neuropathy is equally true for the motor, as well as the sensory changes, and causes atrophy of the intrinsic muscles of the foot (predominantly plantar flexors of the toes), with sparing of the long dorsiflexors. This alters the flexor/extensor balance at the metatarso-phalangeal (mtp) joints and causes clawing of the toes and may be associated with subluxation at the MTP joints. There is a resultant anterior displacement of the submetatarsal fat pads, and indeed reduced subcutaneous tissue thickness at the metatarsal heads has been confirmed in diabetic neuropathy *(28)*. Similar foot deformities are seen in rheumatoid arthritis, and a similar combination of increased foot pressures and reduced subcutaneous tissue thickness has been observed in these patients *(28,29)*. This demonstrates not only that reduced subcutaneous tissue thickness is a key determinant of metatarsal head pressure, but that it is only the combination of high pressure and neuropathy that leads to plantar ulceration—in rheumatoid arthritis, neither insensitivity nor plantar ulceration occur *(29)*.

A further contributing factor to elevated plantar pressure is limited joint mobility. Advanced glycosylation end products are now a well-recognized feature of chronic hyperglycemia, and when glycosylation of collagen occurs the collagen bundles become thickened, cross-linked, and less flexible. This is manifested clinically as thick, tight, waxy skin and restriction of joint movement. Limited joint mobility (LJM) of the subtalar joint alters the mechanics of walking and is strongly associated with high plantar pressure *(30)*. Indeed, this study seemed to suggest that LJM, as assessed in the hands by the prayer sign, was more strongly associated with elevated foot pressures than was neuropathy. Differences in joint mobility have also been suggested as being responsible for the lower pressures and lower ulceration rates seen in black diabetic patients *(31)*. Further support for an alteration in the mechanics of walking in neuropathy comes from our own recent data *(32)* in which peak pressure (the only parameter measured in most previous studies) was found to be much less abnormal than pressure time integrals, indicating an abnormality in the way in which forces are applied through the foot during walking.

Little attention has been paid to understanding the mechanism by which pressure abnormalities lead to tissue damage. Landsmann et al. *(33)* studied the effects of pressure on endothelial cells in culture. Whereas the magnitude of the applied pressure determined cell deformation, it was only the rate of increase of pressure that determined the degree of cellular injury (as measured by intracellular calcium changes). Additionally, older cells (believed to be more analogous to diabetic cells) were more likely to show signs of permanent damage. The clinical implications are not only that diabetic tissue may be more susceptible to the effects of pressure than normal tissue, but that the rate of pressure increase (possibly higher in neuropathic subjects because of weakness of ankle dorsiflexion and resultant "foot slap" during walking) is more important than peak pressure. This remains to be tested clinically.

### *Abnormalities of the Microcirculation*

Thickening of capillary basement membranes is central to the development of diabetic retinopathy and nephropathy, and closely linked with neuropathy. Similar changes can be found in most tissues, and although microvascular disease alone does not cause foot ulceration, it is almost certainly a contributory factor. Evidence of a functional microvascular disorder can be found in uncomplicated diabetes, diabetic neuropathy, and macrovascular disease. The key abnormalities are increased resting microvascular flow, impaired postural vasoconstriction, and a reduced hyperemic response to nociceptive stimulation. In the neuropathic foot, much of the excessive resting flow is through arteriovenous shunt vessels *(34)* and, whereas there is also evidence of increased flow through nutritive skin capillaries, this may not be enough to compensate for the increased metabolic requirements resulting from the higher temperature of the neuropathic foot. When functioning normally, autoregulatory mechanisms maintain a constant flow at varying perfusion pressures, and to achieve this induce vasoconstriction in the foot when the leg is dependent. When this postural vasoconstriction is lost, capillary flow and pressure increase on standing *(35)* and edema may occur. This edema, which is seen in both neuropathy and ulceration, impairs wound healing. Nociceptive stimulation either by iontophoretically applied acetylcholine or by a needle prick results in a flare response that may, in normal subjects, last for 24 h. The loss of this response is particularly marked in neuropathy *(36)* and impairs the capability of the tissue to respond appropriately to trauma, and may also further reduce the patient's already limited ability to detect pain.

### *Other Long-Term Complications*

Patients with retinopathy and nephropathy have been shown to have an increased risk of foot ulceration and amputation *(37–39)*. The pathogenic mechanisms by which these other complications lead to ulceration and amputation are not entirely clear, and none of these studies has corrected for neuropathy and PVD, so it is not possible to judge whether this relationship is indeed causal or just a reflection of the clustering of complications. However, visual impairment makes it more difficult for patients to identify a lesion at an early stage and tissue repair is slow in nephropathy, because of edema, the frequent coexistence of macrovascular disease, and immunological abnormalities. Thus, such patients must always be regarded as being at high risk.

### *Previous Foot Ulceration*

Several studies have confirmed that foot ulceration is more common in those patients with a past history of ulceration or amputation *(20,26)* as well as in patients with a poor social background. In fact, previous ulceration is probably the single most important predictive factor of ulceration.

### *Diabetes Duration and Control*

Several studies, including a recent, large, case-control study from the United States have demonstrated that poor glycemic control as measured by $HbA_1c$, fasting and even a single random blood glucose is strongly predictive of subsequent amputation *(38,39)*. Indeed, among Finnish NIDDM patients, the incidence of amputation was significantly higher among patients with poor control and short-duration diabetes than those with good control and long diabetes duration *(28)*. Most of these studies report amputations occurring over a number of years after the baseline examination and conclude that poor glycemic control leads to a more rapid progression of complications and impairs wound healing. However, glycemic control when specifically examined *(40)*, was not a good predictor of ulcer healing, and furthermore, we have recently found that poor glycemic control also predicts ulceration in the short term (less than 1-yr follow-up) *(41)*, during which time advancement of neuropathy and vascular disease should not be significant. It appears, therefore, that a less enthusiastic approach to personal healthcare is manifest as both poor glycemic control and less diligent footcare.

### *Race*

Lower-extremity amputation rates have been shown to be high among several groups of American Indians *(37,42,43)* and although these studies have not measured the rate among white Americans, comparison with other data indicated an excess risk in most of these populations. This is most marked in the Oklahoma Indians *(43)* whose amputation rate is more than four times higher than that in the general United States diabetic population. Studies in the United Kingdom have shown lower incidences of amputation and foot ulceration in the Asian than the white population *(44,45)*. The data on the rates in black patients are rather scanty. Most and Sinnock reported that amputation was performed more than twice as frequently in black compared to white diabetic patients *(46)*, but Selby recently found no difference in a black population with good access to healthcare *(39)*. Unfortunately, none of the studies of ethnic groups directly addresses the reasons for the reported differences. Access to healthcare seems an unlikely explanation for all of these findings, and biological variation between races is probably important. Nelson speculated *(37)* that among Pima Indians, the earlier onset of NIDDM (and therefore longer diabetes duration in a population matched for age), a tendency to walk barefoot, and the documented high prevalence of medial arterial calcification in the peripheral circulation (itself a strong predictor of amputation in this population) may contribute to the high amputation rates.

### *Cardiovascular Factors*

Several prospective studies have linked hypertension with amputation *(39,43)*, and although this was not confirmed in Pima Indians or middle-aged Finnish subjects *(37,38)*, a similar nonsignificant trend was apparent in both of these populations. It is not clear whether hypertension acts by increasing, either directly or indirectly, the prevalence or severity of peripheral vascular disease, however, neither lipid abnormalities nor, surprisingly, smoking appear to predict amputation, suggesting that the role of hypertension is through a different mechanism.

### *Behavioral/Psychological Factors*

Despite the fact that causal pathways to ulceration are well recognized and many high-risk patients receive education, ulceration remains common. It has been suggested that denial of risk is the main reason for this, and indeed Walsh et al. *(47)* have previously published a series of cases demonstrating extreme denial in foot ulcer patients. However, in our own prospective study of psychological factors in foot ulceration *(41)*, measures of denial have failed to predict ulceration. In contrast, neuropathic patients developing ulcers showed a more negative attitude to the feet, and their belief in the efficacy of advice was lower compared to patients who did not develop ulcers.

### *Wound Healing*

Slow wound healing and increased susceptibility to infection increase the problems of foot ulceration and may predispose to amputation. A number of inherent immunological abnormalities have been documented in diabetes, and several studies have shown an increased infection rate in postoperative wounds *(48)*. Neutrophil function is impaired, with abnormalities of adherence, chemotaxis, phagocytosis, and killing ability *(49)* and these may be partly caused by ascorbic acid transport defects *(50)*. We have recently looked at TGFβ in diabetic foot ulcers, as TGFβ is known to be central to the process of wound healing *(51)*. We observed that there was a failure of upregulation of TGFβ1 in and around diabetic foot ulcers, despite the obvious requirements for tissue repair. There was also a suggestion that TGFβ1 was present at lower levels in diabetic than nondiabetic skin.

Pecoraro et al. looked at factors predicting poor wound healing in diabetic patients with foot ulcers *(40)*, and found that periwound tissue oxygenation was the most important. It was superior to the same measurements carried out on the dorsum of the foot and also to dorsalis pedis arterial pressure. This suggests that local factors, such as impaired microvascular responses to physiological stimuli and tissue edema are at least as important as arterial inflow in determining the adequacy of tissue oxygenation, and hence the ability to mount an adequate healing response.

Another factor that may be important in the development of ulceration is the tissue response to trauma. Recent interesting work *(52)*, has shown microhemorrhages in the subcutaneous tissue around the first metatarsal head in six out of nine patients with previous neuropathic ulceration, but in neither neuropathic nor nonneuropathic controls. This may represent capillary fragility, and an important new step in the pathway to ulceration, as hemorrhage into callus is recognized as commonly preceding ulceration. However, larger prospective studies are required to demonstrate that this is causal of and not secondary to ulceration.

## CHARCOT NEUROARTHROPATHY

A Charcot joint is characterized by the simultaneous presence of bone and joint destruction, fragmentation, and remodelling. It occurs in a wide range of neurological conditions in which sensory loss is an important component. Diabetes is the commonest cause of the Charcot foot and most patients have a dense neuropathy, but good circulation *(53)*. The diagnosis is frequently missed or overlooked and early studies almost certainly underestimated its prevalence. A more recent systematic radiological survey found evidence of Charcot neuroarthropathy in 16% of diabetic patients with a history of neuropathic ulceration *(53)*. Classical textbook descriptions are of a painless deformity, but up to 50% experience some pain and discomfort, although it is never enough to prevent patients from weight bearing. In the early stages, the foot is warm and swollen, and plain radiographs can occasionally be normal, although isotope studies always show a huge increase in the blood flow to the bones of the foot. The midfoot is the most frequently affected site, and progressive joint destruction leads to the collapse of the transverse and longitudinal arches, producing a rocker-bottom foot with bony prominences, and a high risk of ulceration and amputation. The rarer hindfoot Charcot can result in complete erosion of the talus and calcaneum, so that the tibia rests on the ground.

Early animal experiments suggested that simply walking on an insensitive limb could lead to joint destruction *(54)*. Excessive and repetitive stress to bones leads to microfractures, which render the bone more brittle and could lead to joint destruction *(55)*. However, the degree of bone destruction often seen in the absence of major injury has suggested the presence of an underlying bone abnormality, resulting in pathological fractures, with subsequent fragmentation and joint destruction resulting from continued weight bearing on the injured, but insensitive foot. Isotope studies have shown increased blood flow to and vascularity of the bones in the feet of neuropathic patients *(56)*, and this is thought to be because of the arteriovenous shunting seen in autonomic neuropathy. This appears to promote osteoclastic activity and was especially marked in both the affected and unaffected feet of Charcot patients, and might lead to a degree of osteoporosis. Indeed, recently Young has shown a 16% reduction of bone-mineral density in the lower limbs of patients with a Charcot foot, when compared to neuropathic controls *(57)*. This hypothesis, however, remains incomplete, as it is heavily reliant on the role of autonomic neuropathy, which although prominent in many diabetic patients, is not a feature of some of the other neurological conditions associated with Charcot joints. Like other theories, it also fails to explain why the bone destruction is centered around joints and does not affect sites distant to articulations. We have previously reported the presence of periarticular erosions in Charcot feet *(58)*. These appear to precede fractures, and perhaps suggest that an active inflammatory arthropathy (possibly caused by minor trauma), prolonged by continued weight bearing, and characterized by the production of cytokines promoting local bone resorption, erosions, and ultimately fractures, could be a crucial step in the pathogenesis. A full understanding of the pathological process leading to the often dramatic and progressive destruction seen in this condition has not yet been arrived at, and as it is rare and usually presents late, the opportunities for further studies are limited.

## CONCLUSION

Although the roles of peripheral neuropathy and peripheral vascular disease are now well established as the main etiological factors in diabetic foot ulceration, there is much work to be done in both the way in which ulcers develop and the interactions of the main risk factors with each other and with all the other risk factors discussed in this chapter. However, this complexity should not deter the clinician, as it is now very clear that simple clinical tests will identify patients at risk of ulceration and amputation, and appropriate, but simple education about foot care can greatly reduce the likelihood of developing diabetic foot problems.

## REFERENCES


1. Williams DRR. Hospital admissions of diabetic patients: information from hospital activity analysis. Diabetic Med 1985;2:27–32.
2. Bell P. Vascular disease: aetiology and presentation. In: Boulton AJM, Connor H, Cavanagh PR, eds. The Foot in Diabetes, 2nd ed. Wiley, Chichester, UK, 1994, pp. 121–135.
3. Fasching P, Waldhausl W, Wagner OF. Elevated circulating adhesion molecules in NIDDM—potential mediators in diabetic macroangiopathy (letter). Diabetologia 1996;39:1242–1244.
4. Schmidt AM, Crandall J, Hori O, Cao R, Lakatta E. Elevated plasma levels of vascular cell adhesion molecule-1 (VCAM-1) in diabetic patients with microalbuminuria: a marker of vascular dysfunction and progressive vascular disease. Br J Haematol 1996;92:747–750.
5. Abbott RD, Brand FN, Kannel WB. Epidemiology of some peripheral arterial findings in diabetic men and women: experiences from the Framingham Study. Am J Med 1990;88:376–381.
6. Walters DP, Gatling W, Mullee MA, Hill RD. The prevalence, detection and epidemiological correlates of peripheral vascular disease: a comparison of diabetic and non-diabetic subjects in an English community. Diabetic Med 1992;9:710–715.
7. Strandness DE, Priest RE, Gibbons RE, Seattle MD. Combined clinical and pathological study of diabetic and non diabetic peripheral artery disease. Diabetes 1961;13:366–372.
8. King TA, DePalma RG, Rhodes RS. Diabetes mellitus and atherosclerotic involvement of the profunda femoris artery. Surg Gynecol Obstet 1984;159:553–556.
9. Jude E, Shaw J, Chalmers N, Boulton AJM. Peripheral vascular disease (PVD) in diabetic and non-diabetic patients—a comparison. Diabetic Med 1996;13(suppl 7):S47.
10. Osmundson PJ, O'Fallon WM, Zimmerman BR, Kazmier FJ, Langworthy AL, Palumbo PJ. Course of peripheral arterial occlusive disease in diabetes. Vascular laboratory assessment. Diabetes Care 1990;13:143–152.
11. Edmonds ME. Experience in a multi-disciplinary diabetic foot clinic. In: Boulton AJM, Connor H, Ward JD, eds. The Foot in Diabetes, 1st ed. Wiley, Chichester, UK, 1987, pp. 121–133.
12. Thomson FJ, Veves A, Ashe H, Knowles EA, Gem J, Walker MG, Hirst P, Boulton AJM. A team approach to diabetic foot care: the Manchester experience. The Foot 1991;1:75–82.
13. Pecoraro RE, Reiber GE, Burgess EM. Pathways to diabetic limb amputation. Basis for prevention. Diabetes Care 1990;13:513–521.
14. Young MJ, Boulton AJM, MacLeod AF, Williams DRR, Sonksen PH. A multicentre study of the prevalence of diabetic peripheral neuropathy in the United Kingdom hospital clinic population. Diabetologia 1993;36:150–154.
15. Tesfaye S, Stevens LK, Stephenson JM, et al. Prevalence of diabetic peripheral neuropathy and its relation to glycaemic control and potential risk factors: the EURODIAB IDDM complications study. Diabetologia 1996;39:1377–1384.
16. Walters DP, Gatting W, Mullee MA, Hill RD. The prevalence of diabetic distal sensory neuropathy in an English community. Diabet Med 1991;9:349–353.
17. Sosenko JM, Kato M, Soto R, Bild DE. Comparison of quantitative sensory-threshold measures for their association with foot ulceration in diabetic patients. Diabetes Care 1990;13:1057–1061.
18. Boulton AJ, Kubrusly DB, Bowker JH, Gadia MT, Quintero L, Becker DM, Skyler JS, Sosenko JM. Impaired vibratory perception and diabetic foot ulceration. Diabet Med 1986;3:335–337.
19. Young MJ, Breddy JL, Veves A, Boulton AJM. The prediction of diabetic neuropathic foot ulceration using vibration perception thresholds. A prospective study. Diabetes Care 1994;17:557–560.
20. Rith-Najarian SJ, Stolusky T, Ghodes DM. Identifying diabetic patients at high risk for lower-extremity amputation in a primary care setting. Diabetes Care 1992;15:1386–1389.
21. Dyck PJ, Kratz KM, Karnes JL, Litchy WJ, Klein R, Pach JM, Wilson DM, O'Brien PC, Melton LJ. The prevalence by staged severity of various types of diabetic neuropathy, retinopathy and nephropathy in a population-based cohort. Neurology 1993;43:817–824.
22. Uccioli L, Monticone D, Durola J, Russo F, Mormile F, Mennuni G, Menzinger G. Autonomic neuropathy influences great toe blood pressure. Diabetes Care 1994;17:284–287.
23. Ctercteko GC, Dhanendran M, Hutton WC, Le Quesne LP. Vertical forces acting on the feet of diabetic patients with neuropathic ulceration. Br J Surg. 1981;68:608–614.

24. Boulton AJM, Hardisty CA, Betts RP, Franks CI, Worth RC, Ward JD, Duckworth T. Dynamic foot pressure and other studies as diagnostic and management aids in diabetic neuropathy. Diabetes Care 1983;6:26–33.
25. Veves A, Murray HJ, Young MJ, Boulton AJM. The risk of foot ulceration in diabetic patients with high foot pressure: a prospective study. Diabetologia 1992;35:660–663.
26. Murray HJ, Young MJ, Hollis S, Boulton AJM. The association between callus formation, high pressures and neuropathy in diabetic foot ulceration Diabetic Med 1996;13:979–982.
27. Young MJ, Cavanagh PR, Thomas G, Johnson MM, Murray H, Boulton AJM. The effect of callus removal on dynamic plantar foot pressures in diabetic patients. Diabet Med 1992;9:55–57.
28. Young MJ, Coffey J, Taylor PM, Boulton AJM. Weight bearing ultrasound in diabetic and rheumatoid arthritis patients. The Foot 1995;5:76–79.
29. Masson EA, Hay EM, Stockley I, Veves A, Betts RP, Boulton AJM. Abnormal foot pressures alone may not cause ulceration Diabet Med 1989;6:426–428.
30. Fernando DJ, Masson EA, Veves A, Boulton AJM. Relationship of limited joint mobility to abnormal foot pressures and diabetic foot ulceration. Diabetes Care 1991;14:8–11.
31. Veves A, Sarnow MR, Giurini JM, Rosenblum BI, Lyons JE, Chrzan JS, Habershaw GM. Differences in joint mobility and foot pressures between black and white diabetic patients. Diabet Med 1995;12:585–589.
32. Shaw JE, Boulton AJM. Pressure time integrals may be more important than peak pressures in diabetic foot ulceration. Diabetic Med 1996;13(suppl 7):S22.
33. Landsmann AS, Meaney DF, Cargill RS, Macarak EJ, Thibault LE. High strain rate tissue deformation. J Am Podiatr Med Assoc 1995;85:519–527.
34. Flynn MD, Edmonds ME, Tooke JE, Watkins PJ. Direct measurement of capillary blood flow in the diabetic neuropathic foot. Diabetologia 1988;31:652–656.
35. Rayman G, Hassan A, Tooke JE. Blood flow in the skin of the foot related to posture in diabetes mellitus. Br Med J 1986;292:87–90.
36. Parkhouse N, Le Quesne PM. Impaired neurogenic vascular response in patients with diabetes and neuropathic foot lesions. N Engl J Med 1988;318:1306–1309.
37. Nelson RG, Gohdes DM, Everhart JE, Hartner JA, Zwemer FL, Pettitt DJ, Knowler WC. Lower-extremity amputations in NIDDM. 12-yr follow-up study in Pima Indians. Diabetes Care 1988;11:8–16.
38. Siitonen OI, Niskanen LK, Laakso M, Siitonen JT, Pyorala K. Lower-extremity amputations in diabetic and nondiabetic patients. A population-based study in eastern Finland. Diabetes Care 1993;16:16–20.
39. Selby JV, Zhang D. Risk factors for lower extremity amputations in persons with diabetes. Diabetes Care 1995;18:509–516.
40. Pecoraro RE, Ahroni JH, Boyko EJ, Stensel VL. Chronology and determinants of tissue repair in diabetic lower extremity ulcers. Diabetes 1991;40:1305–1313.
41. Vileikyte L, Shaw JE, Kincey J, Carrington AL, Boulton AJM. A Prospective study of neuropathic and psychological factors in foot ulceration. Diabetologia 1996;39(suppl 1):A3.
42. Valway SE, Linkins RW, Gohdes DM. Epidemiology of lower-extremity amputations in the Indian Health Service, 1982–1987. Diabetes Care 1993;16:349–353.
43. Lee JS, Lu M, Lee VS, Russell D, Bahr C, Lee ET. Lower-extremity amputation. Incidence, risk factors, and mortality in the Oklahoma Indian Diabetes Study. Diabetes 1993;42:876–882.
44. Gujral JS, McNally PG, O'Malley BP, Burden AC. Ethnic differences in the incidence of lower extremity amputation secondary to diabetes mellitus. Diabetic Med 1993;10:271–274.
45. Clarke D, Martin K, Kaltas G, Tindall H. Ethnic variation in the diabetic foot clinic. Diabetic Med 1992;9(suppl 1):35A.
46. Most RS, Sinnock P. The epidemiology of lower extremity amputations in diabetic individuals. Diabetes Care 1983;6:87–91.
47. Walsh CH, Soler NG, Fitzgerald MG. Association of foot lesions with retinopathy in patients with newly diagnosed diabetes. Lancet 1975;1:878–880.
48. Grossi EA, Esposito R, Harris LJ, Crooke GA, Galloway AC, Colvin SB, Culliford AT, Baumann FG, Yao K, Spencer FC. Sternal wound infections and use of internal mammary artery grafts. J Thorac Cardiovasc Surg 1991;102:342–346.
49. Sapico FL, Bessman AN. Diabetic foot infections. In: Frykeberg RG, ed. The High Risk Foot in Diabetes Mellitus. Churchill Livingstone, New York, 1991, pp. 197–211.

50. Pecoraro RE, Chen MS. Ascorbic acid metabolism in diabetes mellitus. Ann NY Acad Sci 1987;498:248–258.
51. Shaw JE, Spencer MJ, Herrick SE, Ferguson MWJ, Boulton AJM. Reduced tissue levels of TGFβ1 may contribute to poor healing in diabetic foot ulcers. Diabetologia 1996;39(suppl 1):A4.
52. Brash PD, Foster JE, Vennart W, Daw J, Tooke JE. Magnetic resonance imaging reveals micro-hemorrhages in the feet of diabetic patients with a history of ulceration. Diabetic Med 1996;13:973–978.
53. Cavanagh PR, Young MJ, Adams JE, Vickers KL, Boulton AJM. Radiographic abnormalities in the feet of patients with diabetic neuropathy. Diabetes Care 1994;17:201–209.
54. Elloesser L. On the nature of neuropathic affections of the joints. Ann Surg 1917;66:201–217.
55. Sanders LJ, Frykberg RG. Diabetic neuropathic osteoarthropathy: the Charcot foot. In: Frykberg RG, ed. The High Risk Foot in Diabetes Mellitus. Churchill Livingstone, New York, 1991, pp. 297–338.
56. Edmonds ME, Clarke MB, Newton S, Barrett J, Watkins PJ. Increased uptake of bone radiopharmaceutical in diabetic neuropathy. Q J Med 1985;57:843–855.
57. Young MJ, Marshall A, Adams JE, Selby PL, Boulton AJM. Osteopenia, neurological dysfunction, and the development of Charcot neuroarthropathy. Diabetes Care 1995;18:34–38.
58. Shaw JE, Adams JE, Boulton AJM. Peri-articular abnormalities in neuropathic arthropathy. Diabet Med 1995;12(suppl 2):S43.

# 19 Management of the Diabetic Foot

*John M. Giurini, DPM,*
*Barry I. Rosenblum, DPM,*
*and Thomas E. Lyons, DPM*

***CONTENTS***



## INTRODUCTION

Limb salvage, when dealing with the diabetic foot, deals with the ability to avoid amputation. This goal is carried out through three main aspects of diabetic care: identification of the "at-risk" foot, successful treatment of the acutely involved foot, and prevention of further problems. At each of these junctures patient education plays a vital role. A comprehensive program of diabetic foot management must include each of these aspects to successfully achieve limb salvage.

The development of a limb-salvage team requires its members to be dedicated to the challenge of the diabetic patient whose fears of limb loss rival those of blindness and kidney failure *(1,2)*. Each player must know their role and the availability of consultants in a timely manner is tantamount to success. The members of the team most commonly include a podiatrist, an endocrinologist, a vascular surgeon, and a pedorthist. Other members may include a plastic surgeon, an infectious disease specialist, an orthopedic surgeon, and a teaching nurse as well as any other healthcare provider interested in playing an active role in the care of these difficult patients.

Several grading systems have been described in the literature to classify the varied stages of diabetic foot lesions *(3,4)*. Whereas each system claims to be more complete,

From: *Contemporary Endocrinology: Clinical Management of Diabetic Neuropathy*
Edited by: A. Veves © Humana Press Inc., Totowa, NJ

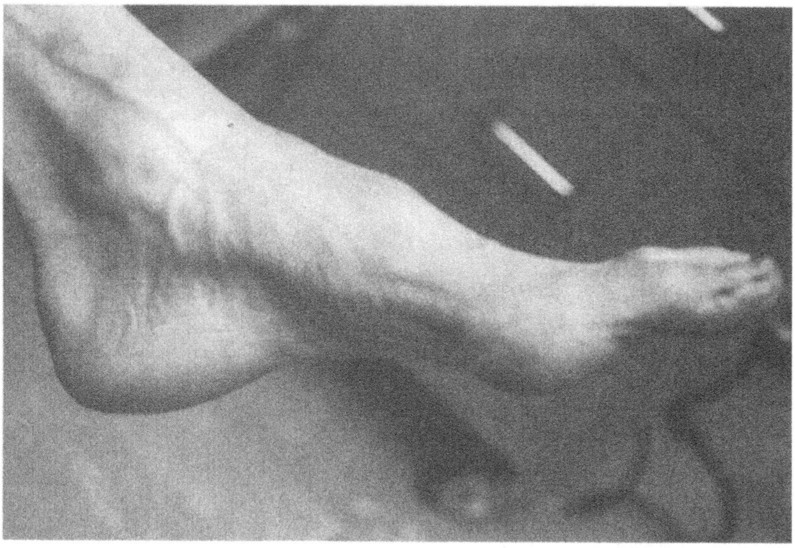

**Fig. 1.** Wasting of intrinsic musculature resulting in prominence of the metatarsal heads makes the Grade-0 foot susceptible to ulcerations.

the main purpose of a classification system is to provide standardized descriptions of the lesion and to formulate treatment algorithms.

## IDENTIFICATION OF RISK FACTORS

Certain clinical features have been identified that predict which patients are at risk of developing a foot ulceration *(5)*. The presence of peripheral sensory neuropathy in the face of unperceived trauma is necessary to proceed down the causal pathway towards ulceration *(6)*. Basic screening tests in clinical practice are adequate to evaluate for the presence of significant sensory loss. A 128-Hz tuning fork and 5.07 Semmes-Weinstein monofilament wire are inexpensive and can be used as screening tools to identify at-risk patients *(7,8)*. Whereas a biothesiometer can provide an objective measurement of vibratory-perception threshold (VPT), this device is often unavailable in the office setting *(9)*. Nerve-conduction studies are rarely necessary to evaluate neuropathy in the diabetic foot.

Foot deformities related to motor neuropathy can put the foot at risk for ulceration. Intrinsic muscle wasting resulting from motor neuropathy will lead to clawing of the digits and plantar flexion deformities of the metatarsal heads, resulting in areas of high focal pressures and possible irritation from footwear dorsally. This has been classically referred to as the "intrinsic minus" foot. Autonomic neuropathy involving the foot most commonly results in dry skin *(10)*. Untreated this can lead to cracking and fissuring, creating a portal of entry for bacteria. (Fig. 1).

Arterial insufficiency can lead to nonhealing of ulcerations once they have developed. Whereas the presence of pedal pulses is probably the most important single indicator of adequate perfusion to the foot, a thorough vascular examination should include measurement of the venous filling time (VFT) and evaluation for dependent rubor and pallor on elevation. Further evaluation may involve noninvasive arterial studies in the form of pulse-volume recordings and the character of the pulse on Doppler (monophasic vs triphasic). Ankle-brachial indices (ABI) are of little value in the diabetic patient. The likelihood of healing should not be based solely on this measurement since it is often falsely elevated. A nonhealing ulceration in the presence of arterial insufficiency warrants a prompt referral to a vascular surgeon *(11)*.

Plantar foot ulcers most commonly occur beneath metatarsal heads that have been identified as having high focal pressures *(12–14)*. Callous under metatarsal heads is characteristic of high foot pressures that can result from plantarly prominent metatarsals as seen in the intrinsic minus foot and when atrophy of the plantar fat pad has occurred *(15,16)*. Recently, the role of limited joint mobility has been described as a potential cause of high plantar foot pressures *(17,18)*. Bone deformities such as bunions, hammertoes, or rockerbottom deformities as seen in Charcot joint disease can also lead to focal areas of high pressure and put the foot at risk for ulceration not only on the plantar surface, but also on the dorsal surface where they come in contact with a shoe. Plantar foot pressures, in the form of vertical load, can be quantitated with computerized pressure sensors *(19)*. However, the Harris mat can provide an inexpensive screening tool that can show areas of high pressures.

The Wagner classification is the most commonly used clinical classification of diabetic foot ulceration. In the following parts of this chapter, the management of each grade of this classification is discussed.

## GRADE-0 FOOT

A Wagner grade-0 foot is the at-risk foot without ulceration *(3)*. The grade-0 foot is characterized by the presence of one or more risk factors. Clinically significant sensory neuropathy may be detected by screening tools such as the Semmes-Weinstein 5.07 monofilament wire or tuning fork *(20)*. Areas of sensory neuropathy should be carefully mapped so as to identify at-risk areas of the foot. Other risk factors may coexist, such as motor neuropathy or high foot pressures. The foot should be closely inspected for corns or calluses as they will identify potentially vulnerable areas. (Fig. 2).

The management of grade-0 lesions is primarily accomplished through a program of education and prevention. Patients should be educated as to the risks associated with the neuropathic foot and the early signs of inflammation, irritation, and infection. They should also be educated as to the early treatment of these conditions. Early treatment involves identifying the cause for these conditions.

Prevention is the hallmark of management of these feet and should include daily inspection of feet by the patient or a family member. Footwear modification should be discussed with the patient when necessary to accommodate bony deformities. High plantar foot pressures can be accommodated with orthoses and padded hosiery *(21,22)*.

An additional technique used to modify pressure points is the habit of changing one's shoes every 4 hours. This has several advantages in preventing ulcerations. Since each shoe has a slightly different pressure point, rotating shoes also rotates pressure points. This prevents the accumulation of pressure over any one area of the foot for extended periods of time. Additionally the outer soles and leather uppers of shoes fatigue with time: The longer one wears a shoe, the less shock absorption and support the shoe will provide. Changing shoes regularly also affords the patient the opportunity to inspect the feet frequently, allowing for the detection of lesions before they become significant problems. This is a recommendation that applies regardless of the grade foot.

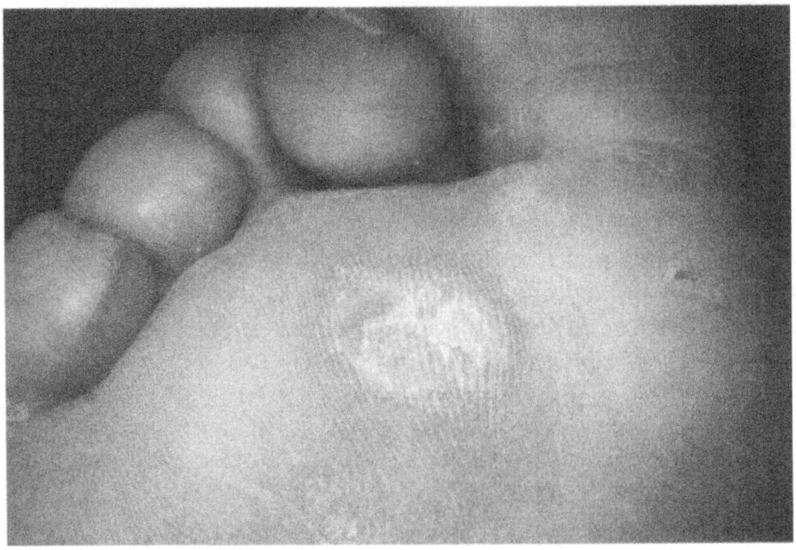

**Fig. 2.** A grade-0 foot with callous formation is indicative of high foot pressures, which requires treatment and accommodation with orthotic devices.

Regular visits to the foot specialist should be part of the patient's routine. The foot should be inspected at every visit. Pulses should be palpated and any lesion should be noted. Any callous should be debrided as these alone can lead to high foot pressures *(23)*. The patient should be instructed on the proper care of the nails and skin. Moisturizing creams should be prescribed for dry, scaly skin so as to avoid fissures. The interdigital spaces should also be inspected for fissures or evidence of tinea pedis.

## GRADE-1 FOOT

A grade-1 ulceration is one that has penetrated beyond the epidermis *(3)*. These ulcerations are indicative of two or more risk factors: peripheral sensory neuropathy and at least one other risk factor. Ulcerations should be evaluated for size, depth, and location. Careful attention should be given to the structures involved as well as to the presence of infection. The presence of and type of drainage should be noted. Cultures are of limited usefulness at this stage as the ulceration will most assuredly be colonized with multiple organisms representing primarily skin flora *(24)*. Typically grade-1 ulcerations have not progressed beyond the dermis. The underlying cause should be identified.

Treatment centers around eliminating all pressure from the site of ulcerations *(5)*. The "gold" standard for eliminating pressure is total nonweightbearing, either with crutches or a walker. However, most patients are unlikely to comply with this regimen entirely. Therefore, several compromise methods for off-loading the foot have been devised. Total contact casting and Scotch boot cast have been described as ways of off-loading the foot and reducing pressures *(25–28)*. The felted-foam dressing is the preferred way of off-loading ulcerations in our institution.

The felted-foam dressing is comprised of a 1/4-inch foam pad with a thin layer of felt laminated onto it. An aperture is fashioned to accommodate the ulceration and through which dressing changes can be performed on a regular basis. This pad is applied to the foot with a self-adhering gauze wrap known as Gauze-Tek. (Fig. 3).

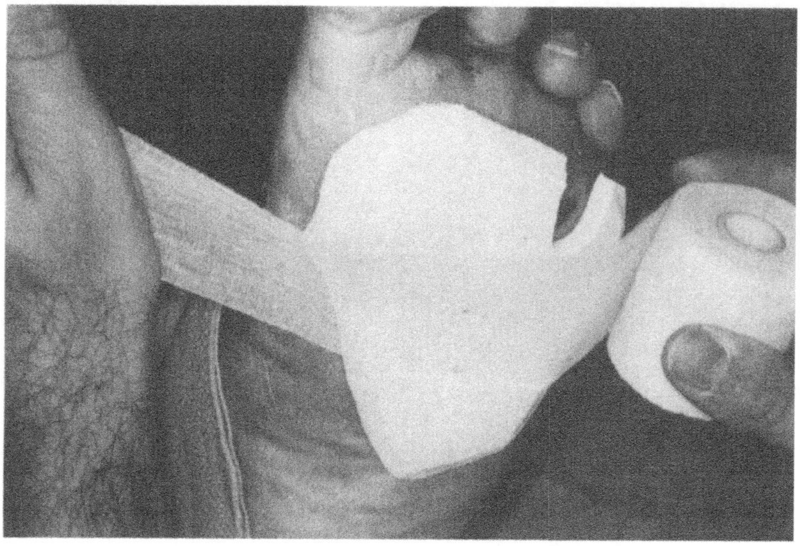

**Fig. 3.** The felted-foam dressing is an effective modality to off-load a grade-1 ulceration.

The ulcer should be debrided to remove any hyperkeratotic tissue surrounding the ulcer and any nonviable, necrotic tissue at the base of the ulceration *(11)*. (Fig. 4). The ulceration is dressed daily to provide a moist environment conducive to wound healing. Harsh, undiluted chemicals should be avoided as they can be toxic to granulation tissue *(29,30)*. Topical antibiotics have limited usefulness in this setting. If an infection is suspected, this is best treated with systemic antibiotics. Oral antibiotics are only recommended when clinical signs of infection are present (i.e., erythema, purulent drainage). Overuse of oral antibiotics may lead to superinfection or development of resistant strains. Exceptions to this rule include patients with severe peripheral vascular disease in whom development of infection may be limb-threatening or patients on immunosuppressive medications as seen in renal transplant patients.

Repeated ulcerations may warrant consideration of surgical correction of any underlying structural deformity. Metatarsal osteotomies, digital arthroplasties, and metatarsal head resections have all proven useful in the prevention of recurrent ulcerations *(31–36)*.

## GRADE-2 FOOT

Continued weightbearing on grade-1 lesions will lead to deepening ulcerations *(3)*. These will go beyond the dermis and can involve deeper structures such as tendons or joint capsule (grade 2) *(3)*. Management of these ulcerations is dependent on accurate assessment of ulcer depth.

The ulcer base should be gently probed with a stainless-steel blunt probe to determine undermining of the ulceration, presence of any penetrating sinus tract, and involvement of deeper structures. This simple technique has an 80% specificity for diagnosing osteomyelitis, avoiding the need for invasive, more expensive diagnostic tests (e.g., bone scans, MRI) *(37)*. The involvement of any of these structures should alert the clinician to the possible need for hospitalization, complete bed rest, and broad-spectrum IV antibiotics (38).

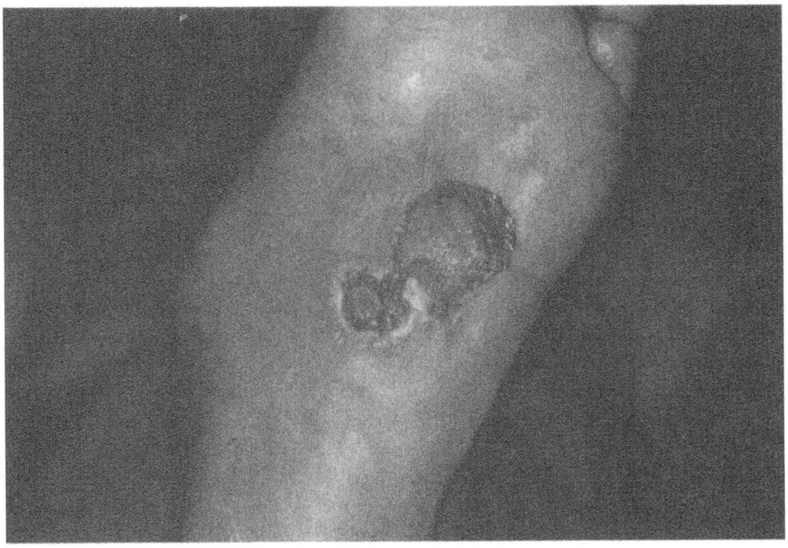

**Fig. 4.** The grade-1 foot is characterized by superficial tissue breakdown involving the epidermis and no deeper structures. Abnormal foot architecture as occurs in Charcot joint disease is a risk for foot ulceration.

Once hospitalized, the foot should be drained dependently and packed open. This can often be performed at the bedside in severely neuropathic patients. However, if the infection is expected to be extensive, the patient should be brought to the operating room where a thorough debridement can be performed *(38)*. Any sinus tract should be explored and drained and all nonviable, necrotic tissue should be debrided, including tendon and/or bone. (Fig. 5). Deep cultures should be taken and iv antibiotics adjusted to cover the offending organism, realizing that the infection may be polymicrobial in nature *(39)*.

Clinicians are often fearful of aggressively debriding a foot with underlying ischemia. Adequate debridement of the infected foot should not be delayed nor compromised over this concern, for delaying surgery may lead to further tissue loss and potential limb loss *(40)*. Once infection is controlled, an arteriogram and lower extremity revascularization should be pursued in the ischemic patient *(41)*.

Radiographs should be taken in all full-thickness ulcerations to evaluate for osteomyelitis *(42,43)*. The use of bone scans, labeled WBC scans, MRIs, and bone biopsies are often recommended for diagnosing osteomyelitis *(44–46)*. However, false positive and false negatives occur with any of these modalities. Our experience has shown the ability to probe bone with a blunt, sterile probe to be reliable and cost-effective in diagnosing osteomyelitis. Dressing changes and packing on a regular basis with bedside debridements as necessary should be performed *(38)*.

Following adequate control of infection and early signs of healing, thought can be given to definitive treatment of the ulceration and underlying bone deformity. Delayed primary closure of the wound will allow for primary wound healing and allow for earlier ambulation. Some clinicians prefer to wait for secondary wound healing to take place, which is perfectly appropriate. This, however, results in prolonged periods of nonweightbearing. It is our tendency to close wounds primarily whenever possible.

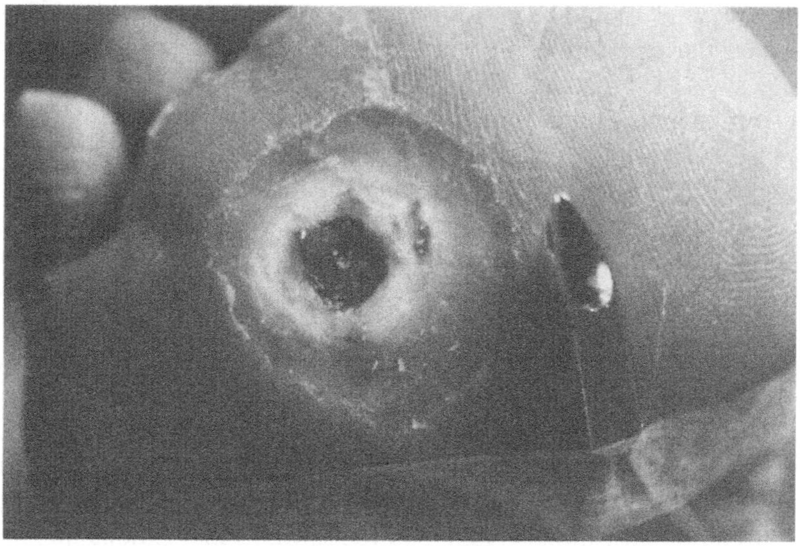

**Fig. 5.** Adequate debridement of ulceration requires removal of all exuberant callous tissue and necrotic tissue, revealing a clean granular base.

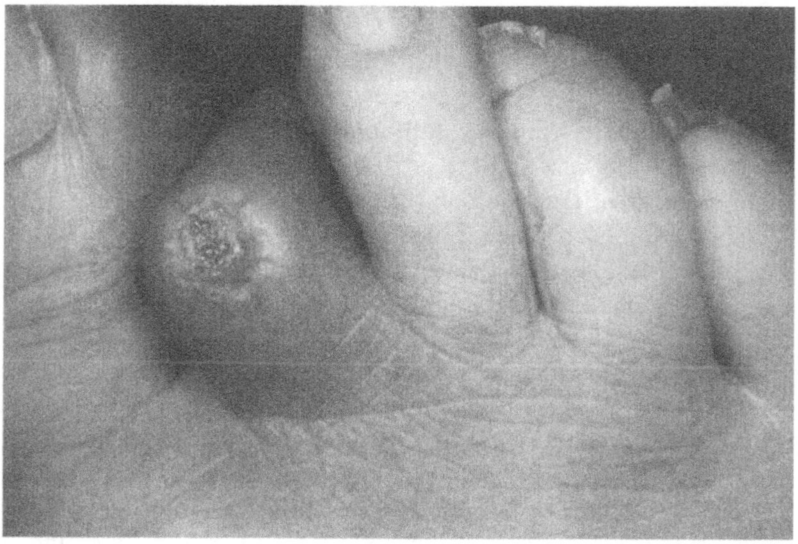

**Fig. 6.** A rigidly contracted digit can be irritated by the toebox of a shoe, creating a grade-2 ulceration.

Not all grade-2 ulcerations require hospitalization *(11)*. (Fig. 6). Although rare, ulcerations over exposed tendon and capsule have the ability to granulate. Outpatient treatment of these lesions must follow the same principles of treating grade-1 ulcerations, namely strict adherence to nonweightbearing. The same strategies to off-load grade-1 ulcerations (i.e., felted-foam dressings, total contact cast, and so on) should be applied to grade-2 ulcerations. Because there tends to be more drainage with these ulcerations, dressings should be performed more regularly, often twice a day. It is often prudent to have these performed by a healthcare professional who is trained in recognition of early signs of infection, such as a visiting nurse. Oral antibiotics, although not often necessary in grade-1 ulcerations, are more commonly prescribed in grade-2 ulcerations because of the depth of the ulcerations, the vital structures involved, and the presence of drainage, creating an ideal environment for bacterial growth. Initially, broad spectrum antibiotics with good *Staphylococcus* coverage (e.g., 1st generation cephalosporins) should be prescribed *(47,48)*. Changes in antibiotics should be based on the results of deep-wound cultures and sensitivity as well as the clinical response of the wound.

The care of the foot following healing is just as important as the care provided to rid the foot of infection. Patients must be followed regularly to assure that an appropriate orthotic device is prescribed. In cases in which metatarsal heads have been resected, either single or multiple, additional pressure can be expected to be transferred to adjacent metatarsal heads *(49)*. Consequently, these should be protected with an orthotic device. Footwear modification is often required as well. Conventional jogging shoes fitted with an orthotic device may often be appropriate. In some cases an extra-depth shoe with a deep toebox may be required. The patient should be educated on the care of the foot and the need for daily inspections. The need for regular visits with a foot specialist for continued monitoring should be impressed upon the patient.

## GRADE-3 FOOT

Deep infection and bone involvement are characteristic of grade-3 ulcerations. These may result from unresponsive grade-2 ulcerations, aggressive bacterial infections or, not uncommonly, puncture wounds resulting in direct inoculation of bone. Because of the depth of these ulcerations and the presence of bone infection, hospitalization and surgical intervention are often required. (Fig. 7).

As with deep infections of grade-2 ulcerations, adequate drainage of infection is key in managing grade-3 lesions *(38)*. Once again, any sinus tract must be explored and any undrained abscess or devitalized tissue must be debrided. In cases of severe infection, open ray amputations may be necessary to control spread of infection.

Following clearing of infection and the appearance of healthy granulation tissue, thought can be given to surgical reconstruction of the wound and foot. This may involve simple delayed primary closure or more complicated reconstructive surgery, including additional bone resections, tissue flaps, or skin grafts *(50)*. No one technique can be applied to all wounds. A flexible approach to wound closure will maximize limb salvage. These lesions will make maximum use of all members of the diabetic foot team *(41,51)*.

The long-term management of the grade-3 foot emphasizes prevention of transfer ulcerations. Because ablative surgery is common in the grade-3 foot, transfer of pressure to adjacent areas of the foot is expected. Prevention of chronically recurrent ulcerations requires the use of appropriate orthoses, prescription footwear, and regular podiatry visits. At each visit, orthoses and shoegear should be inspected for signs of early wear and breakdown. These should be replaced immediately when found to be worn down. The goal of long-term care is to distribute plantar foot pressures more evenly along the entire plantar aspect of the foot, thus avoiding concentration of pressure over any one focal area.

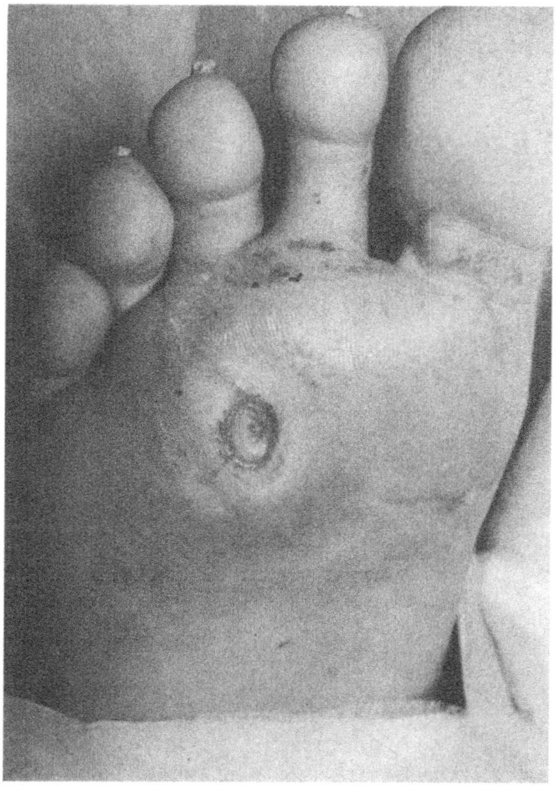

**Fig. 7.** Grade-3 ulcerations are typically characterized by a lesion underlying a metatarsal head involving deep structures such as tendon, joint, capsule, or bone.

## GRADE-4 FOOT

Grade-4 lesions are particularly challenging problems to manage. These patients will often present with a variety of underlying risk factors making overall management difficult. Peripheral vascular disease, osteomyelitis, sepsis, and extensive tissue loss necessitates the cooperation of all members of the limb-salvage team. Consultations with vascular surgeons, podiatrists, plastic surgeons, and orthopedic surgeons are often required. The primary goal in the management of these lesions is to limit tissue loss. Minor trauma in the face of severe arterial insufficiency can result in gangrenous changes of the skin *(6)*. (Fig. 8). This most commonly occurs at the distal end of extremities, since this is where end-arteries are typically found. Lack of adequate perfusion and oxygenation will initially cause focal necrosis that may proceed to cause increasing amounts of tissue loss. These changes are most commonly referred to as dry gangrene.

Overwhelming infection may also result in gangrenous changes either from marked edema of local tissue or from infective vasculitis, both of which result in occlusion of digital arterial branches *(52)*. Infective vasculitis will typically lead to wet gangrene.

Initial therapy of these lesions is dependent on identifying the underlying cause. Gangrene resulting from arterial insufficiency should be treated with immediate vascular assessment and lower extremity revascularization where possible to minimize tissue loss *(40,53)*.

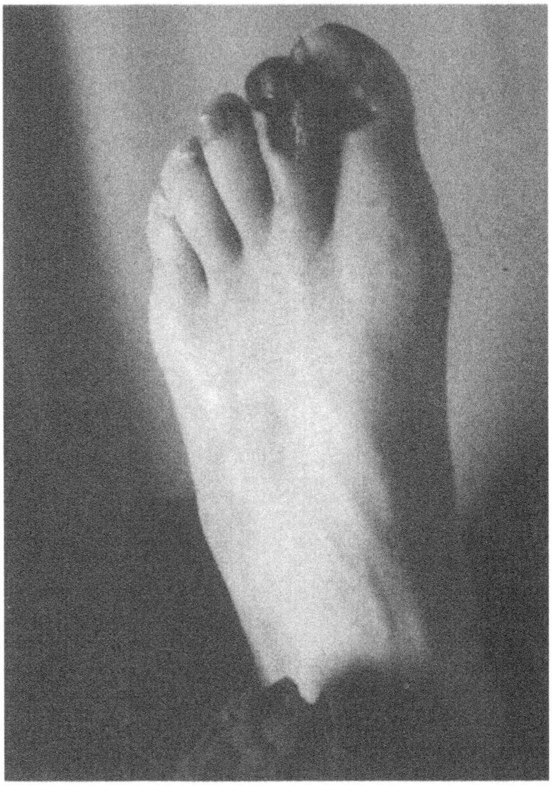

**Fig. 8.** A sock stuffed into the end of a shoe resulted in minor trauma and focal gangrenous changes.

Diabetic vascular disease is characterized by occlusive disease below the popliteal artery, most commonly affecting the anterior and posterior tibial arteries and sparing the foot vessels (i.e., dorsalis pedis) *(54,55)*. This has made distal bypasses possible and effective. This argues against the concept of "small vessel disease" initially proposed in the late 1950s *(56)*. It is now felt that diabetic patients do not suffer from occlusive disease of the digital arteries any more frequently than nondiabetic patients and the concept of "small vessel disease" as a major cause of nonhealing ulcerations in diabetic patients should be put to rest *(57)*.

Arteriography that visualizes the foot vessels should be performed to accurately assess the level of revascularization. The current standard of care dictates the use of digital subtraction angiography (DSA) for adequate vascular evaluation before bypass *(41)*. Following revascularization, amputation should be performed at the most distal level that will support healing. Efforts should be made to preserve as much of the weightbearing surface of the foot as possible. This will allow for more efficient ambulation, better distribution of plantar pressures, and easier shoeing of the foot.

Gangrene resulting from extensive infection will often necessitate immediate incision and drainage, even open amputation. This condition must be readily recognized and treated in an emergent manner as any delay may lead to systemic toxicity. Once the infection has been adequately controlled, attempts should be made to once again salvage as much of the foot as possible. Oxygen consumption increases dramatically with more proximal amputations, increasing work and energy expenditure during ambulation.

## GRADE-5 FOOT

Extensive necrosis of the foot is caused by arterial occlusion and failure of arterial inflow. Primary amputation is the treatment for extensive gangrene. However, these patients should undergo vascular assessment and revascularization when possible to reduce tissue loss and to perform the amputation at the distal most level that will support healing.

### *Care of the Amputated Foot*

The partially amputated foot is particularly vulnerable to further foot problems *(58)*. Loss of the weightbearing surface results in the same forces being distributed over a smaller area, thereby increasing focal pressures. Additionally in certain types of amputations, muscle imbalances and contractures may develop *(59)*. This can also lead to abnormal gait and increased focal pressures. These feet must be adequately protected in orthotic devices and very often therapeutic shoes. Regular inspection and examination by a foot specialist is important in order to detect early signs of breakdown. Any calluses should be trimmed. Likewise, orthoses and shoes must be evaluated regularly for increased wear and loss of support. When this occurs they should be replaced immediately.

## FOOT SURGERY IN THE DIABETIC PATIENT

As little as 10 years ago, most diabetic patients were advised to avoid foot surgery at all cost. Misconceptions and misinformation about healing or small vessel disease prevented many diabetic patients from undergoing potentially limb-sparing local foot procedures. Today, the pendulum has swung towards a more aggressive approach to the care of the diabetic foot and earlier surgical intervention to avoid amputations *(31–36,41,60)*.

Local surgical intervention may be appropriate to correct underlying bone deformities such as hammertoes or plantarflexed metatarsals that pose risks for ulceration. Arthroplasties and metatarsal osteotomies have been shown to be effective procedures to heal ulcerations and to reduce the risk of future ulceration *(32,57,60)*. Local surgical procedures such as metatarsal head resections can be performed to resect localized osteomyelitic bone *(61,62)*. Multiple metatarsal head resections can be performed as an alternative to distal amputation and still leave a functional foot capable of efficient ambulation *(33,34)*. Furthermore, maintaining as much of the plantar weightbearing surface allows for better weight distribution.

In recent years, there has been increasing discussion on the role of prophylactic surgery on the diabetic patient. Some groups define prophylactic surgery as surgery performed to correct an underlying deformity even in the absence of a history of ulceration *(31,60)*. Other groups subscribe to a narrower definition of prophylactic surgery: surgery performed on those deformities having shown a history of ulceration to prevent further ulceration and possible amputation *(35)*.

When surgery is being considered, proper patient selection and preoperative evaluation is tantamount to success. A thorough history and physical examination should be performed with special emphasis on the cardiac and vascular examination. Whenever possible, surgery should be performed under local anesthesia with mild sedation to minimize stress on the heart. Many of these surgical procedures are amenable to this type of anesthesia because of sensory neuropathy *(63)*.

## CHARCOT JOINT DISEASE

Unexplained, nonpainful swelling and erythema of the foot without a portal of entry should be considered Charcot joint disease until proven otherwise. Patients may describe a precedent history of relatively minor trauma. However, the trauma may be so insignificant that the patient has difficulty recalling. Profound sensory neuropathy will render this process relatively painless. Some patients will experience varying degrees of pain. However it is not in proportion with the degree of bone destruction seen on X-rays *(64)*.

Initial evaluation of the Charcot joint requires X-rays. Plain films will often be all that is necessary since the bone destruction is quite obvious. The most common location is Lisfranc's joint (tarsometatarsal articulations) *(65)*. Osseous debris and fragmentation with subluxations of joints are common findings. The degree of fragmentation is variable and is most often related to the particular joints involved and continued ambulation on the fractures. CT scans and MRIs are rarely necessary to make the diagnosis of Charcot joint. CT scans may be useful for preoperative planning if surgical correction of the deformity is being contemplated.

Charcot joint disease is characterized by three clinical phases: acute, coalescence, and reconstruction or remodeling. The acute phase is characterized by edema, localized warmth, erythema, and joint crepitus with range of motion examination. Once appropriate treatment is instituted, edema and erythema reduce rapidly. As Charcot joint progresses to the next phase of coalescence, skin temperature begins to equilibrate and joint crepitus diminishes. The reconstructive or remodeling phase occurs over a period of months and years. During this phase, the joints further stabilize and remodel, eventually leading to a stable foot devoid of significant motion. Unfortunately, the foot can be severely deformed with obvious bony prominences susceptible to ulceration *(64)*.

The treatment of choice for acute Charcot joint disease is total nonweightbearing. This is achieved by the use of crutches, a walker, or, in the event of bilateral involvement, a wheelchair. A walking cast in acute Charcot joint disease is not appropriate treatment. Noncompliance with nonweightbearing in the early stages of this disease will result in further fragmentation of bone, resulting in eventual greater deformity. Casts, splints, or braces may be used for immobilization and to provide stability to the involved joints, but not for weightbearing initially. Our personal preference is use of a removable bivalved cast brace that will allow for regular inspection of the insensate skin *(66)*. There has been much discussion over the use of electrical bone stimulation to enhance healing of these problematic fractures. Isolated reports would appear to favor the use of these devices in Charcot joint disease *(67)*. However, there is a need for a well-designed clinical study to document effectiveness.

Serial X-rays are used in addition to the clinical exam to determine when weightbearing can be instituted. No weightbearing is allowed as long as crepitus and elevated skin temperature persists. These are clinical signs of an active Charcot joint, and ambulation at this stage will exacerbate the disease. Once it is deemed safe to begin weightbearing, this should be done gradually. Typically, weightbearing is begun at 15–20. pounds of weight and is increased in 10-lb increments weekly as long as there are no signs of reactivation (i.e., edema, erythema, warmth). Any signs of reactivation should be followed by a return to nonweightbearing until resolution of symptoms. Initial weightbearing occurs with the brace or cast in place. As weightbearing progresses, the patient is eventually allowed to ambulate short distances without assistive devices.

Whenever possible, conventional footwear is preferred over custom-molded shoes. All shoes should be fitted with a well-molded plastizote orthotic device that will provide support and cushioning to the foot. If severe foot deformity develops, there may be no alternative to a custom-molded shoe that matches the shape of the foot *(68)*.

In recent years, great attention has been given to the surgical reconstruction of the foot deformed by Charcot joint disease *(69–71)*. Severe deformity and instability can result from destruction of the midtarsal, subtalar, or ankle joints. This can lead to a high likelihood for ulceration or difficulty with ambulation. Arthrodesis of the involved joints is attempted to provide a stable platform for ambulation that is resistant to further ulcerations. Patients undergoing joint fusions must be prepared for an extended period of immobilization and nonweightbearing, often as long as 6 months. Strict adherence to the principles of internal fixation is required if an acceptable degree of success is expected.

## FUTURE OF DIABETIC FOOT MANAGEMENT

The last 5 years have resulted in tremendous activity in diabetic foot care. Wound-care centers have been established nationwide to deal with the growing problem of diabetic feet *(72,73)*. More than $200 million in direct hospital costs were spent in 1980 for treatment of diabetic foot complications and amputations *(74)*. Recent cost estimates are not available in the United States. These numbers are expected to grow as our population ages and the incidence of diabetes increases.

Much research has been done in the area of wound healing, having identified several factors important in wound healing *(75,76)*. This research continues today as new topical wound-care agents are being introduced daily. Platelet-derived growth factor using recombinant technology in a gel form is the latest product from the research lab being prepared for clinical use *(77)*. Clinical trials have shown favorable results. This product has recently received FDA approval.

Studies exploring treatment and possible prevention of sensory neuropathy continue. Earlier studies of aldose reductase inhibitors had to be terminated prematurely because of unexpected side effects of the study medications. However, early results showed these agents to hold some promise in the treatment of neuropathy. These studies continue today with modification of these agents. Aldose reductase inhibitors and gamma-linoleic acid, as previously discussed, are few of the modalities already under trial *(78–80)*.

Painful neuropathy (diabetic neuritis) remains a difficult problem to treat. To date there is no one agent universally effective against this complication. Treatment often involves a combination of analgesic agent and tricyclic antidepressant *(81)*. Newer agents are currently being tried. It is too early to comment on their effectiveness.

Further investigation into the underlying cause of Charcot joint disease is needed. Future trials of medications to modulate the Charcot process or medications to strengthen bone may be of clinical benefit *(82)*. Once Charcot joint develops, the use of electrical bone stimulation to achieve more rapid consolidation noninvasively warrants further research *(67)*.

## REFERENCES

1. Thomson FJ, Veves A, Ashe H, Knowles EA, Gem J, Walker MG, Hirst P, Boulton AJM. A team approach to diabetic foot care-the Manchester experience. Foot 1991;1:75–82.

2. Edmonds ME, Blundell MP, Morris HE, Maelor-Thomas E, Cotton LT, Watkins PJ. Improved survival of the diabetic foot: the role of the specialist foot clinic. Q J Med 1986;232:763–771.
3. Wagner FW. The dysvascular foot: a system for diagnosis and treatment. Foot Ankle 1981;2:64–122.
4. Lavery LA, Armstrong DG, Harkless LB. Classification of diabetic foot wounds. J Foot Ankle Surg 1996;35:528–531.
5. Young MJ, Veves A, Boulton AJM. The diabetic foot: aetiopathogenesis and management. Diab/Metab Rev 1993;9:109–127.
6. Pecoraro RE, Reiber GE, Burgess EM. Pathways to diabetic limb amputation: basis for prevention. N Engl J Med 1994;331:854–860.
7. Kumar S, Fernando DJS, Veves A, Knowles EA, Young MJ, Boulton AJM. Semmes-Weinstein monofilaments: a simple, effective and inexpensive screening device for identifying diabetic patients at risk of foot ulceration. Diab Res Clin Pract 1991;13:63–68.
8. Sosenko JM, Kato M, Soto R, Bild DE. Comparison of quantitative sensory-threshold measures for their association with foot ulceration in diabetic patients. Diab Care 1990;13:1057–1061.
9. Young MJ, Breddy JL, Veves A, Boulton AJM. The prediction of diabetic foot ulceration using vibration thresholds: a prospective study. Diabetes Care 1994;17:557–560.
10. Ewing DJ, Martyn CN, Young RJ, Clarke BF. The value of cardiovascular autonomic function tests: 10 years experience in diabetes. Diab Care 1985;8:491–498.
11. Caputo GM, Cavanagh PR, Ulbrecht JS, Gibbons GW, Karchmer AW. Assessment and management of foot disease in patients with diabetes. N Engl J Med 1994;331:854–860.
12. Young MJ, Taylor PM, Boulton AJM. A new, non-invasive technique to predict foot ulcer risk. Diabetes 1993;42(suppl 1):A632.
13. Tovey FE. The manufacture of diabetic footwear. Diab Med 1984;1:69–71.
14. Tovey FE, Moss MJ. Specialist shoes for the diabetic foot. In: Connor H, Boulton AJM, Ward JD, eds. The Foot in Diabetes. Wiley, Chichester, UK, 1987, pp. 97–108.
15. Rosen RC, Davids MS, Bohanski LM. Hemorrhage into plantar callus and diabetes mellitus. Cutis 1985;35:339–341.
16. Harkless LB, Dennis KJ. You see what you look for and recognize what you know. Clin Pod Med Surg 1987;4:331–339.
17. Delbridge L, Perry P, Marr S, Arnold N, Yue DK, Turtle JR, Reeve TS. Limited joint mobility in the diabetic foot: relationship to neuropathic ulceration. Diabetic Med 1988;5:333–337.
18. Fernando DJS, Masson EA, Veves A, Boulton AJM. Relationship of limited joint mobility to abnormal foot pressures and diabetic foot ulceration. Diabetes Care 1991;14:8–11.
19. Veves A, Fernando DJS, Walewski P, Boulton AJM. A study of plantar pressures in a diabetic clinic population. Foot 1991;1:89–92.
20. Olmos PR, Cataland S, O'Dorisio TM, Casey CA, Smead WL, Simon SR. The Semmes-Weinstein monofilament as a potential predictor of foot ulceration in patients with noninsulin-dependent diabetes. Am J Med Sci 1995;309:76–82.
21. Veves A, Masson EA, Fernando DJS, Boulton AJM. Use of experimental padded hosiery to reduce foot pressures in diabetic neuropathy. Diabetes Care 1989;12:653–655.
22. Veves A, Masson EA, Fernando DJS, Boulton AJM. Studies of experimental hosiery in diabetic neuropathic patients with high foot pressures. Diabetic Med 1990;7:324–326.
23. Young MJ, Cavanagh PR, Thomas G, Johnson MM, Murray H, Boulton AJM. The effect of callus removal on dynamic plantar pressures in diabetic patients. Diabetic Med 1992;9:55–57.
24. Joseph WS, Axler DA. Microbiology and antimicrobial therapy of diabetic foot infections. Clin Pod Med Surg 1990;7:467–481.
25. Pollard JP, LeQuesne LP. Methods of healing diabetic forefoot ulcers. Br Med J 1983;286:436–437.
26. Burden AC, Jones GR, Jones R, Blandford RL. Use of the Scotchcast boot in treating diabetic foot ulcers. Br Med 1983;286:1555–1557.
27. Coleman WC, Brand PW, Birke JA. The total contact cast: a therapy for plantar ulcerations on insensitive feet. J Am Podiatry Assoc 1984;74:548–552.
28. Mueller MJ, Diamond JE, Sinacore DR. Total contact casting in treatment of diabetic plantar ulcers. Diab Care 1989;12:384–388.
29. Kucan JO, Robson MC, Heggers JP, Ko F. Comparison of silver sulfadiazine, povidone-iodine and physiologic saline in the treatment of chronic pressure ulcers. J Am Geriatr Soc 1981;29:232–235.
30. Lineweaver W, Howard R, Soucy D, et al. Topical antimicrobial activity. Arch Surg 1985;120: 267–270.

31. Gudas CJ. Prophylactic surgery in the diabetic foot. Clin Podiatr Med Surg 1987;4:445–458.
32. Tillo TH, Giurini JM, Habershaw GM, Chrzan JS, Rowbotham JL. Review of metatarsal osteotomies for the treatment of neuropathic ulcerations. J Am Podiatr Med Assoc 1990;80:211–217.
33. Jacobs RL. Hoffman procedure in the ulcerated diabetic neuropathic foot. Foot Ankle 1982;3:142–149.
34. Giurini JM, Basile P, Chrzan JS, Habershaw GM, Rosenblum BI. Panmetatarsal head resection: a viable alternative to the transmetatarsal amputation. J Am Podiatr Med Assoc 1993;83:101–107.
35. Giurini JM, Rosenblum BI. The role of foot surgery in patients with diabetes. Clin Podiatr Med Surg 1995;12:119–127.
36. Rosenblum BI, Giurini JM, Chrzan JS, Habershaw GM. Preventing loss of the great toe with the hallux interphalangeal joint arthroplasty. J Foot Ankle Surg 1994;33:557–560.
37. Grayson ML, Gibbons GW, Balogh K, Levin E, Karchmer AW. Probing to bone in infected pedal ulcers: a clinical sign of underlying osteomyelitis in diabetic patients. JAMA 1995;273:721–723.
38. Gibbons GW. The diabetic foot: amputations and drainage of infection. J Vasc Surg 1987;5:791–793.
39. Wheat LJ, Allen SD, Henry M, et al. Diabetic foot infections: bacteriologic analysis. Arch Intern Med 1986;146:1935–1940.
40. Taylor LM, Porter JM. The clinical course of diabetic patients who require emergent foot surgery because of infection or ischemia. J Vasc Surg 1987;6:454–459.
41. LoGerfo FW, Gibbons GW, Pomposelli FB Jr, et al. Trends in the care of the diabetic foot: expanded role of arterial reconstruction. Arch Surg 1992;127:617–621.
42. Newman LG, Waller J, Palestro CJ, et al. Unsuspected osteomyelitis in diabetic foot ulcers: diagnosis and monitoring by leukocyte scanning with indium in 111 oxyquinoline. JAMA 1991;266:1246–1251.
43. Keenan AM, Tindel NL, Alavi A. Diagnosis of pedal osteomyelitis in diabetic patients using current scintigraphic techniques. Arch Intern Med 1989;149:2262–2266.
44. Hetherington VJ. Technetium and combined gallium and technetium scans in the neutrophic foot. J Amer Podiatr Assoc 1982;72:458–463.
45. Morrison WB, Schweitzer ME, Wapner KL, Hecht PJ, Gannon FH, Behm WR. Osteomyelitis in feet of diabetics: clinical accuracy, surgical utility, and cost-effectiveness of MR imaging. Radiology 1995;196:557–564.
46. Yuh WTC, Corson JD, Baraniewski HM, Rezai K, Shamma AR, Kathol MH, Sato Y, El-khoury GY, Hawes DR, Platz CE, Cooper RR, Corry RJ. Osteomyelitis of the foot in diabetic patients: evaluation with plain film, Tc-MDP bone scintigraphy, and MR imaging. Am J Roentgen 1989;152:795–800.
47. Jones EW, Edwards R, Finch R, Jeffcoate WJ. A microbiologic study of diabetic foot lesions. Diab Med 1984;2:213–215.
48. Lipsky BA, Pecoraro RE, Wheat LJ. The diabetic foot: soft tissue and bone infection. Infect Dis Clin North Am 1990;4:409–432.
49. Ulbrecht JS, Perry J, Hewitt FG, Cavanagh PR. Controversies in footwear for the diabetic foot at risk. In: Kominsky SJ, ed. Medical and Surgical Management of the Diabetic Foot. Mosby-Year Book, Boston, 1994, pp. 441–451.
50. Attinger CE. Use of soft tissue techniques for the salvage of the diabetic foot. In: Kominsky SJ, ed. Medical and Surgical Management of the Diabetic Foot. Mosby-Year Book, Boston, 1994, pp. 323–366.
51. Gibbons GW, Marcaccio EJ Jr, Burgess AM, et al. Improved quality of diabetic foot care, 1984 vs 1990: reduced length of stay and costs, insufficient reimbursement. Arch Surg 1993;128:576–581.
52. Edmonds M, Foster A, Greenhill M, Sinha J, Philpott-Howard J, Salisbury J. Acute septic vasculitis not diabetic microangiopathy leads to digital necrosis in the neuropathic foot. Diab Med 1992;9 (Suppl 1):P85.
53. Klamer TW, Towne JB, Bandyk DF, Bonner MJ. The influence of sepsis and ischemia on the natural history of the diabetic foot. Am Surg 1987;53:490–494.
54. Pomposelli FB Jr, Jepsen SJ, Gibbons GW, et al. A flexible approach to infrapopliteal vein grafts in patients with diabetes mellitus. Arch Surg 1991;126:724–729.
55. Pomposelli FB Jr, Jepsen SJ, Gibbons GW, et al. Efficacy of the dorsalis pedis bypass for limb salvage in diabetic patients: short term observations. J Vasc Surg 1990;11:745–752.
56. Goldenberg SG, Allen M, Joshi RA, Blumenthal HT. Nonatheromatous peripheral vascular disease of the lower extremity in diabetes mellitus. Diabetes 1959;8:261–273.
57. LoGerfo FW, Coffman JD: Vascular and microvascular disease in the diabetic foot: implications for foot care. N Engl J Med 1984;311:1615–1619.
58. Golner MG. The fate of the second leg in the diabetic amputee. Diabetes 1960;9:100–103.

59. Chang BB, Bock DE, Jacobs RL, Darling RC, Leather RP, Shah DM. Increased limb salvage by the use of unconventional foot amputations. J Vasc Surg 1994;19:341–349.
60. Armstrong DG, Lavery LA, Stern S, Harkless LB. Is prophylactic diabetic foot surgery dangerous?: J Foot Ankle Surg 1996;35:585–589.
61. Rosenblum BI, Pomposelli FB, Giurini JM. Maximizing foot salvage by a combined approach to foot ischemia and neuropathic ulceration in patients with diabetes mellitus: a five year experience. Diabetes Care 1994;17:983–987.
62. Martin JD, Delbridge L, Reeve TS, Clagett GP. Radical treatment of mal perforans in diabetic patients with arterial insufficiency. J Vasc Surg 1990;12:264–268.
63. Frykberg R, Giurini J, Habershaw G, Rosenblum B, Chrzan J. Prophylactic surgery in the diabetic foot. In: Kominsky SJ, ed. Medical and Surgical Management of the Diabetic Foot. Mosby-Year Book, Boston, 1994.
64. Sanders LJ, Frykberg RG. Diabetic neuropathic osteoarthropathy: the Charcot foot. In: Frykberg RG, ed. The High Risk Foot in Diabetes Mellitus. Churchill Livingstone, New York, 1991, pp. 297–338.
65. Sinha S, Munichoodappa C, Kozak GP. Neuroarthropathy (Charcot joints) in diabetes mellitus: clinical study of 101 cases. Medicine 1972;52:191–210.
66. Lesko P, Maurer PC. Talonavicular dislocations and midfoot arthropathy in neuropathic diabetic feet: natural course and principles of treatment. Clin Orthop 1989;240:226.
67. Bier RR, Estersohn HS. A new treatment for Charcot joint in the diabetic foot. JAPMA 1987;77:63–69.
68. Janisse DJ. Prescription insoles and footwear. Clin Podiatr Med Surg 1995;12:41–61.
69. Banks AS, McGlamry ED. Charcot foot. J Am Podiatr Med Assoc 1989;79:213–235.
70. Bono JV, Rogers DJ, Jacobs RL. Surgical arthrodesis of the neuropathic foot: a salvage procedure. Clin Orthop Rel Res 1993;296:14–20.
71. Papa J, Myerson M. Salvage, with arthrodesis, in intractable diabetic neuropathic arthropathy of the foot and ankle. J Bone Joint Surg Am 1993;75:1056–1066.
72. Knighton DR, Fylling CP, Fiegel VD, Cerra F. Amputation prevention in an independently reviewed at-risk diabetic population using a comprehensive wound care protocol. Am J Surg 1990;160:466–472.
73. Steed DL, Edington H, Moosa HH, Webster MW. Organization and development of a university multidisciplinary wound care clinic. Surgery 1993;114:775–779.
74. Kozak GP, Rowbotham JL, Gibbons GW. Diabetic foot disease: a major problem. In: Kozak GD, et al., eds. Management of Diabetic Foot Problems. Saunders, Philadelphia, 1995, pp. 1–9.
75. Bennett NT, Schulz GS. Growth factors and wound healing biomechanical properties of growth factors and their receptors. Am J Surg 1993;165:728–737.
76. Bennett NT, Schulz GS. Growth factors and wound healing: part II. Role in normal wound and chronic wound healing. Am J Surg 1993;166:74–81.
77. Steed DL, Diabetic Ulcer Study Group. Clinical evaluation of recombinant human platelet-derived growth factor for the treatment of lower extremity diabetic ulcers. J Vasc Surg 1995;21:71–81.
78. Boulton AJM, Levin S, Comstock J. A multicentre trial of the aldose reductase inhibitor, tolrestat, in patients with symptomatic diabetic neuropathy. Diabetologia 1990;33:431.
79. Sima AAF, Brill V, Nathaniel T, et al. Regeneration and repair of myelinated fibres in sural nerve biopsy specimens from patients with diabetic neuropathy treated with sorbinil. N Engl J Med 1988;319:548.
80. Keen H, Payan J, Allawi J, et al. Treatment of diabetic neuropathy with γ-linolenic acid. Diabetes Care 1992;16:8.
81. Young RJ, Clarke BF. Pain relief in diabetic neuropathy: the effectiveness of imipramine and related drugs. Diabetes Med 1985;2:262.
82. Selby PL, Young MJ, Boulton AJM. Bisphosphonates: a new treatment for diabetic Charcot neuroarthropathy? Diabetes Med 1994;11:28–31.

# 20 The Impact of Micro- and Macrovascular Disease on Diabetic Neuropathy and Foot Problems

*Cameron M. Akbari,* MD
*and Frank W. LoGerfo,* MD

*CONTENTS*



## INTRODUCTION

Diabetes mellitus is found in as many as 13 million people nationally, or 5.2% of the United States population, and more than 650,000 new cases are diagnosed annually *(1)*. Many of the clinical complications of diabetes may be ascribed to alterations in vascular structure and function, with subsequent end-organ damage and death. Specifically, two types of vascular disease are seen in patients with diabetes: a nonocclusive microcirculatory impairment involving the capillaries and arterioles of the kidneys, retina, and peripheral nerves, and a macroangiopathy characterized by atherosclerotic lesions of the coronary and peripheral arterial circulation *(2–5)*. The former is relatively unique to diabetes, whereas the latter lesions are morphologically similar in both nondiabetic and diabetic patients.

Clinical data linking diabetes to micro- and macrovascular disease are derived from several large epidemiological studies. The Framingham Study of over 5000 subjects demonstrated that diabetes is a powerful risk factor for atherosclerotic coronary and peripheral arterial disease, independent of other atherogenic risk factors, with a relative

From: *Contemporary Endocrinology: Clinical Management of Diabetic Neuropathy*
Edited by: A. Veves © Humana Press Inc., Totowa, NJ

risk averaging twofold in men and threefold for women *(3)*. Retinopathy is the most characteristic complication of diabetes *(4)*, and population-based studies have identified a correlation between its development and the duration of diabetes *(5)*. Similar correlations have been found with nephropathy, neuropathy, and diabetes *(6)*, with perhaps the strongest evidence coming from the Diabetes Control and Complications Trial (DCCT), which showed a delay in the development and progression of these microvascular complications with intensive glycemic control *(7)*. These and other clinical trials have provided the rationale for experimental studies investigating the fundamental pathophysiology of micro- and macrovascular disease in diabetes mellitus.

## MICROVASCULAR DISEASE: OVERVIEW AND ANATOMIC CHANGES

Microvascular dysfunction in diabetes is manifested by an increased vascular permeability and impaired autoregulation of blood flow and vascular tone. These changes culminate into renal failure (nephropathy), loss of vision (retinopathy), neuropathy, and most likely contribute to the cardiovascular complications of diabetes. Although multiple theories have been postulated as to the etiology of accelerated microangiopathy, it is likely that several biochemical derangements exist in the presence of hyperglycemia and diabetes, and that these mechanisms work synergistically to cause microvascular dysfunction. These metabolic alterations produce functional and structural changes at multiple areas within the arteriolar and capillary level, including the basement membrane *(4)*, smooth-muscle cell *(8)*, and, in particular, the endothelial cell *(9)*.

One of the greatest impediments in understanding vascular disease in patients with diabetes is the misconception that they have an untreatable occlusive lesion in the microcirculation *(3)*. This idea originated from a retrospective histologic study demonstrating the presence of PAS-positive material occluding the arterioles in amputated-limb specimens from diabetic patients *(10)*. However, subsequent prospective staining and arterial casting studies *(11,12)* as well as physiological studies *(13)* have demonstrated the *absence* of an arteriolar occlusive lesion.

Whereas there is no occlusive lesion in the diabetic microcirculation, other structural changes do exist, most notably thickening of the capillary basement membrane thickening. This alteration in extracellular matrix may represent a response to the metabolic changes related to diabetes and hyperglycemia. However, the basement membrane thickening does not lead to narrowing of the capillary lumen, and arteriolar blood flow may be normal or even increased despite these changes *(14)*. Capillary basement membrane thickening is the dominant structural change in both diabetic retinopathy and neuropathy. In the kidney, nonenzymatic glycosylation reduces the charge on the basement membrane, which may account for transudation of albumin, an expanded mesangium, and albuminuria *(15)*. Similar increases in vascular permeability occur in the eye and probably contribute to macular exudate formation and retinopathy.

In the diabetic foot, basement membrane thickening may theoretically impair the migration of leukocytes and the hyperemic response following injury, thereby increasing the susceptibility of the diabetic foot to infection *(16,17)*. Although resting total skin microcirculatory flow is similar in both diabetic and nondiabetic patients, the capillary blood flow is reduced in diabetes, indicating a maldistribution and functional ischemia of the skin *(18)*. All of these changes result in an inability to vasodilate and achieve maximal blood flow following injury.

Diabetes also affects the function of the nerve axon reflex. Normally, nociceptive C fiber stimulation (by injury) results in both orthodromic conduction to the spinal cord

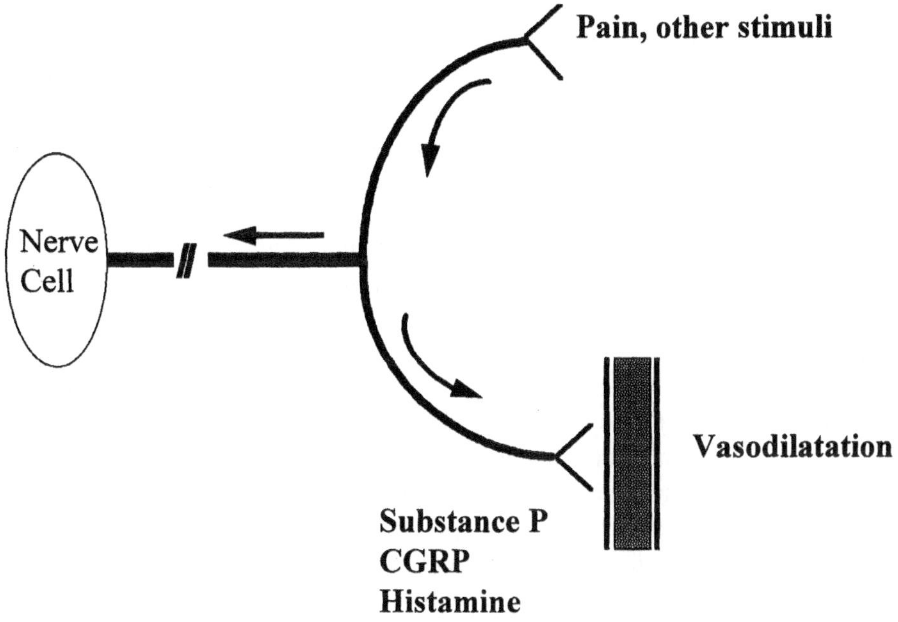


**Fig. 1.** Stimulation of the nociceptive C fiber leads to vasodilation via release of substance P, calcitonin gene-related peptide (CGRP), and histamine. It appears that release of these substances is modulated by acetylcholine.

and antidromic conduction to other axon branches, that is, the axon reflex (Fig. 1). One function of this reflex is the secretion of several active peptides, such as substance P and calcitonin gene related peptide, which cause vasodilation and increased permeability both directly and indirectly (through mast cell release of histamine). This neurogenic vasodilatory response is impaired in diabetes, further reducing the hyperemic response when it is most needed, that is under conditions of injury and inflammation *(19)*.

## PATHOPHYSIOLOGY OF MICROVASCULAR DISEASE AND ENDOTHELIAL DYSFUNCTION IN DIABETES

The normal endothelium plays an important role in blood-vessel wall function and homeostasis by synthesizing and releasing substances, such as prostacyclin, endothelin, prostaglandins, and nitric oxide, which modulate vasomotor tone and prevent thrombosis *(20)*. There is substantial evidence that endothelial function is abnormal in animal models of diabetes mellitus *(21–23)* and in patients with both insulin-dependent and non-insulin-dependent diabetes mellitus *(24,25)* thus directly implicating either hyperglycemia or hyperinsulinemia as a possible mediator of abnormal endothelium-dependent responses. A variety of mechanisms responsible for vascular dysfunction have been proposed, principally abnormalities in the nitric-oxide pathway, abnormal production of vasoconstrictor prostanoids, intracellular signaling, reduction in $Na^+$-$K^+$ ATPase activity, and advanced glycosylated end products *(12,26–28)*.

In 1980, Furchgott and Zawadzki discovered that arterial vasodilation was dependent on an intact endothelium and its release of a substance they called endothelium-derived relaxing factor (EDRF), which causes arterial smooth muscle cell relaxation in response to acetylcholine and other vasodilators *(27)*. Later identified as endothelial-derived nitric oxide (EDNO), it activates vascular smooth-muscle guanylate cyclase, elevates cGMP levels, and may increase $Na^+$-$K^+$ ATPase activity *(28)*. A variety of substances other than acetylcholine may cause EDNO-mediated vasodilation. Several in vivo studies using L-NMMA, an arginine analog and competitive inhibitor of EDNO synthesis, have demonstrated that the vasodilatory effects of insulin are nitric oxide dependent *(29,30)* and that insulin mediates EDNO-dependent vasodilation by modulating the synthesis and release of EDNO. Impaired endothelial-dependent vasodilatation in certain insulin-resistant states may be instrumental in the pathogenesis of atherosclerosis and hypertension and is postulated to be due to diminished insulin-mediated EDNO production and release *(31)*.

Studies by Creager et al. in patients with insulin-dependent and non-insulin-dependent diabetes have demonstrated impaired endothelium-dependent responses to acetylcholine in both groups, but an intact response to exogenous nitric oxide donors (i.e., sodium nitroprusside) in insulin-dependent diabetes only *(24,25)*. It thus appears that abnormal nitric oxide release and/or synthesis predominates in insulin-dependent diabetes, whereas non-insulin-dependent diabetes may be characterized by either a diminished response of smooth muscle to EDNO or increased inactivation of nitric oxide.

Although there is considerable controversy regarding the role of free radicals in diabetic vascular disease *(32)*, an increased production of oxygen-derived free radicals has been described in diabetes and may contribute to endothelial dysfunction *(33)*. In animal models, endothelium-derived free radicals impair EDNO-mediated vasodilatation, and administration of superoxide dismutase and other free-radical scavengers normalizes EDNO-dependent relaxation in diabetic arteries *(34)*.

Advanced glycosylation end products (AGEs) have also been implicated in the pathogenesis of diabetic microvascular complications *(26)*. These are formed from a reversible reaction between glucose and protein to form Schiff bases that then rearrange to form stable Amadori-type early glycosylation products. Some of these reversible early glycosylation products may undergo complex rearrangements to form irreversible AGEs. In experimental diabetes, AGEs impair the actions of EDNO and cause an impaired endothelium-dependent response, which is reversed by administration of an AGE inhibitor *(35)*. AGEs also displace disulfide crosslinkages in collagen and scleral proteins, accounting for the diminished charge in the capillary basement membrane. Moreover, the presence of AGE receptors on both endothelial cells and monocytes, along with AGE deposition in the subendothelium, suggests monocyte deposition into the subendothelial space and secondary complications *(36)*. Makita et al., using a radioreceptor assay for AGEs in serum and arterial wall, have demonstrated higher AGE levels in patients with diabetes compared to nondiabetic controls, with the highest levels occurring among diabetic patients with nephropathy *(37)*. Since at least part of AGE-induced cellular dysfunction is caused by an oxidant-sensitive mechanism, which is inhibited by antioxidants *(38)*, it is likely that both oxygen-derived free radicals and AGEs each contribute to cause impaired EDNO-dependent vasodilation in diabetes.

Experimental studies in diabetic animals have also indicated that abnormal endothelial production of vasoconstrictor prostanoids, notably thromboxane (TX) $A_2$ and prostaglandin (PG) $H_2$, may be a cause of endothelial cell dysfunction. Increased levels of TX $A_2$ have been isolated only from segments of diabetic aortic tissue with an intact endothelium, suggesting that the endothelium is responsible for the increased release, and impaired relaxation to acetylcholine in these segments is restored by treatment with cyclooxygenase inhibitors *(12,29)*. In humans however, the role of vasoconstrictor prostanoids is less clear. Flow-dependent vasodilation in healthy subjects, which may be used as an index of endothelial function, is abolished by L-NMMA but unaffected by aspirin, thus demonstrating that it is entirely mediated by EDNO and independent of vasoactive prostanoids *(39)*. Moreover, the attenuated endothelium-dependent vasodilation following acetylcholine administration which is seen in diabetic patients is not affected by pretreatment with cyclooxygenase inhibitors *(27,28)*.

It, therefore, appears that dysfunction of the microcirculation strongly contributes to the renal, eye, and macrovascular complications of diabetes. Several lines of evidence have indicated that the microcirculation is also implicated in the pathogenesis of diabetic neuropathy, and in fact, the etiology of diabetic neuropathy is a complex interplay between metabolic and microvascular defects. This may provide further insight into the metabolic basis of microvascular and endothelial dysfunction in diabetes.

In addition to the mechanisms described above, attention has centered toward the role of the polyol pathway in diabetic neuropathy. Hyperglycemia induces an increase in the polyol pathway by which glucose is metabolized to sorbitol via aldose reductase. Increased aldose reductase activity impairs myo-inositol uptake that leads to decreased $Na^+$-$K^+$ ATPase activity and loss of electrical conduction in neural tissue *(40)*. This biochemical background serves as the basis for clinical trials using aldose reductase inhibitors and high myo-inositol diets in diabetic neuropathy, the results of which are still inconclusive *(41)*.

Several lines of evidence point toward a relationship between aldose reductase, $Na^+$-$K^+$ ATPase activity, and nitric oxide in the pathogenesis of diabetic neuropathy. First, $Na^+$-$K^+$ ATPase activity in normal arteries is dependent on an intact endothelium, suggesting a stimulatory action by EDNO *(26)*. Second, hyperglycemia causes decreased $Na^+$-$K^+$ ATPase activity in normal rabbit aorta, an effect which is preventable by administering aldose reductase inhibitors or by raising plasma myo-inositol levels *(30)*. Third, administration of L-NMMA, an EDNO inhibitor, decreases $Na^+$-$K^+$ ATPase activity in aortic wall *(24)*. In addition, L-NMMA administration reverses the protective effects of aldose reductase inhibitor treatment on nerve conduction velocity *(43)*. It therefore seems likely that microvascular endothelial dysfunction plays a significant role in the pathogenesis of diabetic neuropathy, and that at least part of this is secondary to the metabolic derangements of diabetes.

Recent clinical studies from our laboratory have helped further define the relationship between the microcirculation, diabetes, and neuropathy *(44)*. In order to determine the effect of neuropathy and hypoxia on the foot microcirculation, we studied five groups of patients: diabetic neuropathic patients (DN), patients with diabetes and Charcot osteoarthropathy (DA), diabetic patients with neuropathy and clinically evident lower-extremity peripheral vascular disease (DV), diabetic patients without complications (DC), and healthy controls (C). The microcirculation was studied in vivo by employing laser Doppler imaging to measure the vasodilatory response to iontophoresis (a noninvasive method of introducing soluble ions into skin) of acetylcholine (endothelium-dependent) and sodium nitroprusside (an exogenous nitric oxide donor, endothelium-independent). Both the direct and indirect (which depends on a normal axon reflex) vasodilatory response were measured. The direct response to acetylcholine, which stimulates the production of nitric oxide, was similarly reduced in DN, DV, and DA compared to DC and C ($p < 0.001$), whereas the direct response to nitroprusside was lowest in DV. The indirect vasodilation during acetylcholine iontophoresis was also reduced in DN, DV, and DA but not in DC and C ($p < 0.0001$). These data suggest that the endothelium-dependent vasodilation and the axon reflex are impaired in the presence of diabetes and neuropathy, but the endothelium-independent response is spared, and that this dysfunction may be attributed to an impaired production of nitric oxide. In addition, it appears that the nerve axon reflex is reduced in diabetic neuropathic patients with and without vascular disease, while it is intact in diabetic patients without neuropathy.

Because of these findings, we also studied the expression of endogenous endothelial nitric oxide synthetase (eNOS) endothelial nitric oxide synthetase (eNOS) activity in the skin taken from the foot of patients in DN, DV, and C *(45)*. Full-thickness skin biopsies from the dorsum of the foot were obtained and immunostained with antiserum to human eNOS, glucose transporter I (GLUT I), and von Willebrand factor, which is an anatomical marker of the endothelium. No differences were found among the three groups in the staining intensity of von Willebrand factor and GLUT I. In contrast, the staining intensity of eNOS was reduced in both diabetic groups compared to controls. Therefore, it appears that in diabetic neuropathic patients, with or without lower-extremity ischemia, the eNOS activity is reduced, despite the fact that the endothelium is anatomically present, and that endothelial functional changes may be related to the development of neuropathy.

## MACROVASCULAR DISEASE AND DIABETES: AN OVERVIEW

There is abundant evidence from several large clinical studies that shows that diabetes is a strong predisposing factor for atherosclerotic macrovascular disease, and that this risk is independent of other accompanying atherogenic factors. Thirty year follow-up from the Framingham study confirmed a higher incidence of coronary heart disease and cardiovascular mortality among diabetic subjects, even when multivariate logistic regression is undertaken to exclude coexisting morbidities *(6,46)*. The Framingham study also confirmed that the risk of stroke is at least 2.5-fold higher in patients with diabetes *(47)*, a finding that has been confirmed in other large epidemiologic studies *(48,49)*. Moreover, diabetes is strongly associated with atherosclerosis of the extracranial internal carotid artery, and thus imparts an additional independent risk of stroke *(49)*.

A variety of mechanisms have been proposed as to the cause of accelerated atherosclerosis in diabetes *(51,52)*. The roles of endothelial dysfunction, advanced glycosylation end products, oxygen-derived free radicals, and vasoactive prostanoids and microvascular disease have already been discussed; it is likely that these also contribute to the pathogenesis of macrovascular atherosclerotic disease. Platelet abnormalities are also seen in diabetes and include increased thromboxane release, increased aggregation, and increased interaction with lipoproteins that may infiltrate the endothelial wall *(53)*. Elevated fibrinogen levels are also more common among diabetic patients and have been associated with a higher incidence of stroke and cardiovascular disease *(54)*. As with microvascular disease, it is likely that all of these mechanisms work together in the pathogenesis of macroangiopathy in diabetes.

## LOWER EXTREMITY ARTERIAL DISEASE AND DIABETES

Lower-extremity arterial disease is more common among patients with diabetes. The presence of diabetes is associated with a two- to threefold excess risk of intermittent claudication compared with its absence *(54)*. Along with neuropathy, ischemia from lower-extremity arterial insufficiency is one of the two principal pathogenic mechanisms in diabetic foot disease, and together they contribute to the sequence of tissue necrosis, ulceration, infection, and ultimately gangrene.

Unlike microvascular disease, which is unique to diabetes and its metabolic alterations, the cause of ischemia is similar in both diabetic and nondiabetic patients and is caused by accelerated atherosclerosis. One notable difference between these populations is the pattern and location of the occlusive atherosclerotic lesion. As noted earlier, there is no evidence for an occlusive lesion at the arteriolar level small-vessel disease ("small-vessel disease") in patients with diabetes. However, diabetic patients are more likely to have atherosclerotic disease affecting the tibial arteries, with sparing of the foot arteries *(12,55)* and thus successful arterial bypass to these distal vessels is often possible.

Because the foot vessels are often patent in the diabetic patient, and because of the success of bypass grafting to these vessels, an appropriate evaluation for ischemia is essential in diabetic patients suspected of having lower extremity arterial disease. The most important observation is the presence or absence of a palpable foot pulse; in simplest terms, if the foot pulses are not palpable, it can be assumed that occlusive disease is present.

Noninvasive arterial tests have several limitations in the presence of diabetes. Medial arterial calcification occurs frequently in diabetic patients. Although it is associated with an increased cardiovascular mortality, it is not part of the occlusive process and not associated with the development of peripheral vascular disease. Calcification of the tibial arteries results in noncompressible vessels and an artifactual elevation of the ankle-brachial pressure index. Lower levels of vessel calcification in the toe vessels supports the use of toe systolic pressures as a more reliable indicator of arterial flow to the foot *(56)*. The use of toe pressures is often limited by the proximity of the foot ulcer to the cuff site, but it is still a valuable addition to the evaluation of foot ischemia in the diabetic patient.

Pulse-volume recordings may also be of value in diabetic patients, since they are unaffected by medial calcification. Limitations are again the presence of ulceration, which precludes forefoot cuff placement, and peripheral edema that often accompanies the infectious process. In addition, the tracings are semiquantitative at best. A flat forefoot tracing is a convincing demonstration of ischemia, but it is difficult to make clinical decisions based upon the magnitude of the waveform. Moreover, an occasional patient with near-normal tracings and a nonhealing ulcer will have significant and correctable distal arterial occlusion by arteriography *(57)*.

Transcutaneous oxygen tension ($TcPO_2$) measurements are also unaffected by medial calcification, and recent reports have noted its reliability in predicting success of diabetic foot ulcer healing *(58)*. Its use is limited however by a lack of equipment standardization, user variability, and a large "gray area" of values in which healing is unpredictable. In addition, $TcPO_2$ measurements are actually higher in diabetic patients with foot ulcers compared to the nondiabetic population, which further compromises the ability to predict ischemia in these patients *(59)*.

The limitations of noninvasive vascular testing in diabetic patients with foot ulceration emphasize the continued importance of a thorough bedside evaluation and sound judgment. We continue to feel that the most important aspect of the physical exam is the status of the foot pulse. In simplest terms, it can be assumed that occlusive disease is present if the foot pulses are not palpable. This finding alone is an indication for contrast arteriography in the clinical setting of tissue loss, poor healing, or gangrene, even if neuropathy may have been the antecedent cause of skin breakdown or ulceration. Importantly, because the foot vessels are often spared by the atherosclerotic occlusive process, even when the tibial arteries are occluded, it is essential that arteriograms not be terminated at the midtibial level. The complete infrapopliteal circulation should be incorporated, including the foot vessels.

## PRINCIPLES OF ARTERIAL RECONSTRUCTION IN THE DIABETIC FOOT

The combination of motor and sensory neuropathy along with loss of the neurogenic inflammatory response and microcirculatory dysfunction results in a biologically compromised foot. Even moderate ischemia may lead to ulceration under these circumstances. Thus the concept of ischemia must be modified in making decisions about arterial reconstruction in the diabetic foot. The biologically compromised foot requires maximum circulation to heal an ulcer.

This leads to three significant principles:

1. All diabetic foot ulcers should be evaluated for an ischemic component.
2. Correction of a moderate degree of ischemia will improve healing.
3. Whenever possible, the arterial reconstruction should be designed to restore normal arterial pressure to the target area.

A complete arteriogram will facilitate choosing an outflow artery that will restore a palpable foot pulse. Proximal bypass to the popliteal or tibio-peroneal arteries may restore foot pulses. More often, however, because of the pattern of occlusive disease in the diabetic patient, bypass grafting to the popliteal or even tibial arteries cannot accomplish this goal, because of more distal obstruction. Similarly, although excellent results have been reported with peroneal artery bypass *(60)*, the peroneal artery is not in continuity with the foot vessels and may not achieve maximal flow to the foot to achieve healing.

Autogenous vein grafting to the dorsalis pedis artery represents a technical advance that provides durable and effective salvage *(61)*. Fundamental to the success of the dorsalis pedis bypass is meticulous technique and its appropriate use. The principal indication for the pedal graft is when there is no other vessel that has continuity with the foot, particularly in cases with tissue loss. Dorsalis pedis bypass is unnecessary when a more proximal bypass will restore foot pulses and should not be done if there is an inadequate length of autogenous vein. In addition, if the dorsum of the foot is extensively infected and the peroneal artery is of good quality on the preoperative arteriogram, preferential choice should be given to peroneal artery bypass.

The distal location of the dorsalis pedis artery theoretically necessitates a long venous conduit, which is often not attainable. However, by using the popliteal or distal superficial femoral artery as an inflow site, a shorter length of vein may be used, with excellent long-term patency *(62)*. This is particularly true in the diabetic patient, again because of the pattern of atherosclerotic disease. In the Deaconess Hospital experience of 384 pedal bypasses over a 7-yr period, 60% of grafts utilized the more distal inflow site, usually the popliteal artery *(63)*. This avoids dissection in the groin and upper thigh, a common location for wound complications. In addition, the shorter length of saphenous vein obviates the need for foot extension of the vein harvest incision, which is parallel to the one required to expose the dorsalis pedis artery; this avoids the resultant skin bridge that may occasionally become ischemic from undue tension. The vein graft to the dorsalis pedis artery can be prepared as an *in situ*, reversed, or nonreversed vein graft, without any significant difference in outcome *(64)*.

Active infection in the foot is not a contraindication to dorsalis pedis bypass, as long as the infectious process is controlled. At the Deaconess Hospital, the results of 56 vein bypasses to the dorsal pedal artery in patients with ischemic foot lesions complicated by infection were recently reviewed *(65)*. Included in this group were 15 patients with severe gangrene, osteomyelitis, and/or deep space abscess. The average duration between admission and bypass was 10 d. Although there was a 12% wound infection rate, the primary graft patency was 92% at 36-mo follow-up. Importantly, this aggressive approach to revascularization in the ischemic and infected foot resulted in a limb salvage rate of 98% at the end of 3 years.

We have recently reported our experience with dorsalis pedis arterial bypass in 367 patients over an 8-yr period *(66)*. Tissue loss was an indication for surgery in almost 85% of patients. The actuarial primary and secondary patency and limb-salvage rates were 68, 82, and 87%, respectively, at 5-yr follow-up. The preoperative digital subtraction arteriogram demonstrated the dorsalis pedis artery in 93% of extremities. In the remaining cases in which no artery was seen but an audible Doppler signal was present, arterial bypass was successful in 57%, emphasizing that blind exploration is reasonable, especially when amputation is the only other option.

This approach to the diagnosis and treatment of lower-extremity arterial disease in patients with diabetes has translated to improved limb salvage. Since 1984, there has been a significant reduction in every category of amputation at the Deaconess Hospital, with an increase in the number of patients undergoing arterial reconstruction, particularly dorsalis pedis bypass grafting. It is hoped that further understanding of the pathophysiology of the micro- and macrocirculation in diabetes mellitus will lead to further improvements in foot care and limb salvage in these patients.

## MACROVASCULAR DISEASE AND DIABETIC NEUROPATHY

As noted elsewhere, current hypotheses regarding the etiology of diabetic neuropathy include a combination of metabolic defects secondary to hyperglycemia and vascular changes which result in nerve hypoxia *(67)*. Evidence for a hypoxic etiology includes reduced endoneurial blood flow, increased vascular resistance *(68,69)*, and decreased endothelial production of nitric oxide *(48)*. Although microvascular dysfunction has been mainly implicated, the role of peripheral vascular disease remains considerable, as it appears likely that a decrease in total limb blood flow would potentiate nerve ischemia. Previous studies in patients with peripheral vascular disease, with or without diabetes, initially showed similar rates of electrophysiologic measurement improvement in diabetic and nondiabetic patients after bypass operation *(70–71)*. However, it is not known whether this improvement is related to functional changes or if it really reflects beneficial changes in the nerve pathology.

Clinical studies from our laboratory have focused on the effect of arterial reconstruction on the natural history of diabetic neuropathy *(72,73)*. Fifty-five patients with diabetes and peripheral vascular disease requiring revascularization were studied. Peroneal nerve conduction velocity was measured prior to arterial bypass, six weeks later and

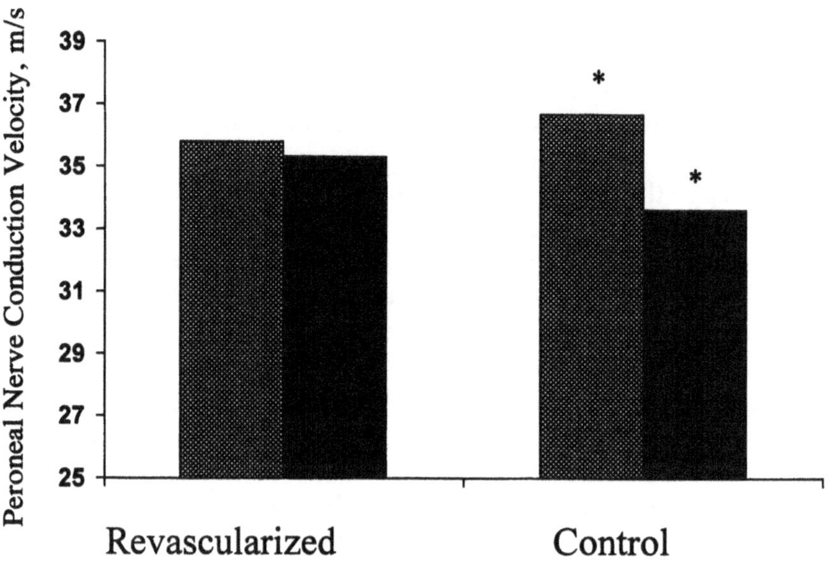


**Fig. 2.** Changes in the postoperative peroneal motor nerve conduction velocity (black bars) compared with the preoperative measurements (gray bars) in the revascularized limbs and limbs not operated on. No difference was found in the revascularized legs, but a significant decrease was found in the control legs (asterisk indicates $p < 0.05$) Ref. 73, reprinted with permission.

then again at a mean follow-up of 19 months. At baseline a significant difference was found between the leg that was scheduled for operation and the contralateral leg in the Neuropathy Disability Score, the Semmes-Weinstein monofilaments and the peroneal nerve conduction velocity. After the revascularization procedure, no difference existed between the operated and the contralateral leg in any nerve-function measurements. However, no significant improvement was found in the operated leg when nerve-function measurements during the second visit were compared to baseline.

In the operated leg, the peroneal nerve conduction velocity remained unchanged during the follow-up period (preoperative 35.79 ± 6.02 vs postoperative 35.33 ± 7.51 m/s, $p$ = NS), but deteriorated in the nonoperated leg (36.68 ± 6.22 vs 33.64 ± 7.30, $p < 0.05$) (Fig. 2). It appears, therefore, that reversal of hypoxia in diabetic patients halts the progression of neuropathy, lending further support to the role of hypoxia in the pathogenesis of nerve dysfunction in diabetes mellitus.

## CONCLUSIONS

Diabetes mellitus is characterized by a variety of microcirculatory abnormalities, which may be instrumental in the pathogenesis of many of the secondary complications. Additionally, a macroangiopathy is also found, manifesting as coronary, extracerebral vascular, and lower-extremity arterial disease. Understanding the complex pathophysiology behind these disorders is the basis of intense ongoing research, and is critical in reducing the overall morbidity and mortality of diabetes.

## REFERENCES


1. American Diabetes Association. Diabetes: 1993 Vital Statistics. 1993.
2. Cameron NE, Cotter MA. The relationship of vascular changes to metabolic factors in diabetes mellitus and their role in the development of peripheral nerve complications. Diabetes Metab Rev 1994;10:189–224.
3. Ruderman NB, Haudenschild C. Diabetes as an atherogenic factor. Prog Cardiovasc Dis 1984;26:373–412.
4. Nathan DM. Long-term complications of diabetes mellitus. N Engl J Med 1993;328:1676–1685.
5. Palmberg P, Smith M, Waltman S, et al. The natural history of retinopathy in insulin-dependent juvenile-onset diabetes. Opthalmology 1981;88:613–618.
6. Pirart J. Diabetes mellitus and its degenerative complications: a prospective study of 4400 patients observed between 1947 and 1973. Diabetes Care 1978;1:168–188, 252–261.
7. DCCT Research Group. The effect of intensive treatment of diabetes on the development and progression of long-term complications in insulin-dependent diabetes mellitus. N Engl J Med 1993;329:977–986.
8. Vanhoutte PM. The endothelium-modulator of vascular smooth-muscle tone. N Engl J Med 1988;319:512–513.
9. Cohen RA. Dysfunction of vascular endothelium in diabetes mellitus. Circulation 1993;87:V67–V76.
10. Goldenberg SG, Alex M. Joshi RA, Blumenthal HT. Nonatheromatous peripheral vascular disease of the lower extremity in diabetes mellitus. Diabetes 1959;8:261–273.
11. Strandness DE Jr, Priest RE, Gibbons GE. Combined clinical and pathologic study of diabetic and nondiabetic peripheral arterial disease. Diabetes 1964;13:366–372.
12. LoGerfo FW. Coffman JD. Vascular and microvascular disease of the foot in diabetes. N Engl J Med 311:1615–1619, 1984.
13. Barner HB, Kaiser GC, Willman VL. Blood flow in the diabetic leg. Circulation 1971;43:391–394.
14. Parving HH, Viberti GC, Keen H, Christiansen JS, Lassen NA. Hemodynamic factors in the genesis of diabetic microangiopathy. Metabolism 1983;32:943–949.
15. Morgensen CE, Schmitz A, Christensen CR. Comparative renal pathophysiology relevant to IDDM and NIDDM patients. Diabetes Metab Rev 1988;4:453–483.
16. Flynn MD, Tooke JE. Aetiology of diabetic foot ulceration: A role for the microcirculation? Diabet Med 1992;8:320–329.
17. Rayman G, Williams SA, Spencer PD, et al. Impaired microvascular hyperaemic response to minor skin trauma in Type I diabetes. Br Med J 1986;292:1295–1298.
18. Jorneskog G, Brismar K, Fagrell B. Skin capillary circulation severely impaired in toes of patients with IDDM, with and without late diabetic complications. Diabetologia 1995;38:474–480.
19. Parkhouse N, LeQueen PM. Impaired neurogenic vascular response in patients with diabetes and neuropathic foot lesions. N Engl J Med 1988;318:1306–1309.
20. Vane JR, Anggard EE, Botting RM. Regulatory functions of the vascular endothelium. N Engl J Med 1990;323:27–36.
21. Gupta S, Sussman I, McArthur CS, Tornheim K, Cohen RA, Ruderman NB. Endothelium-dependent inhibition of $Na^+$-$K^+$ ATPase activity in rabbit aorta by hyperglycemia. Possible role of endothelium-derived nitric oxide. J Clin Invest 1992;90:727–732.
22. Pieper GM, Meier DA, Hager SR. Endothelial dysfunction in a model of hyperglycemia and hyperinsulinemia. Am J Physiol 1995;269:H845–850.
23. Tesfamarian B, Brown ML, Cohen RA. Elevated glucose impairs endothelium-dependent relaxation by activating protein kinase C. J Clin Invest 1991;87:1643–1648.
24. Williams SB, Cusco JA, Roddy M, Johnstone MY, Creager MA. Impaired nitric oxide-mediated vasodilation in patients with non-insulin-dependent diabetes mellitus. J Am Coll Cardiol 1996;27:567–574.
25. Johnstone MT, Creager SJ, Scales KM, Cusco JA, Lee BK, Creager MA. Impaired endothelium-dependent vasodilation in patients with insulin-dependent diabetes mellitus. Circulation 1993;88:2510–2516.
26. Brownlee M, Cerami A, Vlassare H. Advanced glycosylation end products in tissue and the biochemical basis of diabetic complications. N Engl J Med 1988;318:1315–1321.
27. Furchgott RF, Zawadzki JV. The obligatory role of endothelial cells in the relaxation of arterial smooth muscle by acetylcholine. Nature 1980;288:373–376.

28. Palmer RM, Ferrige AG, Moncada S. Nitric oxide release accounts for the biologic activity of endothelium-derived relaxing factor. Nature 1987;327:524–526.
29. Scherrer U, Randin D, Vollenweider P, Vollenweider L, Nicod P. Nitric oxide release accounts for insulin's vascular effects in humans. J Clin Invest 1994;94:2511–2515.
30. Taddei S, Virdis A, Mattei P, Natali A, Ferrannini E, Salvetti A. Effect of insulin on acetylcholine-induced vasodilation in normotensive subjects and patients with essential hypertension. Circulation 1995;92:2911–2918.
31. Baron AD. The coupling of glucose metabolism and perfusion in human skeletal muscle. The potential role of endothelium-derived nitric oxide. Diabetes 1996;45:S105–S109.
32. Oberly LW. Free radicals in diabetes. Free Rad Biol Med 1988;5:113–124.
33. Wolff SP, Dean RT. Glucose autoxidation and protein modification: the role of oxidative glycosylation in diabetes. Biochem J 1987;245:234–250.
34. Diederich D, Skopec J, Diederich A, Dai FX. Endothelial dysfunction in mesenteric resistance arteries of diabetic rats: role of free radicals. Am J Physiol 1994;266:H1153–H1161.
35. Bucala R, Tracey KJ, Cerami A. Advanced glycosylation end products quench nitric oxide and mediate defective endothelium-dependent vasodilatation in experimental diabetes. J Clin Invest 1991;87:432–438.
36. Schmidt AM, Hori O, Brett J, Yan SD, Wautier JL, Stern D. Cellular receptors for advanced glycation end products. Implications for induction of oxidant stress and cellular dysfunction in the pathogenesis of vascular lesions. Arteriosclerosis Thrombosis 1994;14:1521–1528.
37. Makita Z, Radoff S, Rayfield EJ, et al. Advanced glycosylation end products in patients with diabetic nephropathy. N Engl J Med 1991;325:836–842.
38. Wautier JL, Zoukourian C, Chappey O. Receptor-mediated endothelial cell dysfunction in diabetic vasculopathy. Soluble receptor for advanced glycation end products blocks hyperpermeability in diabetic rats. J Clin Invest 1996;97:238–243.
39. Joannides R, Haefeli WE, Linder L, et al. Nitric oxide is responsible for flow-dependent dilatation of human peripheral conduit arteries in vivo. Circulation 1995;91:1314–1319.
40. Greene DA, Lattimer SA, Sima AA. Sorbitol, phosphoinositides, and sodium-potassium ATPase in the pathogenesis of diabetic complications. N Engl J Med 1987;316:599–606.
41. Pfeifer MA, Schumer MP. Clinical trials of diabetic neuropathy: past, present, and future. Diabetes 1995;44:1355–1361.
42. Simmons DA, Winegrad AI. Mechanism of glucose-induced $Na^+$-$K^+$ ATPase inhibition in aortic wall of rabbits. Diabetologia 1989;32:402–408.
43. Stevens MJ, Dananberg J, Feldman EL, et al. The linked roles of nitric oxide, aldose reductase and $Na^+$-$K^+$ ATPase in the slowing of nerve conduction in the streptozotocin diabetic rat. J Clin Invest 1994;94:853–859.
44. Veves A, Akbari CM, Donaghue VM, et al. The effect of diabetes, neuropathy, Charcot arthropathy, and arterial disease on the foot microcirculation. Diabetologia 1996;39(Suppl 1):A3.
45. Veves A, Primavera J, Akbari CM, et al. Expression of endothelial nitric oxide (eNOS) in diabetic neuropathy. Diabetes (in press).
46. Kannel WB, McGee DL. Diabetes and cardiovascular disease. The Framingham Study. JAMA 1979;241:2035–2038.
47. Stokes J, Kannel WB, Wolf PA, Cupples LA, D'Agostino RB. The relative importance of selected risk factors for various manifestations of cardiovascular disease among men and women from 35 to 64 years old: 30 years of follow-up in the Framingham Study. Circulation 1987;75:65–73.
48. Burchfiel CM, Curb JD, Rodriguez BL, Abbott RD, Chiu D, Yano K. Glucose intolerance and 22-year stroke incidence. The Honolulu Heart Program. Stroke 1994;25:951–957.
49. Jorgensen H, Nakayama H, Raaschou HO, Olsen TS. Stroke in patients with diabetes. The Copenhagen Stroke Study. Stroke 1994;25:1977–1984.
50. Yasaka M, Yamaguchi T, Shichiri M. Distribution of atherosclerosis and risk factors in atherothrombotic occlusion. Stroke 1993;24:206–211.
51. Colwell JA, Lopes-Virella MF. A review of the pathogenesis of large vessel disease in diabetes mellitus. Am J Med 1988;85:113–118.
52. Ross R. The pathogenesis of atherosclerosis: an update. N Engl J Med 1986;488–500.
53. Wilhelmsen L, Svardsudd K, Korsan-Bengtsen K, Larsson B, Welin L, Tibblin G. Fibrinogen as a risk factor for stroke and myocardial infarction. N Engl J Med 1984;311:501–505.
54. Brand FN, Abbott RD, Kannel WB. Diabetes, intermittent claudication, and risk of cardiovascular events. The Framingham Study. Diabetes 1989;38:504–509.

55. Menzoian JO, LaMorte WW, Paniszyn CC, et al. Symptomatology and anatomic patterns of peripheral vascular disease: differing impact of smoking and diabetes. Ann Vasc Surg 1989;3:224–228.
56. Young MJ, Adams JE, Anderson GF, et al. Medial arterial calcification in the feet of diabetic patients and matched non-diabetic control subjects. Diabetologia 1993;36:615–621.
57. Pomposelli FB Jr. Noninvasive evaluation of the arterial system in the diabetic lower extremity. In: Kozak GP, Campbell DR, Frykberg RG, Habershaw GM, eds. Management of Diabetic Foot Problems, 2nd ed. W. B. Saunders, Philadelphia, 1995, pp. 138–148.
58. Ballard JL, Eke CC, Bunt TJ, et al. A prospective evaluation of transcutaneous oxygen measurements in the management of diabetic foot problems. J Vasc Surg 1995;22:485–492.
59. Wyss CR, Matsen FA III, Simmons CW, et al. Transcutaneous oxygen tension measurements on limbs of diabetic and nondiabetic patients with peripheral vascular disease. Surgery 1984;95:339–346.
60. Plecha EJ, Seabrook GR, Bandyk DF, et al. Determinants of successful peroneal artery bypass. J Vasc Surg 1993;17:97–106.
61. Pomposelli FB Jr, Jepsen SJ, Gibbons GW, et al. Efficacy of the dorsal pedis bypass for limb salvage in diabetic patients: Short-term observations. J Vasc Surg 1990;11:745–752.
62. Veith FJ, Gupta SK, Samson RH, et al. Superficial femoral and popliteal arteries as inflow sites for distal bypasses. Surgery 1981;90:980–990.
63. Pomposelli FB Jr, Marcaccio EJ, Gibbons GW, et al. Dorsalis pedis arterial bypass: Durable limb salvage for foot ischemia in patients with diabetes mellitus. J Vasc Surg 1995;21:375–384.
64. Pomposelli FB Jr, Jepsen SJ, Gibbons GW, et al. A flexible approach to infrapopliteal vein grafts in patients with diabetes mellitus. Arch Surg 1991;126:724–729.
65. Tannenbaum GA, Pomposelli FB Jr, Marcaccio EJ, et al. Safety of vein bypass grafting to the dorsal pedal artery in diabetic patients with foot infections. J Vasc Surg 1992;15:982–990.
66. LoGerfo FW, Gibbons GW, Pomposelli FB Jr, et al. Trends in the care of the diabetic foot: Expanded role of arterial reconstruction. Arch Surg 1992;127:617–621.
67. Stevens MJ, Feldman EL, Greene DA. The aetiology of diabetic neuropathy: the combined roles of metabolic and vascular defects. Diabet Med. 1995;12:566–579.
68. Tuck RR, Schmelzer JD, Low PA. Endoneurial blood flow and oxygen tension in the sciatic nerves of rats with experimental diabetic neuropathy. Brain 1984;107:935–950.
69. Tesfaye S, Harris N, Jakubowski JJ, et al. Impaired blood flow and arterio-venous shunting in human diabetic neuropathy: a novel technique of nerve photography and fluorescin angiography. Diabetologia 1993;36:1266–1274.
70. Young MJ, Veves A, Walker MG, Boulton AJM. Correlations between nerve function and tissue oxygenation in diabetic patients: further clues to the aetiology of diabetic neuropathy. Diabetologia 1992;35:1146–1150.
71. Young MJ, Veves A, Smith JV, Walker MG, Boulton AJM. Restoring lower limb blood flow improves conduction velocity in diabetic patients. Diabetologia 1995;38:1051–1054.
72. Veves A, Donaghue VM, Sarnow MR, Giurini JM, Campbell DR, LoGerfo FW. The impact of reversal of hypoxia by revascularization in the peripheral nerve function of diabetic patients. Diabetologia 1996;39:344–348.
73. Akbari CM, Gibbons GW, Habershaw GM, LoGerfo FW, Veves A. The effect of arterial reconstruction on the natural history of diabetic neuropathy. Arch Surg 1997;132:148–152.

# INDEX

GPSR Compliance

*The European Union's (EU) General Product Safety Regulation (GPSR) is a set of rules that requires consumer products to be safe and our obligations to ensure this.*

*If you have any concerns about our products, you can contact us on ProductSafety@springernature.com*

In case Publisher is established outside the EU, the EU authorized representative is:

Springer Nature Customer Service Center GmbH
Europaplatz 3
69115 Heidelberg, Germany

**Batch number: 10755805**

Printed by Printforce, the Netherlands